Catheter Interventions for Structural Heart Disease

Editor

RAY V. MATTHEWS

CARDIOLOGY CLINICS

www.cardiology.theclinics.com

Consulting Editors

ROSARIO FREEMAN
JORDAN M. PRUTKIN
DAVID M. SHAVELLE
AUDREY H. WU

August 2013 • Volume 31 • Number 3

ELSEVIER

1600 John F. Kennedy Boulevard • Suite 1800 • Philadelphia, Pennsylvania, 19103-2899

http://www.theclinics.com

CARDIOLOGY CLINICS Volume 31, Number 3

August 2013 ISSN 0733-8651, ISBN-13: 978-0-323-18601-8

Editor: Barbara Cohen-Kligerman

Cardiology Clinics (ISSN 0733-8651) is published quarterly by Elsevier Inc., 360 Park Avenue South, New York, NY 10010-1710. Months of issue are February, May, August, and November. Business and Editorial Offices: 1600 John F. Kennedy Blvd., Ste. 1800, Philadelphia, PA 19103-2899. Customer Service Office: 3251 Riverport Lane, Maryland Heights, MO 63043. Periodicals postage paid at New York, NY and additional mailing offices. Subscription prices are $305.00 per year for US individuals, $508.00 per year for US institutions, $149.00 per year for US students and residents, $373.00 per year for Canadian individuals, $630.00 per year for Canadian institutions, $432.00 per year for international individuals, $630.00 per year for international institutions and $211.00 per year for Canadian and international students/residents. To receive student/resident rate, orders must be accompanied by name of affiliated institution, data of term, and the *signature* of program/residency coordinator on institution letterhead. Orders will be billed at individual rate until proof of status is received. Foreign air speed delivery is included in all *Clinics* subscription prices. All prices are subject to change without notice. **POSTMASTER:** Send address changes to *Cardiology Clinics*, Elsevier Health Sciences Division, Subscription Customer Service, 3251 Riverport Lane, Maryland Heights, MO 63043. **Customer Service: 1-800-654-2452 (U.S. and Canada); 314-447-8871 (outside U.S. and Canada). Fax: 314-447-8029. E-mail: journalscustomerservice-usa@ elsevier.com (for print support); journalsonlinesupport-usa@elsevier.com (for online support).**

Reprints. For copies of 100 or more, of articles in this publication, please contact the Commercial Reprints Department, Elsevier Inc., 360 Park Avenue South, New York, NY 10010-1710. Tel.: 212-633-3812; Fax: 212-462-1935; E-mail: reprints@elsevier.com.

Cardiology Clinics is also published in Spanish by McGraw-Hill Interamericana Editores S. A., P.O. Box 5-237, 06500, Mexico D. F., Mexico; in Portuguese by Reichmann and Alfonso Editores Rio de Janeiro, Brazil; and in Greek by Dimitrios P. Lagos, 8 Pondon Street, GR115-28 Ilissia, Greece.

Cardiology Clinics is covered in *MEDLINE/PubMed (Index Medicus), Excerpta Medica, The Cumulative Index to Nursing and Allied Health Literature* (CINAHL).

Printed and bound by CPI Group (UK) Ltd, Croydon, CR0 4YY

Transferred to digital print 2012

Contributors

EDITORIAL BOARD

ROSARIO FREEMAN, MD, MS, FACC
Associate Professor of Medicine; Director,
Coronary Care Unit; Director,
Echocardiography Laboratory, University of
Washington Medical Center, Seattle,
Washington

JORDAN M. PRUTKIN, MD, MHS, FHRS
Assistant Professor of Medicine, Division of
Cardiology/Electrophysiology, University of
Washington Medical Center, Seattle,
Washington

DAVID M. SHAVELLE, MD, FACC, FSCAI
Associate Professor of Clinical Medicine,
Division of Cardiovascular Medicine, Keck
School of Medicine at USC; Director, Los
Angeles County/USC Cardiac Catheterization
Laboratory; Director, Interventional Cardiology
Fellowship, Los Angeles County/USC Medical
Center, Los Angeles, California

AUDREY H. WU, MD
Assistant Professor, Internal Medicine,
University of Michigan, Ann Arbor, Michigan

EDITOR

RAY V. MATTHEWS, MD
Director of Interventional Cardiology; Professor
of Clinical Medicine, Division of Cardiovascular
Medicine, Keck School of Medicine,
Los Angeles, California

AUTHORS

MEHRA ANILKUMAR, MD
Director of CCU, Department of Cardiology,
LAC-USC Medical Center, Keck School of
Medicine, Los Angeles, California

USMAN BABER, MD, MS
Assistant Professor of Medicine, Cardiac
Catheterization Laboratory, Mount Sinai
Medical Center, New York, New York

JOHN D. CARROLL, MD
Director, Interventional Cardiology; Director,
Division of Cardiology, University of Colorado
Denver, Aurora, Colorado

JOÃO L. CAVALCANTE, MD, FACC, FASE
Assistant Professor of Medicine, Advanced
Cardiovascular Imaging, Heart & Vascular
Institute, University of Pittsburgh Medical
Center, University of Pittsburgh, Pittsburgh,
Pennsylvania

PHILIP B. DATTILO, MD
Fellow, Interventional Cardiology, Division of
Cardiology, University of Colorado Denver,
Aurora, Colorado

CREIGHTON W. DON, MD, PhD, FACC
Assistant Professor of Medicine, Department
of General Internal Medicine, Division of
Cardiology, University of Washington Medical
Center, Seattle, Washington

ANDREW C. EISENHAUER, MD
Assistant Professor of Medicine, Division
of Cardiovascular Medicine, Brigham and
Women's Hospital, Harvard Medical School,
Boston, Massachusetts

CINDY J. FULLER, PhD
Swedish Heart & Vascular Institute, Swedish
Medical Center, University of Washington
Medical Center, Seattle, Washington

STEVEN HADDY, MD, FCCP, FACC
Associate Professor of Clinical Anesthesiology
and Chief of Cardiothoracic Anesthesiology,
Department of Anesthesiology, Keck School of
Medicine, University of Southern California,
Los Angeles, California

PEI-HSIU HUANG, MD
Fellow, Structural Heart and Peripheral
Vascular Interventions, Division of
Cardiovascular Medicine, Brigham and
Women's Hospital, Harvard Medical School,
Boston, Massachusetts

VLADIMIR JELNIN, MD
Department of Structural and Congenital Heart
Disease, Lenox Hill Heart and Vascular
Institute, North Shore/LIJ Health System,
New York, New York

MICHAEL S. KIM, MD
Director, Structural Heart Disease Program,
Division of Cardiology, University of Colorado
Denver, Aurora, Colorado

ANNAPOORNA S. KINI, MD
Associate Professor of Medicine and Director,
Cardiac Catheterization Laboratory, Mount
Sinai Medical Center, New York, New York

CHAD KLIGER, MD
Department of Structural and Congenital Heart
Disease, Lenox Hill Heart and Vascular
Institute, North Shore/LIJ Health System,
New York, New York

ROBERT KUMAR, MD
Department of Structural and Congenital Heart
Disease, Lenox Hill Heart and Vascular
Institute, North Shore/LIJ Health System,
New York, New York

JOHN M. LASALA, MD, PhD
Medical Director of the Cardiac Catheterization
Laboratory; Associate Professor of Medicine
and Director of Interventional Cardiology,
Division of Cardiology, Washington University
School of Medicine, St Louis, Missouri

MING-SUM LEE, MD, PhD
Division of Cardiology, Keck School of
Medicine, University of Southern California,
Los Angeles, California

RAY V. MATTHEWS, MD
Director of Interventional Cardiology; Professor
of Clinical Medicine, Division of Cardiovascular
Medicine, Keck School of Medicine,
Los Angeles, California

PEDRO R. MORENO, MD
Professor of Medicine, Cardiac Catheterization
Laboratory, Mount Sinai Medical Center,
New York, New York

TASNEEM Z. NAQVI, MD, FRCP, MMM
Director, Echocardiography; Senior Associate
Consultant, Mayo Clinic, Scottsdale, Arizona

MARK REISMAN, MD, FACC
Professor of Medicine, Swedish Heart &
Vascular Institute, Swedish Medical Center,
University of Washington Medical Center,
Seattle, Washington

CARLOS E. RUIZ, MD, PhD
Director, Department of Structural and
Congenital Heart Disease, Lenox Hill Heart and
Vascular Institute, North Shore/LIJ Health
System, New York, New York

PAUL SCHOENHAGEN, MD
Cleveland Clinic, Imaging Institute and Heart &
Vascular Institute, Cleveland, Ohio

SAMIN K. SHARMA, MD
Professor of Medicine and Director of
Clinical Cardiology, Cardiac Catheterization
Laboratory, Mount Sinai Medical Center,
New York, New York

DAVID M. SHAVELLE, MD, FACC, FSCAI
Associate Professor of Clinical Medicine,
Division of Cardiovascular Medicine, Keck
School of Medicine at USC; Director, Los
Angeles County/USC Cardiac Catheterization
Laboratory; Director, Interventional
Cardiology Fellowship, Los Angeles
County/USC Medical Center, Los Angeles,
California

ANDRES F. VASQUEZ, MD
Interventional Cardiology Fellow, Division of
Cardiology, Washington University School of
Medicine, St. Louis, Missouri

Contents

Calcific aortic stenosis (AS) is the most frequent expression of aortic valve disease in the Western world, with an increasing prevalence as the population ages. Almost 4% of all adults 75 years of age or older have moderate or severe AS. Many patients do not undergo surgery because of prohibitive comorbidities or other high-risk features. Balloon aortic valvuloplasty (BAV) remains an option for temporary palliation and symptomatic relief in such patients. In addition, BAV continues to serve an important role as a bridge to either surgical or transcatheter aortic valve replacement in certain patients with AS requiring temporary hemodynamic stabilization.

Transcatheter aortic valve replacement has a place in the therapy for valvular aortic stenosis in a selected population of patients with increased risk for standard aortic valve replacement. The SAPIEN family of balloon-expandable transcatheter heart valves is the prototype that initiated this therapy and has undergone rapid development and evolution. The SAPIEN system has taught cardiologists and cardiac surgeons much about the nature of aortic stenosis and the potential for less invasive therapy. This article will review the SAPIEN transcatheter heart valves and the clinical experience.

The treatment of aortic stenosis in high-risk surgical patients is now possible by transcatheter aortic valve replacement. The CoreValve is a new transcatheter valve with a unique design expanding its application in patients with aortic stenosis. The CoreValve is just completing clinical trial in the United States and not yet available for commercial use in the United States but is widely used in Europe.

Occlusion of the left atrial appendage (LAA) may reduce the risk of stroke in patients with atrial fibrillation (AF). Trials comparing LAA occlusion to warfarin anticoagulation in patients with nonvalvular AF showed a reduction in hemorrhagic stroke, although an increase in safety events due to procedural complications. Long-term follow-up suggests possible superiority of LAA occlusion due to fewer strokes and bleeding events. The superior dosing and safety profiles of the novel oral anticoagulants raise the accepted threshold for safety and efficacy of LAA occlusion procedures, and underscore the need for randomized studies comparing LAA occlusion with these newer anticoagulants.

Congenital heart disease accounted for 0.3% of US hospital admissions in 2007, with 48% related to atrial septal defects (ASDs). More than one-fourth of adult congenital heart defects are ASDs, 75% of which are ostium secundum ASDs. The progressive impact of volume overload of the right cardiac chambers can be halted by ASD closure. This review focuses on percutaneous ASD closure.

Patent foramen ovale (PFO) is a common developmental anomaly that allows for the passage of blood and other substances from the venous to the arterial circulation. The study of PFO closure has been challenging due to widely available off-label closures performed outside the clinical trial setting. To date, no study has demonstrated benefit of closure using intention-to-treat analyses. Secondary and subpopulation analyses suggest that there is benefit to closure in patients with atrial septal aneurysms and/or substantial degrees of right-to-left shunting. This article reviews the history, associated technologies, and current data regarding PFO closure.

Patent ductus arteriosus in adults is usually an isolated lesion with a small to moderate degree of shunt, as a larger shunt becomes symptomatic earlier in childhood. The classic murmur of patent ductus arteriosus may be the first clue to its presence, or it may be detected accidently by transthoracic echocardiography, computed tomography, or magnetic resonance angiography for an unrelated condition. The percutaneous approach is safe and effective in more than 98% of patients. Subacute bacterial endocarditis prophylaxis is not indicated routinely except for 6 months following the closure percutaneously or surgically.

Percutaneous paravalvular leak closure is increasingly being performed as an alternative to reoperation in patients with symptomatic prosthetic paravalvular regurgitation. This article reviews the pathogenesis of paravalvular leaks and percutaneous techniques for closure. Newer multimodality imaging techniques, including 3-dimensional (3D) transesophageal echocardiography and 3D/4D computed tomographic angiography, allow improved preprocedural planning and intraprocedural guidance. Specific techniques can be used for challenging patient anatomy and larger paravalvular leaks. Outcomes from experienced centers show acceptable rates of technical and clinical success, with lower procedural morbidity than reoperation.

Echocardiography plays an integral role in the evaluation and treatment of patients undergoing percutaneous interventions for structural heart disease. Preprocedure, accurate echocardiographic assessment of cardiac anatomy is crucial in determining patient eligibility. During catheterization, echocardiography is used for procedural guidance. Postprocedure, echocardiography is used for patient follow-up and determining the effect of device placement on cardiac remodeling. This article provides a practical guide for using echocardiography in common interventional procedures, including percutaneous atrial septal defect closure, transcatheter aortic valve replacement, percutaneous repair of prosthetic valve paravalvular leaks, percutaneous mitral valve edge-to-edge repair, and percutaneous placement of appendage occlusion devices.

Anesthesia for Structural Heart Interventions

Steven Haddy

Surgeries in general and cardiac procedures in particular are increasingly performed using catheter-based or minimally invasive techniques, often with sedation or general anesthesia. These new approaches require close cooperation and communication between the cardiologist and anesthesiologist to ensure patient safety. Anesthesia-related respiratory complications arising in the catheterization laboratory are more frequent and more severe than are seen in the operating room. The principals of safe anesthetic practice as they apply to procedures performed outside the operating room and suggestions to improve safety and outcome are reviewed in this article.

Role of Cross-Sectional Imaging for Structural Heart Disease Interventions

João L. Cavalcante and Paul Schoenhagen

 Video of three-dimensional multi-planar reconstruction/reformatting of the aortic valve with cine loop assessing leaflet motion and aortic valve opening; and a video of dynamic intraprocedural CT angiography with fluoroscopy fusion/overlay allowing best angle assessment for prosthesis deployment accompany this article

With the aging population, significant valvular heart disease is increasingly identified in patients too frail to undergo surgery. Transcatheter therapies for structural heart disease represent an alternative therapeutic approach for these patients. During these procedures, direct visualization of the surgical field is replaced by image guidance for intraprocedural decision making. Advances in percutaneous devices and delivery systems, coupled with enhancements in 3-dimensional imaging with multiplanar reformatting, have allowed these procedures to be performed safely and with excellent results. This article describes the role of cross-sectional imaging for detailed assessment and preprocedural planning of aortic, mitral, and pulmonic valve interventions.

Index

CARDIOLOGY CLINICS

**DOWNLOAD
Free App!**

Review Articles
THE CLINICS

NOW AVAILABLE FOR YOUR iPhone and iPad

Preface
Catheter Intervention in Structural Heart Disease

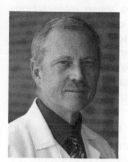

Ray V. Matthews, MD
Editor

The field of interventional cardiology has undergone dramatic change in the last several decades. What began as the practice of enhancing cardiovascular diagnostic capabilities in the catheterization lab in the 1960s has morphed into a major therapeutic arena for a wide variety of cardiac disorders. The initial transition from diagnosis to therapy began with coronary angioplasty in the late 1970s. The simple process of expanding a balloon in the coronary artery to relieve coronary obstruction transformed the specialty of cardiology. Nonetheless, an overwhelming desire to deliver a less invasive therapy drove the rapid adoption of coronary angioplasty. The template for innovation in interventional cardiology was set. Attempts were made to duplicate an invasive surgical therapy with an equally effective percutaneous catheter-based procedure and to do this more rapidly, with less patient discomfort.

Other cardiovascular disorders soon developed percutaneous options. Abdominal aortic aneurysms, atrial septal defects, patent ductus, carotid stenoses, and many other disorders now have catheter-based treatment options. Some have been shown to be comparable to surgical therapies, and some less so. Technologies existing and those developed specifically were employed to explore their benefits for disease processes. Solutions to unblock arteries included elegant devices that cut, drilled, lasered, scored, aspirated, and dilated vessels.

As interventional cardiologists, we became more aware of the engineering of materials as part of the development of new devices. We became knowledgeable in concepts such as radial strength, rotational friction displacement, memory, fatigue, and the like. We also learned of the body's adaptation to implantable devices such as endothelialization and surface clotting. We began to use the concepts learned in one disease for the treatment of another. For example, the concept of an expandable stent is very similar whether applied in a vessel to relieve an obstruction, or in a stenotic aortic valve as a platform to deliver a bioprosthetic valve. The body's response to the stent now becomes the predictable part of the process, whereas previously it was the unknown factor.

An understanding of the biologic response to materials is essential to the advancement of catheter-based therapies. Nitinol is a nickel titanium alloy with a long track record in interventional cardiology. Nitinol has properties that are unique, such as memory and conformability, making it an attractive material to use in many catheter-based therapies. Defect occluders, peripheral stents, stent grafts, vascular filters, appendage occluders, heart valves, IVC filters, and vessel occluders all contain a substantial amount of nitinol. A previously gained understanding of nitinol has allowed the predictable use of this material in subsequent interventional devices through knowledge of its virtues

Cardiol Clin 31 (2013) ix–x
http://dx.doi.org/10.1016/j.ccl.2013.06.001
0733-8651/13/$ – see front matter © 2013 Published by Elsevier Inc.

cardiology.theclinics.com

and its limitations. Thus, we can facilitate device innovation with a limited number of unknowns.

The investigation of catheter-based intervention has changed significantly since the 1970s. Initially the regulatory hurdles were more straightforward and focused principally on safety. Today the burden of proof of utility of devices is immense. In most cases devices must now be proven safe, as effective as or more effective than existing therapy, and be cost effective. Furthermore, this must be done in large, statistically sound clinical trials, often taking years to complete. This burden slows the process of innovation, but some would argue it enhances safety and the scientific process. It is now standard for a new interventional therapy to have survived the scrutiny of a large randomized trial.

Catheter-based intervention for structural heart disease has moved from a specialty limited to a few select clinical investigators to a commonplace occurrence in tertiary referral centers and even present to one degree or another in most

medium-sized community hospitals. The timing of this issue of *Cardiology Clinics* is perfect. This complete and concise issue provides the busy cardiologist the opportunity to gain a complete understanding of the catheter therapy of structural heart disease with maximum efficiency. As the practicing cardiologist sees these interventions happen around him/her, it is incumbent on him/her to have a complete, up-to-date understanding of these therapies to best serve our patients. Most assuredly, there will only be more advances and refinements in catheter-based therapy of structural heart disease in the future.

Ray V. Matthews, MD
Division of Cardiovascular Medicine
Keck School of Medicine
1510 San Pablo Street, Suite 322
Los Angeles, CA 90033, USA

E-mail address:
raymatth@usc.edu

Aortic Stenosis
Role of Balloon Aortic Valvuloplasty

Usman Baber, MD, MS, Annapoorna S. Kini, MD,
Pedro R. Moreno, MD, Samin K. Sharma, MD*

KEYWORDS

- Aortic stenosis • Balloon aortic valvuloplasty • Aortic valve replacement
- Transcatheter aortic valve replacement

KEY POINTS

- Calcific aortic stenosis (AS) is the most frequent expression of aortic valve disease in the Western world, with an increasing prevalence as the population ages.
- Almost 4% of all adults 75 years of age or older have moderate or severe AS.
- Although surgical valve replacement is the definitive treatment of calcific AS, many patients do not undergo surgery because of prohibitive comorbidities or other high-risk features.
- Balloon aortic valvuloplasty (BAV) remains an option for temporary palliation and symptomatic relief in patients who cannot undergo surgical valve replacement.
- BAV also continues to serve an important role as a bridge to either surgical or transcatheter aortic valve replacement in certain patients with AS requiring temporary hemodynamic stabilization.

INTRODUCTION

Aortic valve diseases are among the most common manifestations of cardiac disorder and calcific aortic stenosis (AS) is the leading indication for surgical aortic valve replacement (SAVR) in the United States.[1] Characterized by a long latency period, symptom onset in calcific AS is associated with markedly reduced survival.[2] Three-year survival rates among symptomatic patients with severe AS who do not undergo aortic valve replacement (AVR) may be as low as 25%.[3] With the aging of the population the overall burden and economic impact of AS is expected to increase as disease prevalence increases with age, affecting up to 4% of adults more than 85 years of age.[4,5] Although SAVR remains the definitive treatment of calcific AS,[6] many patients do not realize the benefits of this option because of extensive morbidity or other high-risk clinical

and/or anatomic features.[7,8] Although not an alternative to AVR, balloon aortic valvuloplasty (BAV) provides temporary symptomatic and hemodynamic benefit in select patients with advanced AS. This article provides an overview of calcific AS disorders and assesses the role of BAV in the contemporary treatment of this disease entity.

AS: PATHOLOGIC CONSIDERATIONS

Multiple studies over the last 20 years suggest mechanistic similarities between AS and atherosclerosis. Population-based and epidemiologic studies have shown substantial overlap in risk factors for both diseases.[5,9,10] For example, data from the Cardiovascular Health Study found that older age, male gender, and hypertension were associated with aortic sclerosis.[9] Other studies have identified significant correlations between increased low-density lipoprotein (LDL), smoking,

Disclosures: The authors having nothing to disclose.
Cardiac Catheterization Laboratory, Mount Sinai Medical Center, One Gustave L. Levy Place, New York, NY 10029, USA
* Corresponding author.
E-mail address: samin.sharma@mountsinai.org

Cardiol Clin 31 (2013) 327–336
http://dx.doi.org/10.1016/j.ccl.2013.05.005

diabetes mellitus, and AS.[10] In addition to these clinical associations, there are also similarities in the histopathologic features and clinical manifestation between atherosclerosis and AS. In a landmark pathologic study, Otto and colleagues[11] found that early AS lesions resemble those of atherosclerosis and are characterized by basement membrane disruption, lipid deposition, and a mononuclear cellular infiltrate composed of T cells and macrophages (**Fig. 1**). This shared pathologic substrate translates into a gradual and progressive clinical course across a continuum of disease severity in both AS and atherosclerosis. For example, morphologic changes to the aortic valve leaflets in the initial stages of AS do not result in left ventricular outflow obstruction precluding symptom onset. However, in a subset of patients with aortic sclerosis there is progressive leaflet thickening, commissural fusion, and calcific deposition resulting in the cardinal AS symptoms of angina, syncope, and congestive heart failure.[2] Despite the many similarities in histopathology and clinical factors between atherosclerosis and AS, the association is not causal and important differences exist between the two conditions. For example, calcification tends to occur earlier and is a more prominent feature of AS compared with atherosclerosis. In addition, although smooth muscle cells are prominent in atherosclerosis, fibroblasts, and myofibroblasts are the dominant cell types in AS.

Studies during the last 20 years have shown that endothelial dysfunction, lipid deposition, and chronic inflammation are critical aspects of AS.

Other important pathologic features include an active regulated calcific phenotype in late-stage disease and genetic polymorphisms that increase AS susceptibility.

LIPID DEPOSITION

Although investigators have documented the presence of lipid within stenotic aortic valves for more than 100 years, more recent clinical, histopathologic, and experimental studies have now begun to elucidate the sources and entry mechanisms of these lipoproteins and their subsequent impact on valvular calcification and inflammation. Several clinical studies have consistently shown positive associations between increases in plasma LDL and/or lipoprotein (a) with aortic valve sclerosis or stenosis.[12–14] In a separate report, Pohle and colleagues[15] examined the impact of plasma LDL on the extent and rate of progression of aortic valve calcification among patients with AS. The mean rate of progression of aortic valve calcification over 15 months was substantially higher in those with versus without increased LDL (9% ± 22% vs 43% ± 44%, $P<.001$). Moreover, LDL-C was linearly associated with annualized progression of aortic valve calcification ($r = 0.35$, $P<.001$). Histopathologic studies provide further insight and provide a biological basis for these clinical observations. For example, O'Brien and colleagues[12] were among the first to show that lipoproteins present in stenotic aortic valves contained the atherogenic apolipoproteins (apo) B, apo(a) and apo E. The presence of apo B within

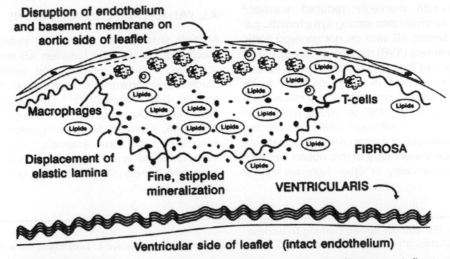

Fig. 1. Early lesion of valvular AS characterized by basement membrane disruption, inflammatory cellular infiltrate, and lipid deposition. (*From* Otto CM, Kuusisto J, Reichenbach DD, et al. Characterization of the early lesion of 'degenerative' valvular aortic stenosis. Histological and immunohistochemical studies. Circulation 1994;90:844–53; with permission.)

aortic valve lesions suggests not only that its source is circulating plasma LDL but also that its entry into the aortic valve may be partially mediated by extracellular matrix proteoglycans, analogous to lipoprotein uptake in atherosclerotic lesions.[16] Lipoproteins bind to proteoglycans via interactions between positively charged basic amino acids on apolipoproteins and negatively charged glycosaminoglycan side chains of proteoglycans.[16] In addition, other studies have colocalized specific apolipoproteins with particular proteoglycans.[17] In a surgical pathologic study, Olsson and colleagues[14] found that oxidized LDL colocalized with areas of inflammation and calcification in stenotic aortic valve specimens. The clinical relevance of these findings is highlighted by oxidized cholesterol stimulating both calcified nodule formation by valve fibroblasts and inflammatory activity.[18] In aggregate, these studies provide a link between increased plasma LDL and lipoprotein (a) and increased AS risk.

CHRONIC INFLAMMATION

Inflammation plays an important role in AS pathogenesis and disease progression. Several reports have documented that inflammatory cells including monocytes and T lymphocytes predominate in early AS lesions.[11,19,20] Monocytes differentiate into macrophages after entering the subendothelium. Other inflammatory cytokines and effector molecules have also been observed in stenotic aortic valves including transforming growth factor beta 1 (TGF-β1),[21] interleukin-1β,[22] tumor necrosis factor alpha,[23] and the terminal complement complex C5b-9.[24] These inflammatory mediators seem to exert their influence largely via regulation of additional enzymes and molecules involved in valvular remodeling and calcification. Additional support for the important role of inflammation in the pathogenesis of AS was recently provided in a histopathologic study by Moreno and colleagues[25] They found a significant increase in both inflammatory cellular infiltration and extent of calcification in bicuspid aortic valve specimens compared with trileaflet aortic valves.[25] Because congenital bicuspid AS is associated with more rapid progression and calcification, these findings provide further evidence for the important overlapping roles of inflammation and calcification in AS.

CALCIFICATION

The pathologic and clinical hallmark of advanced AS is extensive calcification, leading to leaflet rigidity and gradual left ventricular outflow obstruction. The higher prevalence of calcific AS in disease states associated with abnormal bone mineral metabolism, such as Paget disease and advanced chronic kidney disease, provide further evidence for the strong link between calcification and AS.[26,27] The adverse impact of valvular calcification in patients with AS was shown in a landmark report by Rosenhek and colleagues.[28] In this observational study of 128 patients with severe AS, the presence of aortic valve calcification was a robust discriminator of event-free survival because 2-year survival was significantly lower in patients with moderate to severe, versus none or mild, calcification (47% vs 84%, $P<.001$).[28]

Although the presence of calcification in stenotic aortic valves is not a novel finding, recent studies have established that calcific deposition does not occur passively but is an actively regulated process involving multiple cell types and pathways. Mohler and colleagues[18] found that human aortic valve cells in culture were able to differentiate into an osteoblast phenotype capable of mineralization. Moreover, the rate of calcified nodule formation by valvular interstitial cells was enhanced by TGF-β1 and bone morphogenetic protein 2.[18] Extending these observations, Rajamannan and colleagues[29] compared the genetic expression of various bone markers in calcific aortic valves with controls. Results of their ex vivo experiments showed significant upregulation in the diseased valves of genes encoding multiple osteogenic markers including osteocalcin, osteopontin, bone sialoprotein, and the osteoblast-specific transcription factor Cbfa1.[29] Multiple molecular pathways that are the subject of ongoing and intense investigation are involved in the complex regulation of pathologic calcification in advanced AS.[30–32]

TREATMENT OF AS: BAV

SAVR remains the preferred and definitive treatment of severe calcific AS with a class I indication in the most recent American College of Cardiology/American Heart Association valvular guidelines.[33] Relief of left ventricular outflow obstruction via SAVR results in regression of left ventricular hypertrophy, improvement in left ventricular function, and sustained symptomatic benefit.[34–36] Moreover, 1-year survival following SAVR is high, ranging from 92% to 94%.[37,38] However, in the absence of definitive therapy, severe AS is associated with significantly reduced survival, as shown in a retrospective study by O'Keefe and colleagues.[3] In this report, 1-year, 2-year, and 3-year survival rates in patients with untreated severe AS were 57%, 37%, and 25%, respectively.[3]

In contrast, survival rates in age-matched and sex-matched controls were 93%, 85%, and 77%, respectively. Despite the unambiguous benefits of SAVR, many patients are denied surgery either because of high-risk features or patient/physician refusal.[7,39] This was clearly shown in the Euro Heart Survey because approximately 32% of patients with severe valvular heart disease did not undergo surgical treatment.[39] In addition to cardiac causes, the most commonly cited noncardiac reasons for surgical exclusion included old age, chronic obstructive pulmonary disease, renal failure, and short life expectancy. BAV, which involves increasing the aortic valve orifice via balloon dilatation, is a nonsurgical option for patients with severe AS who may be unable or unwilling to undergo surgery.

BAV: TECHNICAL APPROACHES AND COMPLICATIONS

First introduced by Cribier and colleagues[40] in 1986 as a nonsurgical alternative to AVR, percutaneous BAV remains an important therapeutic option for thousands of patients with severe calcific AS who either refuse or are precluded from surgery because of multiple comorbidities. BAV may be performed either using a retrograde (brachial or femoral artery) or anterograde (transseptal) approach. Although much more commonly used and less technically demanding, the retrograde approach requires vascular anatomy suitable for large-bore caliber sheaths, which is a particularly relevant concern in the elderly AS population with multiple comorbid conditions, which often includes peripheral arterial disease. In addition, bleeding complications are greater because of the requirement of an arterial rather than venous access. The most common site of vascular access in the retrograde approach is the common femoral artery. After crossing the valve with a wire in a retrograde fashion, a balloon is then advanced, positioned, and dilated across the stenotic valve. If needed, subsequent dilations may be performed before removing the procedural balloon. After completion, an aortogram is generally performed to assess for any aortic regurgitation.

In contrast, technical challenges of anterograde BAV include transseptal puncture and balloon delivery across the left ventricular apex. Another potential complication of this approach is the creation of an atrial septal defect in up to 5% of patients, resulting in left-to-right shunts.[41] This small increase in cardiac output might result in an erroneous and falsely increased valve area calculation following anterograde BAV.[41] Although there are no randomized comparisons of the two

approaches, observational data suggest similar hemodynamic and clinical results with either technique.[42,43] In the largest series to date, Cubeddu and colleagues[43] conducted a single-center, retrospective analysis of 157 patients with AS who underwent either anterograde (n = 46) or retrograde (n = 111) BAV. Although most baseline characteristics were well balanced in the two groups, the frequency of peripheral arterial disease was significantly higher in those undergoing anterograde BAV (41% vs 18%, P<.01). There were no differences in hemodynamic parameters including mean change in aortic valve area or peak gradient following BAV in the two groups. Despite a higher rate of vascular complications with the retrograde technique, there were no differences in clinical outcomes at 2 years.

Periprocedural complications are common during BAV and reflect both technical complexity and a high-risk patient mix. These complications include, but are not limited to, death, ischemic stroke, bleeding, and acute aortic regurgitation. For example, rates of transfusion, cerebrovascular accident, and mortality in the National Heart, Lung and Blood Institute (NHLBI) balloon valvuloplasty registry were 23%, 3% and 3%, respectively.[44] Although technical improvements and better patient selection have led to a modest reduction in complication rates over the last 20 years,[45] periprocedural morbidity remains high. Balancing immediate procedural risk with any potential symptomatic improvement is therefore a critical component in the evaluation of any patient undergoing BAV.

Despite the high-risk nature of patients undergoing BAV, several studies suggest that use of vascular closure devices (VCD) and/or novel anticoagulants may substantially reduce procedure-related morbidity. High-risk anatomy and the requirement of large-bore arterial sheaths result in a high rate of periprocedural vascular injury, with a reported incidence of 10% to 15%.[44,46,47] In a single-center study, Ben-Dor and colleagues[48] compared vascular complication rates in 333 patients undergoing BAV according to access closure method (manual compression vs suture-mediated vs collaged-based closure device). The overall frequency of vascular complications, defined as vascular perforation, limb ischemia, arteriovenous fistula, pseudoaneurysm requiring intervention, or access site infection, was 8.4% (n = 28). However, risk was significantly reduced with use of VCD compared with manual compression (~6% vs ~17%). Other salutary benefits of VCD use in this study included a lower incidence of transfusion and shorter hospital length of stay compared with manual compression. Concordant findings were recently reported by O'Neill and colleagues[49] in a multicenter retrospective analysis comparing suture-mediated versus manual compression access site closure among patients having BAV. Suture-mediated closure was associated with significant reductions in major bleeding, major adverse cardiovascular events (MACE), and net adverse clinical events (NACE; **Fig. 2**). Moreover, the association between VCD and NACE in this report persisted after multivariable adjustment (odds ratio; 95% confidence interval [CI] 0.38 [0.21–0.58], P<.01).

Major bleeding and/or blood transfusion are also frequent complications of BAV, occurring in up 20% of patients. Although intravenous unfractionated heparin (UFH) remains the standard periprocedural anticoagulant during BAV, recent data suggest that the direct thrombin inhibitor bivalirudin may be a safer and superior alternative. In the percutaneous coronary intervention setting, several studies have shown that bivalirudin results in less bleeding with similar efficacy compared with UFH and provisional glycoprotein IIb/IIIa inhibitor use. Whether or not similar benefits may also be realized among high-risk patients having BAV was recently examined by Kini and colleagues[50] in the 2-center BRAVO (The Effect of Bivalirudin on Aortic Valve Intervention Outcomes) registry. In this pooled analysis, Kini and colleagues found that bivalirudin use was associated with significant reductions in major bleeding (4.9% vs 13.2%, P = .003). Although differences in

MACE were nonsignificant (6.7% vs 11.2%, P = .10), NACE comprising major bleeding or MACE were significantly reduced with bivalirudin compared with UFH (11.2% vs 20.0%, P = .01). These findings led to the ongoing, randomized BRAVO 2.3 study prospectively comparing bivalirudin versus UFH among patients with severe AS undergoing transcatheter AVR (TAVR).[51]

BAV: EARLY HEMODYNAMIC AND CLINICAL IMPACT

Most studies have documented modest but significant improvements in various hemodynamic parameters including transaortic gradient, cardiac output, and aortic valve area (AVA) following BAV.[44,45,52–55] Although results vary according to severity of underlying AS and technique, reductions in peak gradient range between 30% and 40% with similar improvements in AVA. In the NHLBI registry, BAV was associated with a significant reduction in peak aortic gradient from 65 mm Hg to 31 mm Hg (P<.001) and a concordant increase in AVA from 0.5 cm² to 0.8 cm² (P<.001).[44] Agarwal and colleagues[53] similarly reported a significant reduction in peak transaortic gradient from 55 ± 22 to 20 ± 11 mm Hg and an increase in AVA from 0.6 ± 0.2 to 1.2 ± 0.3 cm² in a series of 212 patients with severe AS undergoing BAV. Immediate symptomatic improvement is also common following BAV and is consistent with the favorable changes in postprocedure

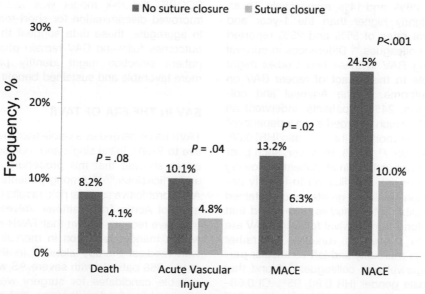

Fig. 2. Impact of suture-mediated closure versus no closure on outcomes during BAV. (*Data from* O'Neill B, Singh V, Kini A, et al. The use of vascular closure devices and impact on major bleeding and net adverse clinical events (NACEs) in balloon aortic valvuloplasty: A sub-analysis of the BRAVO study. Catheter Cardiovasc Interv 2013. [Epub ahead of print].)

hemodynamics. In general, this is reflected as reductions in New York Heart Association (NYHA) functional class. Otto and colleagues, for example, reported that 75% of patients surviving BAV at 30 days improved by at least 1 NYHA functional class.[44]

BAV: LONG-TERM RESULTS AND PREDICTORS OF SURVIVAL

Despite early improvements in clinical and hemodynamic parameters, benefits are not sustained, because mid-term and long-term outcomes following BAV remain poor.[44,55] This finding is attributable both to high rates of restenosis and extensive morbidity in the AS population. Serial echocardiographic and clinical assessments of patients following BAV indicate restenosis rates approaching 60% at 6 months. Among 28 patients who underwent BAV with subsequent echocardiographic follow-up at 3 months, Safian and colleagues[55] reported that the frequency of aortic valve restenosis was 43%. In a larger series, Otto and colleagues compared echocardiographic findings in 187 patients before and 6 months after BAV. Despite an immediate increase in AVA from 0.57 cm^2 to 0.78 cm^2 following BAV, mean AVA at 6 months was reduced to 0.65 cm^2.[44]

Consistent with the high frequency of restenosis, survival after BAV is also expectedly poor.[45,54] Agarwal and colleagues[53] reported 1-year, 3-year, and 5-year survival rates following BAV of 64%, 28%, and 14%, respectively. These rates are slightly higher than the 1-year and 3-year survival rates of 55% and 23% reported by Otto and colleagues.[56] Differences in survival rates following BAV in these two studies might be attributable to the impact of repeat BAV on long-term outcome. In the Agarwal and colleagues[53] report, 24% of patients underwent an additional BAV, which emerged as an independent correlate of lower mortality (hazard ratio [HR] 0.88, 95% CI 0.80–0.95, $P = .02$). However, such poor outcomes are not uniform in all patients following BAV and further risk stratification to identify patients who might realize a greater and sustained benefit is possible. Most studies have found that correlates of long-term survival following BAV are not related to procedural variables but rather reflect baseline morbidity and left ventricular performance. Agarwal and colleagues[53] found that although female gender (HR 0.80, 95% CI 0.68–0.94, $P = .016$) and multiple BAV procedures (HR 0.88, 95% CI 0.80–0.95, $P = .021$) were associated with lower risk after BAV, chronic renal insufficiency (HR 1.30, 95% CI 1.11–1.56, $P = .009$) and

Charlson comorbidity index (HR 1.12, 955 CI 1.03–1.21, $P = .006$) increased mortality risk. Otto and colleagues[56] similarly reported the following clinical, echocardiographic and catheterization predictors of survival: functional status, left ventricular systolic function, cardiac output, cachexia, renal function, mitral regurgitation, and female gender. Several studies with sufficiently large sample sizes have identified strong discriminators of long-term risk following BAV. Klein and colleagues[45] found that the strongest predictor of mortality in 78 patients undergoing BAV was age and that each 10-year increment in age was associated with a 2-fold increase in mortality (relative risk 2.0, 95% CI 1.2–3.3, $P = .005$). There was a substantial difference in median survival in patients younger than, versus older than, 70 years of age (29.3 months vs 5.7 months, $P = .013$). After stratifying patients into low or high levels of risk using baseline assessments of left ventricular function and functional status, Otto and colleagues[56] compared long-term survival between groups. In the low-risk group, 1-year, 2-year, and 3-year survival rates were 76%, 53%, and 36%, respectively. The analogous rates in the high-risk group were 47%, 28%, and 17%. Extending these earlier reports, Elmariah and colleagues[57] proposed a novel algorithm to predict 30-day mortality in patients having BAV. Independent variables that emerged as significant predictors in this model included preprocedural critical status, renal dysfunction, preprocedural right atrial pressure, and cardiac output. Compared with the EuroSCORE, the risk model was associated with improved discrimination for short-term mortality. In aggregate, these data suggest that, although outcomes following BAV remain poor, improved patient selection might identify patients with more favorable and sustained benefit.

BAV IN THE ERA OF TAVR

TAVR has emerged as a viable therapeutic alternative to SAVR. Initial single and multicenter experiences showed that this procedure is both safe and efficacious.[58,59] Among patients with severe AS at prohibitive surgical risk, results of The Placement of Aortic Transcatheter Valves (PARTNER) trial have recently shown that TAVR is associated with a marked reduction in mortality compared with medical therapy alone.[60] In this landmark study, 358 patients with severe AS who were not suitable candidates for surgery were randomly allocated to standard therapy, including BAV, or transfemoral TAVR. BAV was performed in all patients before TAVR and in 84% of patients receiving standard therapy. All-cause mortality at

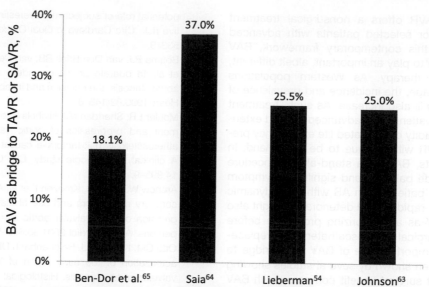

Fig. 3. Proportion of BAV procedures performed as bridge to TAVR or SAVR in selected registries.

1 year was significantly reduced with TAVR (30.7% vs 50.7%, *P*<.001). Results of the PARTNER B trial similarly showed that TAVR was noninferior to SAVR among eligible, albeit high-risk, surgical candidates with severe AS.[61]

Despite the apparent benefits and large number of potentially eligible patients for TAVR, many patients are initially denied this procedure for clinical, hemodynamic, or anatomic reasons. At a single center participating in a TAVR trial, Ben-Dor and colleagues[62] reported that, among 469 patients with severe AS screened for participation, 363 (77.1%) were excluded. In general, TAVR exclusions may be attributable to permanent (ie, lack of suitable vascular access) or temporary (ie, low cardiac output, hemodynamic instability) causes. It is within this latter context that BAV may serve a novel and therapeutic role in the management of patients with severe AS, namely as a bridge to TAVR. In support of this emerging role for BAV, several studies have shown that patients initially considered too high-risk for AVR were able to successfully undergo TAVR or SAVR following BAV as a bridging procedure. Although the frequency varies, approximately 20% to 30% of all BAV procedures are performed as a bridge indication (**Fig. 3**).[63] In a single-center study, Saia and colleagues[64] reported that, among 210 consecutive patients referred for BAV, 78 (37%) underwent BAV as a bridge before TAVR. Following BAV, 36 patients (46%) underwent TAVR, whereas 22 (28%) improved sufficiently to undergo SAVR. There were no differences in 30-day mortality between patients undergoing initial TAVR versus TAVR after bridging BAV (*P* = .74). BAV as a bridge

to TAVR/SAVR is associated with markedly improved outcomes compared with BAV alone.[52,65] For example, Ben-Dor and colleagues[65] reported significant and large reductions in mortality among patients with severe AS undergoing BAV as a bridge versus BAV alone (22.3% vs 55.2%, *P*<.001). Similar findings have previously been reported in the pre-TAVR era when comparing outcomes between patients undergoing BAV alone BAV as bridge to SAVR.[54]

With ongoing evolution of this technology and its active evaluation in low-risk patients, the scope and applicability of TAVR are expected to grow. Although current guidelines endorse a limited and largely palliative role for the use of BAV,[33] the introduction of TAVR has spurred greater enthusiasm for this procedure.[52] In one large-volume center, the number of annual BAV procedures almost tripled from 54/y to 130/y in a 2-year period after the introduction of TAVR.[52] In part, this reflects the need for a BAV in many patients before performing TAVR. These results indicate that BAV, either performed as an adjunctive or bridge procedure, remains relevant in the treatment of severe calcific AS.

SUMMARY

Pathophysiologic insights and treatment approaches to severe calcific AS have undergone substantial changes over the last 20 to 30 years. No longer considered an inevitable or degenerative process of aging, calcific deposition of the aortic valve is now understood to be an actively regulated process similar to atherosclerosis. In addition, TAVR offers a nonsurgical treatment alternative for selected patients with advanced AS. Within this contemporary framework, BAV will continue to play an important, albeit different, role in AS therapy. As Western populations continue to age, the incidence and prevalence of calcific AS will also increase. As such, treatment options for patients with advanced AS and extensive comorbidity or truncated life expectancy precluding TAVR will continue to be in demand. In such patients, BAV as a stand-alone procedure might provide palliative and significant symptom relief. Many patients with AS with hemodynamic instability or rapid clinical deterioration might also require BAV as a temporizing procedure before definitive surgical or transcatheter valve replacement. The important role of BAV as a bridge to AVR has been shown by several studies showing a significant survival benefit compared with BAV alone. Ongoing studies will continue to enhance understanding of AS and further refine the role of BAV in the TAVR era.

REFERENCES

1. Lindroos M, Kupari M, Heikkila J, et al. Prevalence of aortic valve abnormalities in the elderly: an echocardiographic study of a random population sample. J Am Coll Cardiol 1993;21:1220–5.
2. Ross J Jr, Braunwald E. Aortic stenosis. Circulation 1968;38:61–7.
3. O'Keefe JH Jr, Vlietstra RE, Bailey KR, et al. Natural history of candidates for balloon aortic valvuloplasty. Mayo Clin Proc 1987;62:986–91.
4. Nkomo VT, Gardin JM, Skelton TN, et al. Burden of valvular heart diseases: a population-based study. Lancet 2006;368:1005–11.
5. Stewart BF, Siscovick D, Lind BK, et al. Clinical factors associated with calcific aortic valve disease. Cardiovascular Health Study. J Am Coll Cardiol 1997;29:630–4.
6. Bonow RO, Carabello BA, Chatterjee K, et al. 2008 Focused update incorporated into the ACC/AHA 2006 guidelines for the management of patients with valvular heart disease: a report of the American College of Cardiology/American Heart Association Task Force on Practice Guidelines (Writing Committee to Revise the 1998 Guidelines for the Management of Patients with Valvular Heart Disease). endorsed by the Society of Cardiovascular Anesthesiologists, Society for Cardiovascular Angiography and Interventions, and Society of Thoracic Surgeons. J Am Coll Cardiol 2008;52: e1–142.
7. Bach DS, Siao D, Girard SE, et al. Evaluation of patients with severe symptomatic aortic stenosis who do not undergo aortic valve replacement: the potential role of subjectively overestimated operative risk. Circ Cardiovasc Qual Outcomes 2009;2:533–9.
8. Bouma BJ, van Den Brink RB, van Der Meulen JH, et al. To operate or not on elderly patients with aortic stenosis: the decision and its consequences. Heart 1999;82:143–8.
9. Mohler ER, Sheridan MJ, Nichols R, et al. Development and progression of aortic valve stenosis: atherosclerosis risk factors–a causal relationship? A clinical morphologic study. Clin Cardiol 1991;14:995–9.
10. Aronow WS, Ahn C, Kronzon I, et al. Association of coronary risk factors and use of statins with progression of mild valvular aortic stenosis in older persons. Am J Cardiol 2001;88:693–5.
11. Otto CM, Kuusisto J, Reichenbach DD, et al. Characterization of the early lesion of 'degenerative' valvular aortic stenosis. Histological and immunohistochemical studies. Circulation 1994;90:844–53.
12. O'Brien KD, Reichenbach DD, Marcovina SM, et al. Apolipoproteins B, (a), and E accumulate in the morphologically early lesion of 'degenerative' valvular aortic stenosis. Arterioscler Thromb Vasc Biol 1996;16:523–32.
13. Walton KW, Williamson N, Johnson AG. The pathogenesis of atherosclerosis of the mitral and aortic valves. J Pathol 1970;101:205–20.
14. Olsson M, Thyberg J, Nilsson J. Presence of oxidized low density lipoprotein in nonrheumatic stenotic aortic valves. Arterioscler Thromb Vasc Biol 1999;19:1218–22.
15. Pohle K, Maffert R, Ropers D, et al. Progression of aortic valve calcification: association with coronary atherosclerosis and cardiovascular risk factors. Circulation 2001;104:1927–32.
16. Skalen K, Gustafsson M, Rydberg EK, et al. Subendothelial retention of atherogenic lipoproteins in early atherosclerosis. Nature 2002;417:750–4.
17. O'Brien KD, Olin KL, Alpers CE, et al. Comparison of apolipoprotein and proteoglycan deposits in human coronary atherosclerotic plaques: colocalization of biglycan with apolipoproteins. Circulation 1998;98:519–27.
18. Mohler ER 3rd, Chawla MK, Chang AW, et al. Identification and characterization of calcifying valve cells from human and canine aortic valves. J Heart Valve Dis 1999;8:254–60.
19. Olsson M, Dalsgaard CJ, Haegerstrand A, et al. Accumulation of T lymphocytes and expression of interleukin-2 receptors in nonrheumatic stenotic aortic valves. J Am Coll Cardiol 1994;23:1162–70.
20. Olsson M, Rosenqvist M, Nilsson J. Expression of HLA-DR antigen and smooth muscle cell differentiation markers by valvular fibroblasts in degenerative aortic stenosis. J Am Coll Cardiol 1994;24:1664–71.

21. Anger T, Pohle FK, Kandler L, et al. VAP-1, Eotaxin3 and MIG as potential atherosclerotic triggers of severe calcified and stenotic human aortic valves: effects of statins. Exp Mol Pathol 2007;83:435–42.

22. Kaden JJ, Dempfle CE, Grobholz R, et al. Interleukin-1 beta promotes matrix metalloproteinase expression and cell proliferation in calcific aortic valve stenosis. Atherosclerosis 2003;170:205–11.

23. Kaden JJ, Dempfle CE, Grobholz R, et al. Inflammatory regulation of extracellular matrix remodeling in calcific aortic valve stenosis. Cardiovasc Pathol 2005;14:80–7.

24. Helske S, Oksjoki R, Lindstedt KA, et al. Complement system is activated in stenotic aortic valves. Atherosclerosis 2008;196:190–200.

25. Moreno PR, Astudillo L, Elmariah S, et al. Increased macrophage infiltration and neovascularization in congenital bicuspid aortic valve stenosis. J Thorac Cardiovasc Surg 2011;142:895–901.

26. Maher ER, Pazianas M, Curtis JR. Calcific aortic stenosis: a complication of chronic uraemia. Nephron 1987;47:119–22.

27. Strickberger SA, Schulman SP, Hutchins GM. Association of Paget's disease of bone with calcific aortic valve disease. Am J Med 1987;82:953–6.

28. Rosenhek R, Klaar U, Schemper M, et al. Mild and moderate aortic stenosis. Natural history and risk stratification by echocardiography. Eur Heart J 2004;25:199–205.

29. Rajamannan NM, Subramaniam M, Rickard D, et al. Human aortic valve calcification is associated with an osteoblast phenotype. Circulation 2003; 107:2181–4.

30. Caira FC, Stock SR, Gleason TG, et al. Human degenerative valve disease is associated with up-regulation of low-density lipoprotein receptor-related protein 5 receptor-mediated bone formation. J Am Coll Cardiol 2006;47:1707–12.

31. Kaden JJ, Bickelhaupt S, Grobholz R, et al. Receptor activator of nuclear factor kappaB ligand and osteoprotegerin regulate aortic valve calcification. J Mol Cell Cardiol 2004;36:57–66.

32. Steinmetz M, Skowasch D, Wernert N, et al. Differential profile of the OPG/RANKL/RANK-system in degenerative aortic native and bioprosthetic valves. J Heart Valve Dis 2008;17:187–93.

33. Bonow RO, Carabello BA, Chatterjee K, et al. 2008 Focused update incorporated into the ACC/AHA 2006 guidelines for the management of patients with valvular heart disease: a report of the American College of Cardiology/American Heart Association Task Force on Practice Guidelines (Writing Committee to Revise the 1998 Guidelines for the Management of Patients With Valvular Heart Disease): endorsed by the Society of Cardiovascular Anesthesiologists, Society for Cardiovascular Angiography and Interventions, and Society of Thoracic Surgeons. Circulation 2008;118:e523–661.

34. Croke RP, Pifarre R, Sullivan H, et al. Reversal of advanced left ventricular dysfunction following aortic valve replacement for aortic stenosis. Ann Thorac Surg 1977;24:38–43.

35. Kennedy JW, Doces J, Stewart DK. Left ventricular function before and following aortic valve replacement. Circulation 1977;56:944–50.

36. Pantely G, Morton M, Rahimtoola SH. Effects of successful, uncomplicated valve replacement on ventricular hypertrophy, volume, and performance in aortic stenosis and in aortic incompetence. J Thorac Cardiovasc Surg 1978;75:383–91.

37. Jacobs JP, Edwards FH, Shahian DM, et al. Successful linking of the Society of Thoracic Surgeons database to social security data to examine survival after cardiac operations. Ann Thorac Surg 2011;92:32–7 [discussion: 38–9].

38. Kvidal P, Bergstrom R, Horte LG, et al. Observed and relative survival after aortic valve replacement. J Am Coll Cardiol 2000;35:747–56.

39. Iung B, Baron G, Butchart EG, et al. A prospective survey of patients with valvular heart disease in Europe: the Euro Heart Survey on Valvular Heart Disease. Eur Heart J 2003;24:1231–43.

40. Cribier A, Savin T, Saoudi N, et al. Percutaneous transluminal aortic valvuloplasty using a balloon catheter. A new therapeutic option in aortic stenosis in the elderly. Arch Mal Coeur Vaiss 1986;79: 1678–86 [in French].

41. Feldman T. Transseptal antegrade access for aortic valvuloplasty. Catheter Cardiovasc Interv 2000;50: 492–4.

42. Block PC, Palacios IF. Comparison of hemodynamic results of anterograde versus retrograde percutaneous balloon aortic valvuloplasty. Am J Cardiol 1987;60:659–62.

43. Cubeddu RJ, Jneid H, Don CW, et al. Retrograde versus antegrade percutaneous aortic balloon valvuloplasty: immediate, short- and long-term outcome at 2 years. Catheter Cardiovasc Interv 2009;74:225–31.

44. Percutaneous balloon aortic valvuloplasty. Acute and 30-day follow-up results in 674 patients from the NHLBI Balloon Valvuloplasty Registry. Circulation 1991;84:2383–97.

45. Klein A, Lee K, Gera A, et al. Long-term mortality, cause of death, and temporal trends in complications after percutaneous aortic balloon valvuloplasty for calcific aortic stenosis. J Interv Cardiol 2006;19:269–75.

46. McKay RG. The Mansfield Scientific Aortic Valvuloplasty Registry: overview of acute hemodynamic results and procedural complications. J Am Coll Cardiol 1991;17:485–91.

47. Witzke C, Don CW, Cubeddu RJ, et al. Impact rapid ventricular pacing during percutaneous balloon aortic valvuloplasty in patients with critical aortic stenosis: should we be using it? Catheter Cardiovasc Interv 2010;75:444–52.

48. Ben-Dor I, Looser P, Bernardo N, et al. Comparison of closure strategies after balloon aortic valvuloplasty: suture mediated versus collagen based versus manual. Catheter Cardiovasc Interv 2011; 78:119–24.

49. O'Neill B, Singh V, Kini A, et al. The use of vascular closure devices and impact on major bleeding and net adverse clinical events (NACEs) in balloon aortic valvuloplasty: a sub-analysis of the BRAVO study. Catheter Cardiovasc Interv 2013. [Epub ahead of print].

50. Kini A Li YJ, Cohen M et-al. Results of a Two Center Registry. Bivalirudin versus Unfractionated Heparin During Aortic Valvuloplasty 2013. [Epub ahead of print].

51. Sergie Z, Lefevre T, Van Belle E, et al. Current peri-procedural anticoagulation in transcatheter aortic valve replacement: could bivalirudin be an option? Rationale and design of the BRAVO 2/3 studies. J Thromb Thrombolysis 2013. [Epub ahead of print].

52. Ben-Dor I, Pichard AD, Satler LF, et al. Complications and outcome of balloon aortic valvuloplasty in high-risk or inoperable patients. JACC Cardiovasc Interv 2010;3:1150–6.

53. Agarwal A, Kini AS, Attanti S, et al. Results of repeat balloon valvuloplasty for treatment of aortic stenosis in patients aged 59 to 104 years. Am J Cardiol 2005;95:43–7.

54. Lieberman EB, Bashore TM, Hermiller JB, et al. Balloon aortic valvuloplasty in adults: failure of procedure to improve long-term survival. J Am Coll Cardiol 1995;26:1522–8.

55. Safian RD, Warren SE, Berman AD, et al. Improvement in symptoms and left ventricular performance after balloon aortic valvuloplasty in patients with aortic stenosis and depressed left ventricular ejection fraction. Circulation 1988;78:1181–91.

56. Otto CM, Mickel MC, Kennedy JW, et al. Three-year outcome after balloon aortic valvuloplasty. Insights into prognosis of valvular aortic stenosis. Circulation 1994;89:642–50.

57. Elmariah S, Lubitz SA, Shah AM, et al. A novel clinical prediction rule for 30-day mortality following balloon aortic valvuloplasty: the CRRAC the AV score. Catheter Cardiovasc Interv 2011;78:112–8.

58. Himbert D, Descoutures F, Al-Attar N, et al. Results of transfemoral or transapical aortic valve implantation following a uniform assessment in high-risk patients with aortic stenosis. J Am Coll Cardiol 2009; 54:303–11.

59. Webb JG, Altwegg L, Boone RH, et al. Transcatheter aortic valve implantation: impact on clinical and valve-related outcomes. Circulation 2009;119: 3009–16.

60. Leon MB, Smith CR, Mack M, et al. Transcatheter aortic-valve implantation for aortic stenosis in patients who cannot undergo surgery. N Engl J Med 2010;363:1597–607.

61. Smith CR, Leon MB, Mack MJ, et al. Transcatheter versus surgical aortic-valve replacement in high-risk patients. N Engl J Med 2011;364:2187–98.

62. Ben-Dor I, Pichard AD, Gonzalez MA, et al. Correlates and causes of death in patients with severe symptomatic aortic stenosis who are not eligible to participate in a clinical trial of transcatheter aortic valve implantation. Circulation 2010;122: S37–42.

63. Johnson RG, Dhillon JS, Thurer RL, et al. Aortic valve operation after percutaneous aortic balloon valvuloplasty. Ann Thorac Surg 1990;49:740–4 [discussion: 744–5].

64. Saia F, Marrozzini C, Moretti C, et al. The role of percutaneous balloon aortic valvuloplasty as a bridge for transcatheter aortic valve implantation. Eurointervention 2011;7:723–9.

65. Ben-Dor I, Maluenda G, Dvir D, et al. Balloon aortic valvuloplasty for severe aortic stenosis as a bridge to transcatheter/surgical aortic valve replacement. Catheter Cardiovasc Interv 2012. [Epub ahead of print].

Transcatheter Aortic Valve Replacement Using the Edwards SAPIEN Transcatheter Heart Valves

Pei-Hsiu Huang, MD, Andrew C. Eisenhauer, MD*

KEYWORDS

- Aortic stenosis • Transcatheter aortic valve replacement • Edwards SAPIEN • Paravalvular leak
- Atrioventricular block

KEY POINTS

- The SAPIEN family of balloon-expandable transcatheter heart valves is the prototype device that initiated the widespread adoption transcatheter aortic valve replacement (TAVR).
- TAVR results in a definitive survival benefit compared with standard medical therapy and balloon aortic valvuloplasty.
- TAVR provides an alternative to surgical aortic valve replacement in high-risk patients.
- TAVR is associated with a range of potentially serious complications that affect clinical outcomes.
- With increasing dissemination of transcatheter valve technology, careful patient selection remains key to positive clinical outcomes.

INTRODUCTION

The prevalence of aortic stenosis continues to increase at a time when life expectancy exceeds 75 years for much of the developed world.[1] Described as early as the 1960s, the prognosis of patients with aortic stenosis remains favorable over a long latent phase. With the inevitable progression of aortic stenosis, survivability declines precipitously after the onset of symptoms. Although medical therapy can achieve modest symptomatic improvement, it does not alter the natural history of the disease. Definitive treatment involves replacement of the diseased aortic valve, which has historically been performed by open surgery and requires accepting the inherent risks of operating on this population of elderly individuals.

Transcatheter aortic valve replacement (TAVR) was introduced in 2002 as an alternative treatment to the standard surgical aortic valve replacement (SAVR) and has quickly become an accepted treatment of the patient at increased surgical risk. Transcatheter heart valve (THV) technology continues to advance leading to improved clinical outcomes and expanded adoption. Many new valve systems that are in various stages of development will debut in the coming years. This article reviews TAVR using the Edwards SAPIEN THV (Edwards Lifesciences, Irvine, CA).

Disclosures: P-H Huang, no relevant disclosures. A.C. Eisenhauer, grant support from Edwards Lifesciences, Advisory Board, Cardiosolutions Inc.
Division of Cardiovascular Medicine, Brigham and Women's Hospital, Harvard Medical School, 75 Francis Street, Boston, MA 02115, USA
* Corresponding author.
E-mail address: aeisenhauer@partners.org

BEFORE THE SAPIEN VALVES

In 1989, Andersen and colleagues[2] developed a bioprosthetic heart valve designed for transcatheter deployment. The valve consisted of a porcine aortic valve sewn onto a stainless steel frame fashioned from surgical wires. The assembly was carefully compressed onto a balloon catheter and deployed in various positions via endovascular insertion in several pigs.[2,3] This work showed the feasibility of transcatheter valve delivery and would become the foundation for future transcatheter valve systems.

A decade later, Cribier and colleagues[4] reported the development a new percutaneous heart valve for the treatment of native aortic valve stenosis based on the Andersen valve concept. Unpublished autopsy studies suggested that the valve could be effectively expanded and stabilized within a stenotic native aortic valve without impinging on the mitral valve or coronary ostia. The device used a balloon-expandable stainless steel stent frame supporting 3 bovine pericardial valve leaflets. Like the Andersen valve, this THV was crimped onto a balloon catheter that was then advanced into position across the aortic valve and deployed via inflation of the balloon catheter, displacing the native leaflets to allow function of the new valve leaflets.

FIRST-IN-HUMAN EXPERIENCE

Cribier and colleagues[5] performed the first human implantation of a THV for the treatment of aortic stenosis on April 16, 2002. The patient was a 57-year-old man with severe aortic stenosis, among other comorbidities, presenting in cardiogenic shock. The patient first underwent balloon aortic valvuloplasty after several surgeons declined to perform aortic valve replacement because of his clinical status. Despite initial improvement, his clinical status deteriorated again over the following week and, as a last-resort treatment, he underwent implantation of a THV with a dramatic improvement over the following days. The THV continued to function appropriately 17 weeks after implantation, when the patient died of infection of an amputation site.

SAPIEN THVS
SAPIEN

Continued development of this valve technology, subsequently acquired by Edwards Lifesciences Corporation, led first to the Cribier-Edwards design, which then evolved further to the SAPIEN THV. The SAPIEN valve (**Fig. 1**A) carries over the bovine pericardial valve leaflet design used in the Carpentier-Edwards PERIMOUNT surgical valve, mounting them on a balloon-expandable stainless steel stent frame. A polyethylene terephthalate (PET) fabric skirt covered the bottom inner portion of the stent frame to seal the aortic annulus from paravalvular leak (PVL). The SAPIEN THV is available in 23-mm and 26-mm sizes for transfemoral (TF) delivery through sheaths with internal diameters of 22 French (Fr) and 24 Fr, respectively (**Table 1**). In Europe, the SAPIEN THV received CE Mark approval on September 5, 2007. The United States Food and Drug Administration (FDA) approved the SAPIEN THV for clinical use in patients not eligible for SAVR on November 2, 2011, and expanded the indications to include very-high-risk surgical patients on October 19, 2012.

SAPIEN XT

The next-generation SAPIEN XT THV (**Fig. 1**B) alters the design of the earlier-generation valve through the use of a cobalt chromium stent frame to increase radial strength and new leaflet geometry to optimize function and coaptation. These changes allowed a reduction in the insertion profile such that the 23-mm and 26-mm valves could be delivered through sheaths with internal diameters of 18 Fr and 19 Fr, respectively. A larger 29-mm SAPIEN XT was recently introduced to treat annulus sizes up to 27 mm. The availability of an

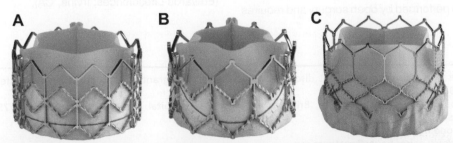

Fig. 1. Edwards SAPIEN family of THVs: The SAPIEN (*A*), SAPIEN XT (*B*), and SAPIEN 3 (*C*). (*Courtesy of* Edwards Lifesciences, LLC, Irvine, CA.)

Table 1
SAPIEN THV systems and delivery sheath sizes

Valve System	Indicated Annulus Size (mm)	TF Sheath ID (Fr)		Minimum Vessel Diameter	TA/TAo Sheath ID (Fr)
SAPIEN					
23 mm	18–22	22		7	26[a]
26 mm	21–25	24		8	26[a]
SAPIEN XT			(eSheath)		
23 mm	18–22	18	16	6	24
26 mm	21–25	19	18	6.5	24
29 mm	24–27	—	20	7	26
SAPIEN 3			(eSheath)		
20 mm	16–19	—	14	5.5	18
23 mm	18–22	—	14	5.5	18
26 mm	21–25	—	14	5.5	18
29 mm	24–28	—	16	6	21

Abbreviations: Fr, French; ID, internal diameter; TA, transapical; TAo, transaortic.
[a] Transaortic delivery not indicated with this system.

expandable introducer sheath (eSheath) further reduced the insertion profile to allow delivery of the SAPIEN XT valves through even smaller 16-Fr, 18-Fr, and 20-Fr sheaths (**Fig. 2**). Transapical (TA) and transaortic (TAo) delivery are also possible. The SAPIEN XT received CE Mark approval on March 2, 2010. This device is currently available as an investigational device in the United States.

SAPIEN 3

The SAPIEN 3 (see **Fig. 1**C) represents the continued evolution of the SAPIEN valve systems. The cobalt chromium stent frame and bovine pericardial leaflets use a new design that allow an insertion profile as small as 14 Fr. In addition to the inner PET skirt, a new outer PET skirt provides a second seal to minimize PVL. The SAPIEN 3 will be available in sizes of 20 mm, 23 mm, 26 mm, and 29 mm to treat annulus diameters between 16 mm and 28 mm. As of this writing, the SAPIEN 3 is only

available outside the United States as an investigational device. Among the 15 patients receiving the SAPIEN 3 THV in the initial feasibility study, there were no deaths, strokes, vascular complications, or more than mild PVL at 30 days.[6]

DELIVERY SYSTEMS
TF Systems

The RetroFlex delivery system consists of a balloon catheter wrapped within a deflectable catheter (**Fig. 3**). The deflectable catheter serves to stabilize and push the valve so that it does not slip off the balloon catheter as it is advanced into place, and to facilitate movement through the aortic arch by deflecting the distal tip of the inner balloon catheter, guiding the valve around the arch. Subsequent iterations of this TF delivery system retained the same basic design. The addition of a nose cone on the RetroFlex 2 helped delivery of the THV across the native valve. The RetroFlex

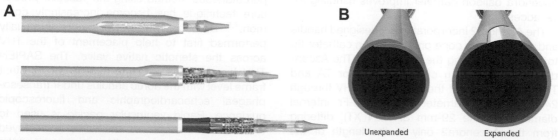

Unexpanded   Expanded

Fig. 2. The eSheath expands as the transcatheter valve is passed through the sheath and recoils to a smaller diameter after the valve has passed through (*A*). A cross-sectional view of the unexpanded and expanded eSheath (*B*). (*Courtesy of* Edwards Lifesciences, LLC, Irvine, CA.)

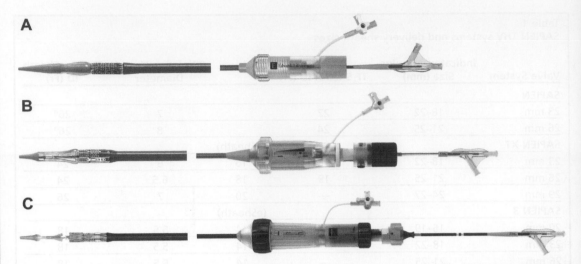

Fig. 3. TF delivery systems: The RetroFlex 3 (*A*), NovaFlex+ (*B*), and Commander (*C*). (*Courtesy of* Edwards Lifesciences, LLC, Irvine, CA.)

3, the system used with the SAPIEN THV, simplified the proximal end of the catheter and shortened the nose cone to reduce left ventricular (LV) damage.

The NovaFlex+ system is used with the SAPIEN XT. In this system, the valve is crimped onto the thinner balloon catheter shaft proximal to the balloon rather than on the balloon directly and then aligned to the balloon in the descending aorta before delivery. This design reduces the delivery profile, allowing the use of a smaller diameter sheath.

The newest Commander delivery catheter used with the SAPIEN 3 THV incorporates a more flexible catheter and the ability to finely adjust the valve position in the aortic annulus.

TA and TAo Systems

The Ascendra system allows TA implantation of the SAPIEN THV through a sheath with an internal diameter of 26 Fr (**Fig. 4**). The short length of the Ascendra balloon catheter improves handling for TA access.

The Acendra2 incorporates a redesigned handle and adds a nose cone on the balloon catheter tip to facilitate crossing the native valve. The Ascendra+ is the system currently used for TA and TAo implantation of the SAPIEN XT THV through 24-Fr internal diameter sheath (26-Fr internal diameter for the 29-mm SAPIEN XT), differing from the Ascendra2 only in the length of the balloon catheter.

The Certitude system, used with the SAPIEN 3 THV, integrates a valve pusher with the balloon

to simplify deployment and flexes to allow better valve alignment during TAo implantation.

IMPLANTATION TECHNIQUE

Initially, TAVR utilized an antegrade approach in which the valve was introduced into the femoral vein, advanced through a transseptal puncture across the mitral valve and turned into the aortic annulus. The technical complexity along with the added risk of the transseptal puncture and the need to traverse the mitral valve led operators to abandon this as the standard approach. Retrograde transarterial delivery via the femoral artery (**Fig. 5**) became the typical route as refinement in equipment facilitated transport of the THV around the aortic arch and across the stenotic native valve. The common femoral artery is cannulated and dilated to allow placement of the large-diameter delivery sheath into the descending aorta. Although surgical cutdown was the original method of accessing the femoral artery, a fully percutaneous method using the vascular preclosure technique has become increasingly common.[7,8] Balloon aortic valvuloplasty is usually performed first to help placement of the THV across the stenotic native valve. The SAPIEN THV is positioned with the midline of the stent frame level with the aortic annulus under transesophageal echocardiographic and fluoroscopic guidance. Rapid ventricular pacing is used to abate cardiac output as the valve is deployed (**Fig. 6**). The catheters are then removed and the femoral arteriotomy repaired. Temporary balloon occlusion of the iliofemoral vessels aids closure

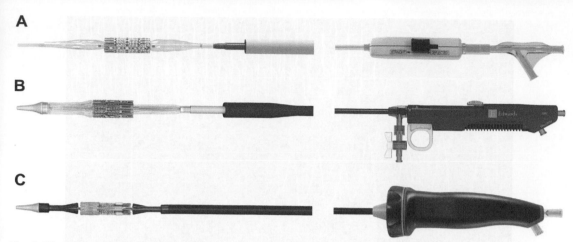

Fig. 4. TA delivery systems: The Ascendra (*A*), Ascendra+ (*B*), and Certitude (*C*). (*Courtesy of* Edwards Lifesciences, LLC, Irvine, CA.)

of the arterial access in fully percutaneous procedures.[9–11]

ALTERNATIVE ACCESS SITES

Alternative access sites allow TAVR in patients without adequate iliofemoral vessel anatomy for TF delivery.

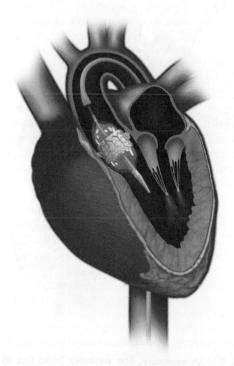

Fig. 5. TAVR via TF access. (*Courtesy of* Edwards Lifesciences, LLC, Irvine, CA.)

TA Access

Feasibility of direct LV apex cannulation through a small thoracotomy for THV delivery (**Fig. 7**) was shown in the mid-2000s.[12–15] Potential advantages to this approach are better control of valve position because of the proximity of the native aortic valve to the access site and ease of crossing the stenotic native valve in the antegrade direction. Complications of this access relate to closure of the LV apex and myocardial injury from puncture of the LV apex, which may result in impairment of LV function.[16,17] Compared with TF access, there seems to be an additional periprocedural hazard, although without effect on the long-term outcomes.[18–20] TA access similarly had no benefit on quality of life compared with SAVR because of potentially significant postoperative discomfort.[21]

TAo Access

This mode of access presents several potential advantages, including the need for a smaller surgical exposure, less impairment of pulmonary function, and avoidance of myocardial injury from LV puncture. TAo procedures involve surgical exposure through a hemisternotomy or second intercostal space thoracotomy (**Fig. 8**). The initial experience with this access has been favorable and it has rapidly gained popularity as an alternative access site.[22,23]

Other Access

Although the Edwards SAPIEN THV systems are not approved for other access routes, some have reported experience with transubclavian/transaxillary delivery.[24,25] More recently, one center reported a series of 3 patients who underwent

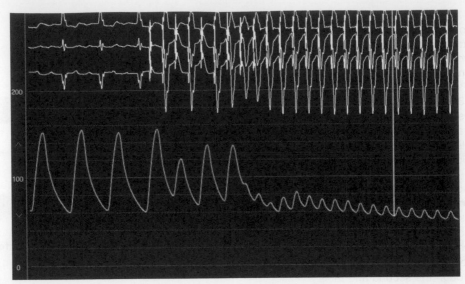

Fig. 6. Rapid ventricular pacing minimizes pulsatility and abates cardiac output to allow precise placement during valve deployment.

transcarotid TAVR using the Edwards SAPIEN valve.[26]

CLINICAL EXPERIENCE
PARTNER Trial

Early clinical experience with the SAPIEN THVs came from small clinical series and registries. The Placement of AoRtic TraNscathetER

(PARTNER) trial was the first randomized trial comparing TAVR with standard medical therapy or SAVR in 2 patient cohorts. The PARTNER cohort B consisted of 358 patients ineligible for SAVR because of excessive surgical risk randomized to TF-TAVR or standard therapy including balloon aortic valvuloplasty performed in 84% of

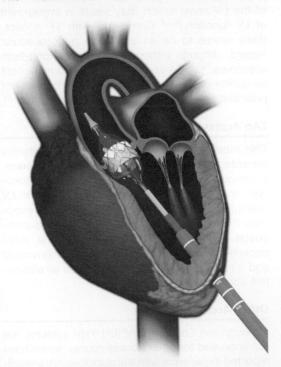

Fig. 7. TAVR via TA access. (*Courtesy of* Edwards Lifesciences, LLC, Irvine, CA.)

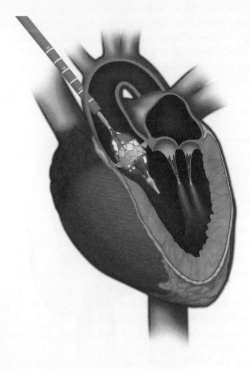

Fig. 8. TAo exposure. The patient's head lies to the left of the figure, feet to the right. (*Courtesy of* Edwards Lifesciences, LLC, Irvine, CA).

patients. The overall Society of Thoracic Surgeons (STS) score of 11.6% ± 6.0% reflected the high-risk status of this cohort. At 1 year, the TAVR group had a markedly lower rate of all-cause mortality than the standard-therapy group (30.7% vs 50.7%, P<.001).[27] This effect was sustained at 2 years (43.3% vs 68%, P<.001) and 3 years (54.1% vs 80.9%, P<.0001).[28,29] The TAVR group also had a dramatically lower rate of cardiovascular mortality (41.4% vs 74.5%, P<.0001) and rehospitalization (42.3% vs 75.7%, P<.0001) than the standard-therapy group at 3 years. However, the high incidence of stroke in the TAVR group compared with the standard-therapy group (15.7% vs 5.5% at 3 years, P = .0094) raised significant concern. Although much of the stroke risk developed early in the periprocedural period, the difference between the two groups continued to widen through the second and third years.

Cohort A included 699 patients who were operable, albeit at high surgical risk (STS score ≥10%). These patients were randomized to TAVR (either TF or TA depending on the possible access), or SAVR. Although the SAVR group sustained a higher rate of all-cause mortality than the TAVR group at 30-days (6.5% vs 3.4%, P = .07), there was no difference between TAVR and SAVR at 1 year (24.2% vs 26.8%, P = .44), 2 years (35.0% vs 33.9%, P = .78), and 3 years (44.2% vs 44.8%, P = .48), suggesting that the higher initial mortality reflected the risk from the surgery.[18,30,31] Other clinical outcomes also highlighted the differences in periprocedural risk between the two procedures. For example, the TAVR group had a reduction in symptoms at 30 days compared with the SAVR group, although the difference diminished by 1 year and remained similar between the 2 groups out to 3 years. Major vascular complications occurred more frequently at 3 years with TAVR (12.5% vs 3.8%, P<.001) but SAVR carried a higher risk of major bleeding (31.5% vs 20.8%, P = .003). Moderate to severe PVL also occurred more frequently at 2 years after TAVR than after SAVR (6.9% vs 0.9%, P<.001). The combined rate of all strokes and transient ischemic attacks was higher in the TAVR group than in the SAVR group at 30 days (5.5% vs 2.4%, P = .04) and 1 year (8.3% vs 4.3%, P = .04). However, the incidence of stroke did not differ between TAVR and SAVR out to 3 years despite the early periprocedural hazard.

The first PARTNER trial teaches several important lessons in addition to showing the effectiveness of TAVR compared with standard medical therapy and as an alternative to SAVR. Despite aggressive contemporary medical therapy, which included balloon aortic valvuloplasty in most patients, survival remained poor for patients who did not undergo TAVR. However, patients continued to have high mortality after TAVR, showing the importance of aggressively treating comorbid illnesses. Complications such as strokes, vascular access site difficulties, and PVL contribute to significant morbidity and suggest an opportunity for further improvement as the technology evolves.

PARTNER Nonrandomized Continued Access Registry

The nonrandomized continued access (NRCA) registry captured data from an additional 1017 high-risk and inoperable patients undergoing TF-TAVR and 988 high-risk patients undergoing TA-TAVR after closure of enrollment for the PARTNER study.[32,33] Comparisons were made with the respective TF and TA-TAVR cohorts from the randomized trial (TF-RCT and TA-RCT). Patients in the TF-NRCA were older but had fewer comorbid illnesses, reflected by lower STS scores and logistic EuroSCOREs, than TF-RCT. Outcomes at 30 days did not differ between the TF-RCT and TF-NRCA, but 1-year mortality was significantly lower in the TF-NRCA than in the TF-RCT (19.9% vs 25.4%). The 1-year incidence of cardiovascular death, stroke, and rehospitalization did not differ between the TF cohorts. The TF-NRCA group had fewer major vascular complications (5.5% vs 15.4%, P<.0001) and major bleeding complications (6.8% vs 15.3%, P<.0001) than the TF-RCT cohort, although the TA-NRCA patients had a similar risk profile to the TA-RCT patients. Mortality at 2 years was similar between the two groups (TA-NRCA 33.6% vs TA-RCT 40.7%, P = .160). There was a marked reduction in the rate of stroke in the TA-NRCA at the end of the first year (3.8% vs 9.6%, P = .01). Although the absolute incidence of complications remains significant, these results suggest that outcomes improve with increasing procedural experience.

PARTNER II

The PARTNER II trial builds on the first series in a few important ways. The trial evaluates the newer-generation SAPIEN XT THV and exemplifies the continued evolution of TAVR. The trial includes lower-risk patients, Ao alternative access, and the expansion of indications with the valve-in-valve registry. Like the first trial, PARTNER II studies 2 cohorts. The inoperable cohort compares use of the SAPIEN valve with the SAPIEN XT valve. The operable cohort compares TAVR with SAVR in intermediate-risk patients (STS score ≥4%). The design also incorporates 6 registries for inoperable patients to study those with small iliofemoral vessels, TA, and TAo access, the larger 29-mm THV, and treatment of degenerated bioprosthetic valves.

The results of the randomized inoperable cohort were recently presented.[34] The primary composite end point of all-cause mortality, disabling stroke, and rehospitalization for symptoms of aortic stenosis or complications of the valve procedure was not different between the SAPIEN and SAPIEN XT at 1 year (34.7% vs 33.9%, P [noninferiority] = 0.0034) and the individual end point components also did not differ between groups. However, the lower-profile SAPIEN XT resulted in fewer 30-day major vascular complications (9.6% vs 15.5%, P = .04). Enrollment for the intermediate-risk operable cohort is expected to conclude in 2014.

STACCATO

The STACCATO trial attempted to compare TA-TAVR with SAVR in a lower-risk population and originally intended to randomize 200 patients enrolled from multiple sites in Denmark to either TA-TAVR or SAVR.[35] Eligible patients were 75 years old or older with severe aortic stenosis but were excluded for a variety of comorbidities. As a result, 87% of patients assessed for eligibility failed to enter the trial and 70 patients were ultimately randomized before the trial was prematurely terminated because of excessive adverse outcomes in the TA-TAVR cohort. The mean STS score of patients receiving TA-TAVR was 3.1 ± 1.5 and 3.4 ± 1.2 for patients having SAVR, reflecting the low surgical risk of the study population. Among the 34 patients randomized to and undergoing TA-TAVR, 2 deaths, 3 strokes, and 1 case of renal failure requiring dialysis occurred at 30 days. In addition, 7 patients required SAVR or reoperation for anatomic limitation to TA-TAVR (1), left coronary artery occlusion (2), aortic rupture (1), severe PVL (2), or postoperative bleeding (1). By comparison, 3 events occurred among the 36 patients in the SAVR group including 1 major stroke and 1 instance of reoperation for bleeding. Although STACCATO received much criticism for its design and execution, these results reemphasize the point that, with the current THV technology, SAVR should remain the standard treatment rather than TA-TAVR, or perhaps TAVR in general, in low-risk patients.

Registry Data

Several large registries provide insight on the real-world use of THVs.[36–47] Select registries capturing data on the Edwards SAPIEN THV are presented in

Table 2. Overall, the short-term and long-term survival, as well as the rates of other outcomes including stroke, vascular complications, and PVL, were similar across registries. Registries capturing data on both SAPIEN and CoreValve did not find significant differences between the two valves except for the higher rate of heart block and need for a pacemaker after TAVR.

COMPLICATIONS

Worldwide experience with TAVR has uncovered a range of potentially serious complications that may affect patient outcomes. These complications are important to examine in detail and they must be considered carefully when counseling patients on their options for treatment of aortic stenosis. Further development of this technology could reduce the incidence of PVL and vascular access complications, for example. Other complications such as stroke may relate more to comorbid disease and continue to challenge clinicians. At first, rates of complications were difficult to compare across TAVR studies, in large part because of the nonstandard definitions. In order to understand these issues with more precision, the Valve Academic Research Consortium (VARC) proposed standardized definitions of various clinical end points followed in TAVR trials to facilitate comparison across trials.[48]

Vascular Access Complications

The need to insert large-bore arterial access sheaths for TF-TAVR places patients at risk for vascular access complications. Among patients undergoing TF-TAVR in the PARTNER trial, 15.3% had a major vascular complication and 11.9% had a minor vascular complication within 30 days of the procedure.[49] Contemporary TAVR registries report major vascular complication rates of 2.7% to 14%.[37–40,43,44] Patients with major vascular complications also had higher rates of major bleeding, transfusion, renal failure, and significantly higher rates of death at 30 days and 1 year. Although the risk of vascular complications is associated with various clinical and procedural factors such as female gender, iliofemoral artery size, and arterial calcifications, the importance of procedural experience must not be overlooked.[49,50] Early center experience was recognized to increase the risk of major vascular complications 3.7-fold.[50] Patients undergoing TF-TAVR in the PARTNER NRCA registry had a significantly lower rate of major vascular complications (5.5%) compared with TF-TAVR in those enrolled in the randomized cohorts (15.4%).[32] Increasing procedural experience along with the shift from the early-generation

Table 2
Select national TAVR registries

Registry	N	Device	Age (y)	Male (%)	LES	Follow-up	Death (%)	Stroke (%)	Vascular Complications (%)	>Mod AI (%)	PPM (%)
Germany[36]	697	MCV, ES	81.4 ± 6.3	44.2	20.5 ± 13.2	30 d	12.4	2.8	4	2.3	39.3
UK TAVI[37]	870	MCV, ES	81.9 ± 7.1	52.4	18.5	2 y	26.3	4.1	6.3	13.6	16.3
FRANCE II[40]	3195	MCV, ES	82.7 ± 7.2	51	21.9 ± 14.3	1 y	24	4.1	4.7	16.5 (30 d)	15.6
Belgian[42]	881	MCV, ES	83 ± 6	47	27 ± 16	1 y	10	6	—	—	17
PARTNER EU[43]	130	ES	82.1 ± 5.5	44.6	30 ± 13.7	1 y	49.3	8.5	10.7 (30 d)	—	2.5
Milan[44]	400	MCV, ES	79.4 ± 7.4	50.6	24.2 ± 17	30 d	4.7	1.0	13.5	—	—
Canadian[45]	339	ES	81 ± 8	44.8	9.8 ± 6.4[a]	30 d	10.4	2.3	—	—	4.9

Abbreviations: AI, aortic insufficiency; ES, Edwards SAPIEN; LES, Logistic EuroScore; MCV, Medtronic CoreValve; PPM, permanent pacemaker.
[a] Society of Thoracic Surgeons risk score.

SAPIEN to the smaller-profile SAPIENT XT was shown to lower the rate of major vascular complications from 8% to 1%.[8] The results of the PARTNER II inoperable cohort showed a similar decrease in the rate of major vascular complications (9.6% vs 15.5%) with the newer lower-profile SAPIENT XT compared with the SAPIEN.[34] Thus, progressive decline in vascular access complications is likely the result of both technical experience, improved patient selection, and smaller-diameter access equipment.

PVL

In contrast to SAVR, PVL occurs frequently after TAVR. In the PARTNER trial, 66% of patients had trace or mild and 12% had moderate or severe PVL after TAVR.[18,27] This rate compares well with registry reports in which the incidence of moderate or severe PVL after TAVR with the Edwards balloon-expandable valves ranges between 2.3% and 13.9%.[37,38,40,44] In the recently presented PARTNER II inoperable cohort, 22.5% of patients had moderate or severe PVL after TAVR.[34]

Compared with the CoreValve THV (Medtronic, Inc, Minneapolis, MN), there seems to be a lower rate of PVL after implantation of the Edwards THV in the FRANCE II registry. Over time, most case series show that PVL seems to remain stable or even improve in a small percentage of patients.[19,51–53] In the PARTNER study, PVL worsened by at least 1 grade in 22.4% of patients but remained unchanged or improved by at least 1 grade in 46.2% and 31.5% of patients at 2 years.[30] At 3 years, roughly 50% of patients continued to have at least mild PVL without significant change from 2 years.[31]

The significance of the presence of PVL, or any aortic regurgitation, is its association with worse clinical outcomes. Several studies have shown that moderate or severe PVL conferred an additional risk of both short-term and long-term mortality. Even mild PVL after TAVR was associated with a 17.1% increase in mortality at 3 years, as shown in the PARTNER trial.[31]

The mechanism for TAVR-associated PVL differs from that after SAVR. Although surgical prostheses develop leak due to dehiscence of the sewing ring from the annular tissue caused by, factors such as suturing technique, suture rupture, infection, or annular calcification, the primary mechanism of PVL after TAVR relates to the incomplete seal at the separation of the aortic and LV cavities by the prosthesis. Of the common factors associated with PVL after TAVR, improper valve sizing is strongly associated with PVL.[54]

Recent studies have shown that the aortic annulus is not circular, and demonstrated the superiority of computed tomography imaging compared with either transthoracic or transesophageal echocardiography for measuring its size.[55,56] Appropriate valve sizing in turn reduced the incidence of PVL after TAVR.[57,58]

Stroke

When the first PARTNER trial was reported, one of the major concerns was the rate of stroke among those who underwent TAVR. Inoperable patients consistently had higher rates of stroke at 2 years after TAVR compared with standard medical therapy (13.8% vs 5.5%, $P = .01$).[28] Although the rate of stroke remained steady in the standard-treatment group, an excess of strokes within the first 30 days was seen in those undergoing TAVR, most occurring within the first 48 hours after the procedure. A greater number of ischemic strokes were seen within the first 30 days but the late increase in stroke beyond 30 days was caused by a similar percentage of ischemic and hemorrhagic strokes. In the high-risk surgical patients, cohort A, the rate of stroke with TAVR was twice that of SAVR both at 1 year (6.0% vs 3.2%, $P = .08$) and 2 years (7.7% vs 4.9%, $P = .17$) but did not reach significance.[30] Similar to TAVR in cohort B, there was an early hazard of stroke with TAVR versus SAVR (4.6% vs 2.4%, $P = .12$). PARTNER II cohort B results showed a similar overall rate of stroke at 30 days at 4.1% with no difference between the rates of either the SAPIEN or SAPIEN XT groups.[34] These rates of stroke were consistent with those reported by large multicenter or national registries 0.6% to 5% (see **Table 2**).

There seem to be 2 distinct phases of stroke: the early phase relating to the TAVR or SAVR procedure, and the late phase caused more by patient-related and disease-related factors.[59] This finding has been corroborated by transcranial Doppler studies showing that the highest embolic load was seen during wire manipulation in the aortic arch and insertion and deployment of the valve.[60–62] There was no difference in the cerebral embolic load between the TA or TF access routes.

In order to reduce the risk of cerebral emboli, there are several embolic protection devices under development. These devices, including the Embol-X (Edwards Lifesciences, Irvine, CA),[63] TriGuard (Keystone Heart Ltd, Israel),[64] and Claret CE Pro (Claret Medical, Inc, Santa Rosa, CA),[65] have been investigated in small clinical series and shown to reduce the number of embolic lesions detected on post-TAVR magnetic resonance imaging.

Atrioventricular Block

Implantation of a THV in the aortic annulus can also potentially injure the LV conduction system, resulting in atrioventricular block and the need for a pacemaker. In the PARTNER trial, the incidence of new pacemaker placement was 5% to 7% at 2 years.[28,30] The PARTNER II cohort A showed a similar rate of pacemaker placement of 6% with no difference between groups receiving the SAPIEN or the SAPIEN XT valves.[34] Although no study has directly compared the SAPIEN THVs with the CoreValve system, higher rate of atrioventricular block requiring new pacemaker implants after CoreValve (up to 49%) is frequently cited as one of the distinguishing outcomes.[66,67] The reason for this difference may relate to the Core-Valve design, which sits lower in the LV outflow tract after implantation and exerts an outward radial force on the aortic annulus and LV outflow tract because of its self-expanding stent frame.[68] However, the observation that many patients develop conduction blocks before deployment of the valve suggests that other mechanisms of conduction system injury may be the cause.[69] New left bundle branch block (LBBB) occurs in up to 18% of patients after placement of a SAPIEN THV, but pre-procedural LBBB did not predict the need for a pacemaker after TAVR.[66] However, preexisting right bundle branch block (RBBB) was a predictor of post-TAVR complete heart block requiring a pacemaker.[66] New-onset LBBB after TAVR has also been associated with an absolute 13.8% increase (37.8% vs 24%, $P = .0002$) in mortality and independently predicts death.[70] Therefore, atrioventricular block after TAVR should be regarded as more than a simple nuisance event.

PATIENT SELECTION

As worldwide experience with TAVR grows, it has become increasingly apparent that appropriate patient selection can significantly improve procedure outcomes. Patients being considered for TAVR often have several comorbidities that make their care difficult. In evaluating patients for TAVR, the first consideration is to determine whether or not aortic valve replacement will benefit the patient in terms of mortality or quality of life. In elderly patients, it is important to recognize that quality of life may be of equivalent or even more significant outcome than mortality. Then there are those whose clinical condition has deteriorated to the degree that aortic valve replacement by any means is thought to have no benefit or perhaps even cause harm to the patient, as was shown in the first PARTNER trial, in which inoperable patients with an STS risk greater than or equal to 15% had no survival benefit compared with standard medical therapy.[28]

The impact of frailty on outcomes after TAVR remains poorly understood as well. In the first PARTNER trial, 18.4% of patients were determined to be frail, although its association with clinical outcomes in the trial has not been reported. Two small studies showed that frailty increased the risk of mortality after TAVR 4-fold.[71,72] However, a third and larger study showed no difference in survival between frail and nonfrail patients.[45] The discrepancy may be related to the different definitions of frailty. The on-going PARTNER II trial incorporates more rigorous measures of frailty and may bring more clarity to this issue.

SUMMARY

TAVR has attained a place in the therapy for valvular aortic stenosis in a selected population of patients with increased risk for standard aortic valve replacement surgery. The SAPIEN family of balloon-expandable THVs is the prototype that initiated this therapy and, despite (or perhaps because of) its initial success, has undergone rapid development and evolution. The SAPIEN system has taught cardiologists and cardiac surgeons much about the nature of this disease and the potential for less invasive and equally or more effective therapy for it. However, this knowledge has come at the price of also learning about the complications and limitations of the therapy. There are multiple additional platforms in varying stages of development and, as knowledge and technology evolve, it is not certain which will emerge as the new standard for this therapy. What is certain is that the therapeutic landscape will continue to change rapidly and that equipment and practice in 5 years will look very different from the current situation.

REFERENCES

1. United Nations Statistics Division - Demographics and Social Statistics. 2013 [Internet]. Available at: http://unstats.un.org/unsd/demographic/products/socind/. Accessed May 13, 2013.
2. Andersen HR, Knudsen LL, Hasenkam JM. Transluminal catheter implantation of a new expandable artificial cardiac valve (the stent–valve) in the aorta and the beating heart of closed chest pigs [abstract]. Eur Heart J 1990;11(Suppl):224a.
3. Andersen HR, Knudsen LL, Hasenkam JM. Transluminal implantation of artificial heart valves. Description of a new expandable aortic valve and initial results with implantation by catheter

technique in closed chest pigs. Eur Heart J 1992; 13(5):704–8.

4. Cribier A, Eltchaninoff H, Borenstein N, et al. Transcatheter implantation of balloon-expandable prosthetic heart valves: early results in an animal model [abstract]. Circulation 2001;104(Suppl II): II-552.

5. Cribier A, Eltchaninoff H, Bash A, et al. Percutaneous transcatheter implantation of an aortic valve prosthesis for calcific aortic stenosis: first human case description. Circulation 2002;106(24):3006–8.

6. Binder RK, Rodés-Cabau J, Wood DA, et al. Transcatheter aortic valve replacement with the SAPIEN 3: a new balloon-expandable transcatheter heart valve. JACC Cardiovasc Interv 2013;6(3):293–300.

7. Davidson MJ, Welt FG, Eisenhauer AC. Percutaneous balloon-expandable aortic valve implantation: transfemoral. Operat Tech Thorac Cardiovasc Surg 2011;16(1):30–40.

8. Toggweiler S, Gurvitch R, Leipsic J, et al. Percutaneous aortic valve replacement: vascular outcomes with a fully percutaneous procedure. J Am Coll Cardiol 2012;59(2):113–8.

9. Sharp AS, Michev I, Maisano F, et al. A new technique for vascular access management in transcatheter aortic valve implantation. Catheter Cardiovasc Interv 2010;75(5):784–93.

10. Généreux P, Kodali S, Leon MB, et al. Clinical outcomes using a new crossover balloon occlusion technique for percutaneous closure after transfemoral aortic valve implantation. JACC Cardiovasc Interv 2011;4(8):861–7.

11. Buchanan GL, Chieffo A, Montorfano M, et al. A "modified crossover technique" for vascular access management in high-risk patients undergoing transfemoral transcatheter aortic valve implantation. Catheter Cardiovasc Interv 2013; 81(4):579–83.

12. Webb JG, Munt B, Makkar RR, et al. Percutaneous stent-mounted valve for treatment of aortic or pulmonary valve disease. Catheter Cardiovasc Interv 2004;63(1):89–93.

13. Huber CH, Cohn LH. Direct-access valve replacement: a novel approach for off-pump valve implantation using valved stents. J Am Coll Cardiol 2005; 46(2):366–70.

14. Ye J, Cheung A, Lichtenstein SV, et al. Transapical aortic valve implantation in humans. J Thorac Cardiovasc Surg 2006;131(5):1194–6.

15. Lichtenstein SV, Cheung A, Ye J, et al. Transapical transcatheter aortic valve implantation in humans: initial clinical experience. Circulation 2006;114(6): 591–6.

16. Kempfert J, Rastan A, Holzhey D, et al. Transapical aortic valve implantation: analysis of risk factors and learning experience in 299 patients. Circulation 2011;124(Suppl 11):S124–9.

17. Barbash IM, Dvir D, Ben-Dor I, et al. Impact of transapical aortic valve replacement on apical wall motion. J Am Soc Echocardiogr 2013;26(3):255–60.

18. Smith CR, Leon MB, Mack MJ, et al. Transcatheter versus surgical aortic-valve replacement in high-risk patients. N Engl J Med 2011;364(23):2187–98.

19. Ewe SH, Delgado V, Ng AC, et al. Outcomes after transcatheter aortic valve implantation: transfemoral versus transapical approach. Ann Thorac Surg 2011;92(4):1244–51.

20. Johansson M, Nozohoor S, Kimblad PO, et al. Transapical versus transfemoral aortic valve implantation: a comparison of survival and safety. Ann Thorac Surg 2011;91(1):57–63.

21. Reynolds MR, Magnuson EA, Wang K, et al. Health-related quality of life after transcatheter or surgical aortic valve replacement in high-risk patients with severe aortic stenosis: results from the PARTNER (Placement of AoRtic TraNscathetER Valve) Trial (Cohort A). J Am Coll Cardiol 2012;60(6):548–58.

22. Bapat V, Khawaja MZ, Attia R, et al. Transaortic transcatheter aortic valve implantation using Edwards Sapien valve: a novel approach. Catheter Cardiovasc Interv 2012;79(5):733–40.

23. Lardizabal JA, O'Neill BP, Desai HV, et al. The transaortic approach for transcatheter aortic valve replacement: initial clinical experience in the United States. J Am Coll Cardiol 2013;61(23):2341–5.

24. Cioni M, Taramasso M, Giacomini A, et al. Transaxillary approach: short- and mid-term results in a single-center experience. Innovations (Phila) 2011;6(6):361–5.

25. Sharp AS, Michev I, Colombo A. First trans-axillary implantation of Edwards Sapien valve to treat an incompetent aortic bioprosthesis. Catheter Cardiovasc Interv 2010;75(4):507–10.

26. Guyton RA, Block PC, Thourani VH, et al. Carotid artery access for transcatheter aortic valve replacement (TAVR). Cathet Cardiovasc Diagn 2012. [Epub ahead of print].

27. Leon MB, Smith CR, Mack M, et al. Transcatheter aortic-valve implantation for aortic stenosis in patients who cannot undergo surgery. N Engl J Med 2010;363(17):1597–607.

28. Makkar RR, Fontana GP, Jilaihawi H, et al. Transcatheter aortic-valve replacement for inoperable severe aortic stenosis. N Engl J Med 2012;366(18): 1696–704.

29. Tuzcu EM. PARTNER cohort B three year: clinical and echocardiographic outcomes from a prospective, randomized trial of transcatheter aortic valve replacement in "inoperable" patients. Transcatheter Cardiovascular Therapeutics (TCT). Miami (FL), 2012.

30. Kodali SK, Williams MR, Smith CR, et al. Two-year outcomes after transcatheter or surgical aortic-valve replacement. N Engl J Med 2012;366(18): 1686–95.

31. Thourani VH. Three-year outcomes after transcatheter or surgical aortic valve replacement in highrisk patients with severe aortic stenosis. American College of Cardiology 62nd Annual Scientific Session (ACC.13). San Francisco, 2013.

32. Fearon WF. New data from the PARTNER Non-randomized Continued Access registry: outcomes after transfemoral transcatheter aortic valve replacement. American College of Cardiology 62nd Annual Scientific Session (ACC.13). San Francisco, 2013.

33. Dewey TM. New data from PARTNER continued access (non-randomized): transapical outcomes after TAVR. Transcatheter Cardiovascular Therapeutics (TCT). Miami (FL), 2012.

34. Leon MB. A randomized evaluation of the SAPIEN XT transcatheter valve system in patients with aortic stenosis who are not candidates for surgery: PARTNER II, inoperable cohort. American College of Cardiology 62nd Annual Scientific Session (ACC.13). San Francisco, 2013.

35. Nielsen HH, Klaaborg KE, Nissen H, et al. A prospective, randomised trial of transapical transcatheter aortic valve implantation vs. surgical aortic valve replacement in operable elderly patients with aortic stenosis: the STACCATO trial. EuroIntervention 2012;8(3):383–9.

36. Zahn R, Gerckens U, Grube E, et al. Transcatheter aortic valve implantation: first results from a multi-centre real-world registry. Eur Heart J 2011;32(2): 198–204.

37. Moat NE, Ludman P, de Belder MA, et al. Long-term outcomes after transcatheter aortic valve implantation in high-risk patients with severe aortic stenosis: the U.K. TAVI (United Kingdom Transcatheter Aortic Valve Implantation) Registry. J Am Coll Cardiol 2011;58(20):2130–8.

38. Wendler O. The multicenter SOURCE XT TAVR Registry. Transcatheter Valve Therapies. Seattle (WA), 2012.

39. Rodés-Cabau J, Webb JG, Cheung A, et al. Long-term outcomes after transcatheter aortic valve implantation: insights on prognostic factors and valve durability from the Canadian multi-center experience. J Am Coll Cardiol 2012; 60(19):1864–75.

40. Gilard M, Eltchaninoff H, Iung B, et al. Registry of transcatheter aortic-valve implantation in high-risk patients. N Engl J Med 2012;366(18):1705–15.

41. Ussia GP. TAVI with self-expanding prosthesis: 3-year outcomes from Italian registry. EuroPCR. Paris (France), 2012.

42. Bosmans J. Procedural 30-day, 6-month and 1-year outcome following TAVI: results of the Belgian registry. EuroPCR. Paris (France), 2012.

43. Lefevre T, Kappetein AP, Wolner E, et al. One year follow-up of the multi-centre European PARTNER transcatheter heart valve study. Eur Heart J 2011; 32(2):148–57.

44. Buchanan GL. Valve academic research consortium outcomes following TAVI with two available devices: 30-day and 1-year results from the Milan registry. EuroPCR. Paris (France), 2012.

45. Rodés-Cabau J, Webb JG, Cheung A, et al. Transcatheter aortic valve implantation for the treatment of severe symptomatic aortic stenosis in patients at very high or prohibitive surgical risk: acute and late outcomes of the multicenter Canadian experience. J Am Coll Cardiol 2010; 55(11):1080–90.

46. Wendler O, Walther T, Schroefel H, et al. Transapical aortic valve implantation: mid-term outcome from the SOURCE registry. Eur J Cardiothorac Surg 2013;43(3):505–11 [discussion: 511–2].

47. Thomas M, Schymik G, Walther T, et al. One-year outcomes of cohort 1 in the Edwards SAPIEN Aortic Bioprosthesis European Outcome (SOURCE) registry: the European registry of transcatheter aortic valve implantation using the Edwards SAPIEN valve. Circulation 2011;124(4):425–33.

48. Leon MB, Piazza N, Nikolsky E, et al. Standardized endpoint definitions for transcatheter aortic valve implantation clinical trials: a consensus report from the Valve Academic Research Consortium. J Am Coll Cardiol 2011;57:253–69.

49. Généreux P, Webb JG, Svensson LG, et al. Vascular complications after transcatheter aortic valve replacement: insights from the PARTNER (Placement of AoRTic TraNscathetER Valve) Trial. J Am Coll Cardiol 2012;60(12):1043–52.

50. Hayashida K, Lefevre T, Chevalier B, et al. Transfemoral aortic valve implantation new criteria to predict vascular complications. JACC Cardiovasc Interv 2011;4(8):851–8.

51. Webb JG, Altwegg L, Boone RH, et al. Transcatheter aortic valve implantation: impact on clinical and valve-related outcomes. Circulation 2009; 119(23):3009–16.

52. Ye J, Cheung A, Lichtenstein SV, et al. Transapical transcatheter aortic valve implantation: follow-up to 3 years. J Thorac Cardiovasc Surg 2010;139(5): 1107–13, 1113.e1.

53. Godino C, Maisano F, Montorfano M, et al. Outcomes after transcatheter aortic valve implantation with both Edwards-SAPIEN and CoreValve devices in a single center: the Milan experience. JACC Cardiovasc Interv 2010;3(11):1110–21.

54. Détaint D, Lepage L, Himbert D, et al. Determinants of significant paravalvular regurgitation after transcatheter aortic valve: implantation impact of device and annulus discongruence. JACC Cardiovasc Interv 2009;2(9):821–7.

55. Jabbour A, Ismail TF, Moat N, et al. Multimodality imaging in transcatheter aortic valve Implantation

and post-procedural aortic regurgitation: comparison among cardiovascular magnetic resonance, cardiac computed tomography, and echocardiography. J Am Coll Cardiol 2011;58(21):2165–73.

56. Gurvitch R, Webb JG, Yuan R, et al. Aortic annulus diameter determination by multidetector computed tomography: reproducibility, applicability, and implications for transcatheter aortic valve implantation. JACC Cardiovasc Interv 2011;4(11):1235–45.

57. Jilaihawi H, Kashif M, Fontana G, et al. Cross-sectional computed tomographic assessment improves accuracy of aortic annular sizing for transcatheter aortic valve replacement and reduces the incidence of paravalvular aortic regurgitation. J Am Coll Cardiol 2012;59(14):1275–86.

58. Willson AB, Webb JG, Labounty TM, et al. 3-Dimensional aortic annular assessment by multidetector computed tomography predicts moderate or severe paravalvular regurgitation after transcatheter aortic valve replacement: a multicenter retrospective analysis. J Am Coll Cardiol 2012; 59(14):1287–94.

59. Miller DC, Blackstone EH, Mack MJ, et al. Transcatheter (TAVR) versus surgical (AVR) aortic valve replacement: occurrence, hazard, risk factors, and consequences of neurologic events in the PARTNER trial. J Thorac Cardiovasc Surg 2012; 143(4):832–43.e13.

60. Erdoes G, Basciani R, Huber C, et al. Transcranial Doppler-detected cerebral embolic load during transcatheter aortic valve implantation. Eur J Cardiothorac Surg 2012;41(4):778–83 [discussion: 783–4].

61. Szeto WY, Augoustides JG, Desai ND, et al. Cerebral embolic exposure during transfemoral and transapical transcatheter aortic valve replacement. J Cardiovasc Surg 2011;26(4):348–54.

62. Kahlert P, Al-Rashid F, Döttger P, et al. Cerebral embolization during transcatheter aortic valve implantation: a transcranial Doppler study. Circulation 2012;126(10):1245–55.

63. Etienne PY, Papadatos S, Pieters D, et al. Embol-X intraaortic filter and transaortic approach for improved cerebral protection in transcatheter aortic valve implantation. Ann Thorac Surg 2011; 92(5):e95–6.

64. Onsea K, Agostoni P, Samim M, et al. First-in-man experience with a new embolic deflection device in transcatheter aortic valve interventions. EuroIntervention 2012;8(1):51–6.

65. Naber CK, Ghanem A, Abizaid AA, et al. First-in-man use of a novel embolic protection device for patients undergoing transcatheter aortic valve implantation. EuroIntervention 2012;8(1):43–50.

66. Erkapic D, De Rosa S, Kelava A, et al. Risk for permanent pacemaker after transcatheter aortic valve implantation: a comprehensive analysis of the literature. J Cardiovasc Electrophysiol 2012;23(4): 391–7.

67. Généreux P, Head SJ, van Mieghem NM, et al. Clinical outcomes after transcatheter aortic valve replacement using valve academic research consortium definitions: a weighted meta-analysis of 3,519 patients from 16 studies. J Am Coll Cardiol 2012;59(25):2317–26.

68. Welt FG, Davidson MJ, Eisenhauer AC. The transcatheter valve revolution: time for a compensatory pause. Circulation 2012;126(6):674–6.

69. Nuis RJ, van Mieghem NM, Schultz CJ, et al. Timing and potential mechanisms of new conduction abnormalities during the implantation of the Medtronic CoreValve System in patients with aortic stenosis. Eur Heart J 2011;32(16):2067–74.

70. Houthuizen P, Van Garsse LA, Poels TT, et al. Left bundle-branch block induced by transcatheter aortic valve implantation increases risk of death. Circulation 2012;126(6):720–8.

71. Ewe SH, Ajmone Marsan N, Pepi M, et al. Impact of left ventricular systolic function on clinical and echocardiographic outcomes following transcatheter aortic valve implantation for severe aortic stenosis. Am Heart J 2010;160(6):1113–20.

72. Green P, Woglom AE, Généreux P, et al. The impact of frailty status on survival after transcatheter aortic valve replacement in older adults with severe aortic stenosis: a single-center experience. JACC Cardiovasc Interv 2012;5(9):974–81.

Transcatheter Aortic Valve Replacement with CoreValve

Ray V. Matthews, MD*, David M. Shavelle, MD

KEYWORDS

- CoreValve • TAVR • TAVI • Percutaneous • Heart valve • Aortic stenosis

KEY POINTS

- The treatment of aortic stenosis in high-risk surgical patients is now possible by transcatheter aortic valve replacement.
- The CoreValve is a new transcatheter valve with a unique design expanding its application in patients with aortic stenosis.
- The CoreValve is just completing clinical trial in the United States and not yet available for commercial use in the United States but is widely used in Europe.

INTRODUCTION

Few developments in contemporary medicine have captured the imagination as thoroughly as the promise of percutaneous implantation of a heart valve. This promise has evolved into reality as more than 50,000 patients worldwide have now received a percutaneous valve.[1] For adult cardiologists the first valve to explore percutaneous replacement was the aortic valve. Degenerative or senile aortic stenosis (AS) is a disease of the elderly and the most common cause for aortic valve replacement.[2] The outcome of patients with symptomatic AS is poor, with approximately 50% dying within 2 years of the diagnosis.[3] Despite many similarities to atherosclerosis, there are currently no effective medical therapies that have been shown to reduce disease progression and/or delay the need for surgical valve replacement.[4] Balloon aortic valvuloplasty (BAV) introduced by Cribier and colleagues[5] in 1982 was an initial attempt at a nonsurgical treatment option. Subsequent randomized clinical trials showed high rates of restenosis without an improvement in long-term survival (see "Balloon Aortic Valvuloplasty" in this issue).[6] Given that degenerative AS occurs in the elderly, many patients have increased surgical risks because of their advanced age and associated comorbid medical conditions. Recent studies have found that as many as 30% of elderly patients with symptomatic AS are not offered surgical aortic valve replacement (SAVR) due to the perceived excessive morbidity and mortality.[7,8] The development of percutaneous valves has enabled aortic valve replacement to be applied successfully to a subgroup of patients previously thought to be too ill to receive therapy.

The evolution of Transcatheter Aortic Valve Replacement (TAVR) has involved several investigators. Andersen and coworkers[9] were among the first to investigate TAVR using an early prototype in animal models. Bonhoeffer and colleagues[10] explored the use of a bovine valve in a lamb in the pulmonic position. Cribier and coworkers[11] are credited with the first implant in a human using a prototype balloon-expandable valve successfully deployed into a man with critical AS in 2002. Leon and colleagues[12] subsequently developed what would eventually be the first commercially available percutaneous aortic

Disclosures: The authors have nothing to disclose.
Division of Cardiovascular Medicine, Keck School of Medicine, 1510 San Pablo Street, Suite 322, Los Angeles, CA 90033, USA
* Corresponding author.
E-mail address: raymatth@usc.edu

Cardiol Clin 31 (2013) 351–361
http://dx.doi.org/10.1016/j.ccl.2013.05.007
0733-8651/13/$ – see front matter © 2013 Elsevier Inc. All rights reserved.

valve. The Edwards Sapien valve (described in detail in article entitled,) marketed, manufactured, and distributed by Edwards Life Sciences (Irvine, CA, USA) is a bovine pericardial valve sewn to a balloon-expandable stainless steel stent frame. The second percutaneous aortic valve to undergo clinical evaluation is the CoreValve from Medtronic, Inc (Minneapolis, MN, USA). This valve is constructed on a self-expanding stent platform, making it distinctly different from the Edwards Sapien valve. In this article, the CoreValve, the implant procedure, ongoing and future clinical studies evaluating its use for treatment of AS, and procedural complications are discussed in detail.

THE COREVALVE DESIGN

The CoreValve stent platform is constructed of nitinol, which is a nickel-titanium alloy that has been extensively studied in human vascular applications and has several properties that make it uniquely suited for a valve-stent system. Nitinol is manufactured so that it exhibits the property of memory. Therefore, it can be constrained within a sheath delivery system and, when released, will expand to a predetermined size. Furthermore, nitinol has the peculiar but useful property of being more malleable at cool temperatures and more firm when warmed. Therefore, at body temperature it is possible to amplify its radial strength, which is potentially valuable in valve applications.

The nitinol cage itself is constructed to provide optimal radial strength at the distal skirt, which abuts the aortic annulus and enlarges in a "mushroom"-like shape to contact the ascending aorta (**Fig. 1**). The proximal aortic end of the CoreValve is much larger, to allow the valve to "center" itself in the aortic annulus, using the proximal ascending aorta. The nitinol cage struts are more closely spaced distally near the annulus and more widely spaced proximally. Because the cage covers the aortic sinuses and the coronary ostia, this wide spacing helps preserve coronary artery access for intervention either acutely or at a later date. At the proximal end of the cage are 2 eyelet holes positioned 180° apart to hold the valve securely in contact with the delivery system until final deployment.

The other key component of the valve system is the leaflets. The CoreValve leaflets are constructed of porcine pericardial tissue that is hand sewn onto the struts of the cage. The leaflets are also treated with a proprietary process to resist calcification. The leaflets are suspended with a portion of the pericardial tissue commissure, sewn high up on the cage, giving it the look of a suspension bridge. The suspension of the commissures in this way is designed to reduce stress and improve the valve's longevity. The CoreValve is currently available in 4 sizes: 23 mm, 26 mm, 29 mm, and 31 mm (see **Fig. 1**). Each size is designed to be used in a native annulus slightly smaller than the valve cage diameter to insure proper annular contact and sealing. The self-expanding design of the CoreValve allows it to conform to the aortic annulus, which is most often elliptical, as opposed to circular, making the annulus perimeter an important parameter to assess preprocedure. Adequate coronary sinus dimensions are necessary to accommodate the displaced aortic leaflets and still allow normal coronary blood flow. **Table 1** is the sizing chart for the

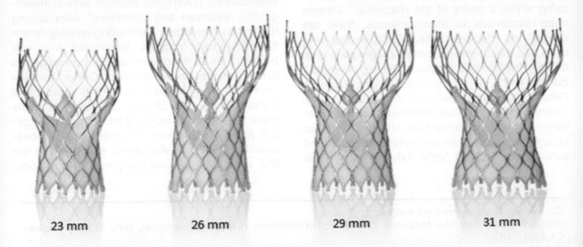

23 mm   26 mm   29 mm   31 mm

Fig. 1. Currently available CoreValve sizes. (*Courtesy of* Medtronic, Inc., Minneapolis, MN. The CoreValve® System is not commercially available in all countries and is an investigational device in other countries such as the US. CoreValve is a registered trademark of Medtronic CV Luxembourg S.a.r.l.).

Table 1
Currently available CoreValve sizes and the required anatomic measurements used to select valve size

Valve Size (mm)	Aortic Annulus Diameter (mm)	Ascending Aorta Diameter (mm)	Sinus of Valsalva Diameter (mm)	Native Leaflet to Sinotubular Junction Length (mm)	Aortic Annulus Perimeter (mm)
23	18–20	≤34	≥25	≥15	56.5–62.8
26	20–23	≤40	≥27	≥15	62.8–72.3
29	23–27	≤43	≥29	≥15	72.3–84.8
31	26–29	≤43	≥29	≥15	81.6–91.1

CoreValve with size ranges given for each of the key anatomic measurements. This chart is the basis for choosing a specific valve size; patients with anatomy outside of these parameters cannot receive the CoreValve.

COREVALVE DEPLOYMENT

Deployment of the CoreValve involves the following procedural steps: (1) loading of the valve into the delivery sheath; (2) placement of an 18-Fr sheath within the common femoral artery, subclavian artery, or ascending aorta (direct aortic access); (3) BAV; and (4) delivery, positioning, and release of the valve.

Loading

The valve is removed from its factory packing in solution. It is then immersed into iced sterile saline. This cold temperature immersion increases the deformability of the nitinol and assists in the loading process. Loading is performed entirely by hand just before implantation. The device is hooked onto the connection eyes and the sheath is slowly advanced over the cage with a tool to compress the frame during this action. The delivery system is 18 Fr and consists of a retractable sheath over the distal 6 cm only, to limit forward motion of the valve during sheath retraction. The delivery system has ports to flush and de-air the system and a delivery rotating knob to allow for precise deployment (**Fig. 2**).

Balloon Aortic Valvuloplasty

BAV is typically performed before valve deployment, but may not be mandatory in all patients.

The decision to perform BAV is related to the amount of leaflet and annular calcification, the severity of AS, and the clinical status of the patient. The presence of significant and deep annular calcification may increase the risk of annular rupture during BAV. BAV is usually performed during rapid right ventricular pacing to reduce cardiac output to achieve a decrease in systolic blood pressure to less than 60 mm Hg and a decrease in pulse pressure to less than 10 mm Hg. Failure to achieve significant reduction in cardiac output during BAV suggests higher pacing rates are needed and is helpful to determine before implantation of the CoreValve prosthesis.

Delivery and Deployment

The delivery system containing the loaded valve is advanced through an 18-Fr sheath and over a stiff 0.035-in guidewire located in the left ventricular apex. The valve and delivery sheath are advanced across the aortic valve to a position 2 to 4 mm below the inferior margin of the aortic annulus/ aortic cusp plane (**Fig. 3**). Depth of deployment is assessed in real time with small injections of contrast into the aortic cusps from a catheter that has been positioned from the contralateral femoral artery. The alignment angle of the aortic cusps is usually predetermined by computed tomographic (CT) scanning[13] but can also be determined using various fluoroscopic imaging algorithms.[14] Rapid right ventricular pacing is frequently used to reduce cardiac output transiently and limit valve motion during the few seconds that the valve cage is beginning to open. Rapid right ventricular pacing is usually initiated at the point of annular contact of the CoreValve

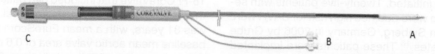

Fig. 2. CoreValve delivery system. (A) Distal retractable sheath housing the constrained valve. (B) Flush ports. (C) Rotating deployment knob. (*Courtesy of* Medtronic, Inc., Minneapolis, MN. The CoreValve® System is not commercially available in all countries and is an investigational device in other countries such as the US. CoreValve is a registered trademark of Medtronic CV Luxembourg S.a.r.l.).

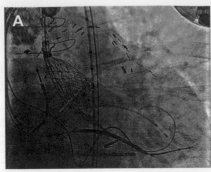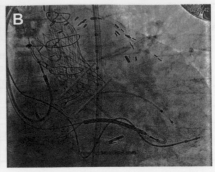

Fig. 3. Positioning of CoreValve. (*A*) CoreValve being positioned within aortic valve, device not yet released. Dotted red line shows annulus plane. (*B*) CoreValve released from the delivery system. Double arrows show implant depth that is the distance from annulus plane (*dotted red line*) to the inferior portion of the valve cage (*solid red line*); implant depth in this case is approximately 3 cm.

frame as it begins to "flower" from the sheath. At two-thirds of the deployment, the valve is functional and can be pulled out of the annulus in the case of low deployment; however, no other manipulations can be accomplished at this time. Although it is not possible to resheath the Core-Valve, if necessary, there are methods to remove the valve from the body at two-thirds of deployment, involving dragging the two-thirds deployed valve over the aortic arch and into the 18-Fr sheath that is positioned within the abdominal aorta. This maneuver carries the risk of emboli from aortic debris and should be avoided unless no other alternative is available. The final release of the cage allows the valve to achieve final orientation (see **Fig. 3**). Position, depth of implant, and final hemodynamics are confirmed with aortic angiography, transesophageal echocardiography, and simultaneous measurement of the left ventricular and aortic pressures.

CLINICAL DATA

The first-in-man CoreValve was performed in 2004 by Laborde in India on a 62-year-old man with critical AS, lung cancer, and chronic renal failure.[15] The procedure was performed under general anesthesia with femoral cardiopulmonary bypass. Although the implantation procedure was successful, the patient subsequently died because of multiorgan failure 4 days later.

Soon thereafter, other single-center experiences were initiated. Twenty-five patients with severe AS who were deemed high risk for SAVR were implanted in Sieberg, Germany in 2006 by Grube and associates.[16] These patients were implanted with general anesthesia and cardiopulmonary bypass. Implantation success was 88% and in-hospital mortality was 20% during this early experience. These initial implants required a 21-Fr

or 24-Fr sheath and surgical cut down of the common femoral, common iliac, and subclavian arteries.

Subsequent CoreValve design generations 2 and 3 reduced the delivery sheath size to 21 Fr and then to 18 Fr, thus allowing fewer patients to require cardiopulmonary bypass and a surgical cut down of the access vessels. Grube and co-workers[17] reported the Sieburg experience in 86 patients in 2006 that were sicker by EuroScore assessment using both the newer devices. The implantation success was similar to the previous series, but 30-day mortality was improved to 12%.

Given the larger initial delivery sheaths and frequent use of cardiopulmonary bypass, it became increasingly clear that a multidisciplinary team of cardiac surgeons and interventional cardiologists were required. Reports of the surgical role in these procedures began to appear as well.[18] Series from European centers showed improving results with the third-generation CoreValve.[19] Implantation success rates achieved greater than 90% and 30-day mortality was now less than 10%.

In May, 2007 CoreValve received Conformite Europeene (CE) Mark approval in Europe. As this occurred, many high-volume centers began using CoreValve throughout Europe. In addition, some of the centers involved in the initial registries combined the experience of multiple centers. Piazza and colleagues[20] in 2008 reported a European multicenter experience of the third-generation 18-Fr CoreValve that included 646 patients enrolled the year following CE Mark approval. Mean age was 81 years, with a mean EuroScore of 23 and a baseline mean aortic valve area of 0.6 cm². Procedural success was 97% and all-cause 30-day mortality was 9%, which demonstrated the feasibility of widespread application of this technology with excellent results in an extremely ill patient group.

The French Aortic National CoreValve and Edwards 2 registry was a national registry of the 33 centers approved by the French government to perform TAVR and both Sapien and CoreValve devices were included.[1] One thousand forty-three CoreValve implants between January 2010 and October 2011 performed throughout France were reported. All patients had severe AS and were refused SAVR and no patients were excluded from participation in this registry based on comorbid conditions, age, or procedural results. The Society of Thoracic Surgery and Logistic EuroScores were both elevated, confirming the high-risk nature of this group: 14.2 ± 11.2 and 21.3 ± 14.3, respectively. Overall procedural success for CoreValve was excellent at 97.6%; 30-day all-cause mortality was 9.4%, and 1-year all-cause mortality was 23.7%.

Intermediate and long-term data on the CoreValve are available from the United Kingdom Transcatheter Aortic Valve Implantation (TAVI UK) Registry reported in 2011.[21] In this registry, 870 patients were included with 2-year follow-up. Of the entire group, 452 patients (52%) were implanted with the CoreValve. For the CoreValve patients, all-cause mortality at 30 days, 1 year, and 2 years was 5.8%, 21.7%, and 23.9%, respectively. Multivariate predictors of death at 2 years were ejection fraction less than 30%, moderate to severe aortic regurgitation, and severe chronic obstructive pulmonary disease.

The results of the ADVANCE Registry were reported at the 2012 Euro PCR meeting.[22] A total of 1015 patients from 44 centers throughout Europe, Asia, and South America were enrolled from March 2010 to July 2011. The mean age was 81 years and the mean logistic EuroScore was 19.2%. Procedural success in this contemporary group of patients in experienced implanting centers was 97.8%. The 6-month all-cause mortality was 12.8% and cardiovascular mortality was 8.4%. The 6-month major stroke rate was 3.4%. The ADVANCE Registry represents the most contemporary information regarding outcomes of the CoreValve prosthesis.

Despite the extensive worldwide experience with both the Sapien valve and the CoreValve, no randomized comparison of the 2 valves has been performed. To conduct such a trial with each valve continually undergoing design improvements would be problematic. In the absence of a randomized controlled clinical trial, the use of a statistical method called propensity matching allows the most accurate comparison of both valves. The Pooled-RotterdAm-Milano-Toulouse In Collaboration (PRAGMATIC) Plus Initiative pooled TAVI data from 4 experienced centers on 793 patients

(453 CoreValve and 340 Sapien).[23] The authors performed propensity matching of baseline patient characteristics between those implanted with CoreValve and the Sapien valve. The 30-day all-cause mortality for CoreValve versus Sapien was 8.8% versus 6.4%, cardiovascular mortality 6.9% versus 6.4%, stroke 2.9% versus 1.0%, vascular complications 9.3% versus 12.3%, and 1-year cardiovascular mortality 8.3% versus 7.4%. For all of these outcome events, there was no statistically significant difference between the 2 valves. However, need for permanent pacing was 22.5% with CoreValve and 5.9% with Sapien ($P<.001$).

CoreValve had received widespread application in Europe since CE Mark approval in 2007 with over 30,000 implants by 2011. CoreValve began its approval process in the United States by initiating a large multicenter, randomized clinical trial in December of 2010. The template for such a trial was largely established by the US Food and Drug Administration (FDA) during execution of the Placement of AoRTic TraNscathetER Valve (PARTNER) trial, which was the Sapien valve's pivotal trial.[12,24] Similar to the PARTNER trial, the CoreValve Pivotal trial includes 2 patient groups: one group considered to be at prohibitive risk for SAVR, called the "extreme-risk" group; the other group were those deemed at "high risk" for SAVR (**Fig. 4**). The high-risk group was randomized to SAVR versus TAVR. The extreme-risk group did not require randomization given that a similar group of patients included in the PARTNER trial was clearly shown to benefit from TAVR. The FDA considered randomization of the extreme-risk group to medical therapy (with or without BAV) to be unethical and allowed patients to be enrolled in a registry, with all patients in this group receiving CoreValve.

Enrollment in the extreme-risk group was completed in January 2012 and enrollment in the high-risk randomized group was completed in October 2012. As these arms completed, enrollment plans to launch additional registries began. These registries were designed to evaluate the use of the CoreValve in previously excluded subgroups including those with severe mitral and tricuspid regurgitation, end-stage renal disease, bicuspid aortic valves, low-gradient normal ejection fraction, and failing aortic bioprosthetic valves (valve-in-valve). Commercial availability of CoreValve in the United States will not likely occur until 2014. Approval will be sought for the first group to have completed enrollment, the extreme-risk group.

As with most new medical devices, as experience with implantation grew so did a greater appreciation of the nuances of appropriate device

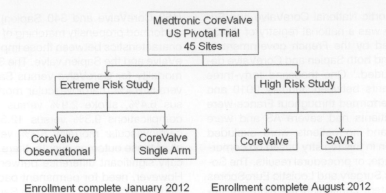

```
                    ┌─────────────────────┐
                    │  Medtronic CoreValve │
                    │   US Pivotal Trial   │
                    │       45 Sites       │
                    └─────────────────────┘
              ┌──────────────┴──────────────┐
      ┌───────────────┐              ┌───────────────┐
      │ Extreme Risk  │              │  High Risk    │
      │    Study      │              │    Study      │
      └───────────────┘              └───────────────┘
       ┌──────┴──────┐                ┌──────┴──────┐
  ┌──────────┐  ┌──────────┐    ┌──────────┐  ┌──────┐
  │ CoreValve│  │ CoreValve│    │ CoreValve│  │ SAVR │
  │Observ-   │  │Single Arm│    └──────────┘  └──────┘
  │ational   │  └──────────┘
  └──────────┘
```

Enrollment complete January 2012   Enrollment complete August 2012

Study Sample ~ 1600

Fig. 4. CoreValve United States pivotal trial study design.

selection and procedural complications. Aortic annulus sizing and the degree and location of calcification as assessed by CT allowed for predictions regarding perivalvular aortic regurgitation (perivalvular leak) and procedural success.[25] Because the valve leaflets are not removed as in SAVR, there must be space within the aorta when the leaflets are pinned open by the percutaneous valve cage. Failure to account for this can potentially result in coronary ostial occlusion from valve leaflet calcium and/or bulky valve leaflets. Therefore, the width of the coronary sinuses and the height of the coronary ostial origins from the aortic annulus are crucial measurements and part of the preprocedure CT planning.[26–28]

FEMORAL ACCESS

Vascular access with 18-Fr sheaths requires the operator to assess the likelihood of access success and risk of complications before the TAVR procedure. The common femoral vessels are the favored and most common route of arterial access. The vessel caliber, the amount and distribution of calcification, and the degree of tortuosity all contribute to the likelihood of safely advancing and removing the 18-Fr sheath. Although angiography and intravascular ultrasound have been used to evaluate the femoral access vessels, CT angiography provides the most comprehensive and precise assessment **(Fig. 5).**[28]

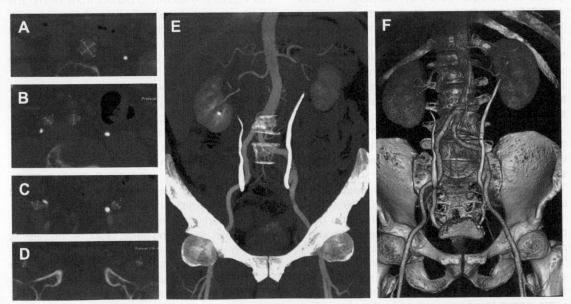

Fig. 5. CT angiography of the aorta and peripheral vessels. (*A–D*) Axial CT images. (*A*) Aorta. (*B*) Common iliac arteries. (*C*) External iliac arteries. (*D*) Common femoral arteries. (*E*) Maximum intensity projection imaging of aorta, iliac, and common femoral arteries. (*F*) Volume-rendering imaging of aorta, iliac, and common femoral arteries.

Not only placement of the 18-Fr sheath but also percutaneous repair of the puncture site are important and may represent the most common source of vascular-related complications. Although surgical cut down and direct closure of the access vessels were initially used, nearly all implants now use percutaneous suture-based closure with the Prostar XL or the Perclose Proglide devices (Abbott Vascular Mountain View, CA, USA). Using these techniques, van Mieghem and colleagues[29] reported on 99 consecutive CoreValve 18-Fr cases from 2006 to 2009 that were closed or attempted to be closed percutaneously. Thirteen cases (13%) had a vascular complication requiring either percutaneous or surgical repair and 8% required a blood transfusion. Other centers have since reported similar outcomes.[29,30] Data from the more recent CoreValve ADVANCE Registry suggest the rate of vascular complications is even lower: 10.7% among 996 patients using the more strict Valve Academic Research Consortium definitions.[22,31] Life-threatening and major bleeding events in the ADVANCE Registry were 4% and 9.7%, respectively.

ALTERNATIVE VASCULAR ACCESS

During the initial TAVR experience, it became apparent that the 18-Fr sheath platform of the CoreValve was small enough to explore use in sites other than the femoral arteries (**Fig. 6**). With a limited cut down in the upper left chest, the subclavian and axillary arteries can also be accessed.[32–35] This access site can be used in cases of femoral and/or iliac peripheral vascular disease as the subclavian and axillary arteries tend to be less affected than the lower extremity arteries. The angle of entry to the aortic valve from the left subclavian artery is similar to that from the femoral approach, so the remainder of the implant procedure is similar.

In patients with extensive peripheral vascular disease or patients of small body habitus, both the iliac and the subclavian artery luminal dimensions may be too small to accommodate the 18-Fr sheath. In these cases, a direct aortic approach into the ascending aorta is desirable (**Fig. 7**).[36] Adapting the surgical technique of minimally invasive SAVR, an incision is made in the upper right chest, with the right lung deflated after dual lumen endotracheal intubation, and the ascending aorta is exposed. Purse-string sutures allow the 18-Fr sheath to be held in place following aortic puncture under direct visualization. At the end of the procedure, the sheath is removed and the sutures are tied. The incision is closed and a chest tube is used to re-expand the right lung.

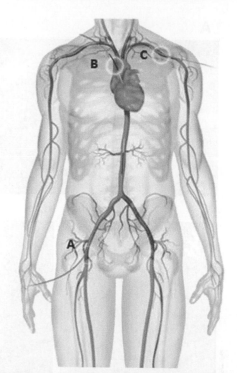

Fig. 6. CoreValve arterial access options. (A) Femoral artery. (B) Direct aortic access. (C) Subclavian artery. (*Courtesy of* Medtronic, Inc., Minneapolis, MN. The CoreValve® System is not commercially available in all countries and is an investigational device in other countries such as the US. CoreValve is a registered trademark of Medtronic CV Luxembourg S.a.r.l.).

Alternative incisions may be used for the direct aortic approach, such as a left chest approach or an upper third mini-sternotomy. However, the right chest approach is optimal in most cases.

The angle of entry into the aortic valve is more central from the direct aortic approach, making CoreValve deployment more uniform in most cases. Furthermore, steep angulations between the aortic valve and the ascending aorta can make the TAVR femoral approach impossible because the valve deploys tipped at an angle relative to the valve annulus. The direct aortic approach can be modified to select the puncture location on the ascending aorta to optimize CoreValve orientation within the valve annulus. The distance from the aortic annulus to the aortic puncture must be long enough to allow release of the valve from containment within the sheath, usually approximately 6 cm.

PERMANENT PACING

Anchoring of the CoreValve into the aortic annulus involves continuous outward expansion of the nitinol frame into a roughened, irregular, and

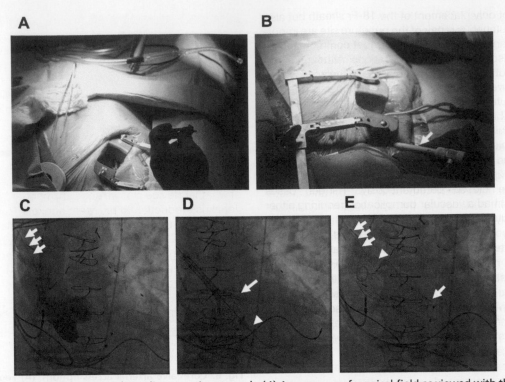

Fig. 7. Implant of CoreValve from direct aortic approach. (*A*) Appearance of surgical field as viewed with the patient's head at bottom of the screen. Four-inch hemi-sternotomy with direct visualization of the ascending aorta. (*B*) Eighteen-French delivery sheath has been placed directly into the aorta through the hemi-sternotomy. (*C*) Position of 18-Fr delivery sheath (*multiple arrows*) within the ascending aorta. Note the coaxial alignment of delivery sheath with the aortic annulus. (*D*) Release of the distal portion of CoreValve (*arrow*) with the left ventricular outflow tract; arrowhead shows nosecone of delivery system. (*E*) CoreValve has been released from delivery system. Arrow shows distal portion of valve frame; arrowhead shows proximal portion of valve frame, just outside of delivery sheath (*multiple arrows*).

calcified aortic annulus. The area of contact of the valve includes the aortic annulus and 3 to 4 mm below the annulus into the left ventricular outflow tract. The valve can also function correctly even if placed slightly higher or lower than this position. On the left ventricular surface of the interventricular septum lies the left bundle. Compression of the left bundle can thus cause a left bundle branch block, or in the case of a pre-existing right bundle branch block, complete heart block. Given the advanced age of implanted patients and the increased incidence of pre-existing conduction abnormalities in AS patients, there may be a need for a permanent pacemaker after TAVR. Given the position of the CoreValve prosthesis within the subannular position, the need for a permanent pacemaker following valve deployment is not unexpected.[37–39]

In the PARTNER trial of the balloon-expandable Sapien valve, the incidence of permanent pacemaker implantation was 3.8% at 30 days in the high-risk group randomized to TAVR.[24] This rate seems reasonable given that this valve does not

normally anchor below the annulus. In contrast, the incidence of permanent pacemaker implantation in the CoreValve ADVANCE registry was 26%.[22] In the TAVI UK Registry in 452 patients implanted with CoreValve, the permanent pacemaker rate was 24%.[21] Jilaihawi and coworkers[40] reported in a recent meta-analysis of 5024 TAVR cases, including both the Sapien and the CoreValve, that the mean new pacemaker rate was 5.9% for Sapien and 24.5% for Corevalve. However, implantation of a permanent pacemaker has not been shown to alter the outcome in TAVR patients.[41] At this time, the primary issue with permanent pacemaker implantation seems to be the added cost of the device and the additional pacemaker follow-up required.

STROKE

The risk of major disabling stroke after TAVR has emerged as the single most important concern for this emerging therapy. In the PARTNER inoperable (cohort B) patients, the major stroke rate at

1 year was 7.8% for the TAVR patients compared with 3.9% for those managed conservatively.[12] The stroke rate of those patients undergoing TAVR in the PARTNER randomized high risk (cohort A) was 5.1%, compared with those randomized to SAVR 2.4%.[24]

Several issues emerged from the early TAVR experience regarding stroke. The mechanisms of stroke remain unclear. Possibilities included the following: (1) forcible implantation of a percutaneous valve in the native calcified aortic valve resulting in the embolization of valve debris and/or calcium; (2) advancement of a large-bore delivery sheath and device through the aortic arch in elderly patients with advanced atherosclerosis; or (3) embolization of material from the newly implanted prosthesis. An evaluation of the PARTNER high-risk group that did not have femoral access (due to peripheral vascular disease) provides information on the issue of device advancement through the aortic arch. Patients randomized to the apical implant TAVR approach were compared with SAVR.[24] The 1-year stroke rate remained higher in the apical TAVR patients compared with SAVR, 12% versus 4.3% for SAVR, respectively, suggesting that mechanistically more was at play than aortic debris from catheter advancement in the arch. Others have suggested that patients with no femoral access were at higher stroke risk because of severe underlying peripheral vascular disease. This concept is supported by the on-going increase in stroke out to 2 years observed in the apical TAVR patients compared with the femoral TAVR or the SAVR patients.[42]

The risk of stroke with the CoreValve prosthesis has been much less well studied. The only large, multicenter, randomized trial designed to gain insight into the stroke rate is the CoreValve pivotal US trial, particularly the high-risk arm. Although the results of this subgroup are not yet available, they should be reliable as the definition of stroke was required to be determined by an independent neurologist as part of an FDA-mandated neurologic substudy. The incidence of major stroke as adjudicated by a neurologist in the ADVANCE CoreValve registry was 3.4% at 6 months.[22] Thirty-day stroke rates in the PRAGMATIC Plus registry were 2.9% for CoreValve and 1.0% for Sapien, which was not statistically different.[43]

Distal protection devices to catch or filter debris destined for the cerebral circulation are being developed; as of now, none are available for use in the United States.[44,45] In the absence of a clear understanding of the mechanism of stroke during TAVR, distal protection devices run the risk of needlessly complicating the TAVR procedure. However, diffusion-weighted MRI studies before and immediately after TAVR have demonstrated new subclinical defects in most patients, suggesting embolism is at least a component of the problem.[46]

SUMMARY

The CoreValve expands the application of TAVR through its unique self-expanding design, low-delivery profile, and wide range of valve sizes. Early-generation devices have been safe and effective at treating patients with AS who are at high or prohibitive surgical risk. The US Pivotal CoreValve trial will provide clinical data needed for FDA approval and eventual commercial availability. Future design modifications will likely add to the deliverability and further enhance device safety. These changes in the CoreValve and the development of other designs by competing entities make the future of TAVR for those who suffer from AS promising.

REFERENCES

1. Gilard M, Eltchaninoff H, Iung B, et al. Registry of transcatheter aortic-valve implantation in high-risk patients. N Engl J Med 2012;366(18):1705–15.
2. Bonow RO, Carabello BA, Chatterjee K, et al. 2008 focused update incorporated into the ACC/AHA 2006 guidelines for the management of patients with valvular heart disease: a report of the American College of Cardiology/American Heart Association Task Force on Practice Guidelines (Writing Committee to revise the 1998 guidelines for the management of patients with valvular heart disease). Endorsed by the Society of Cardiovascular Anesthesiologists, Society for Cardiovascular Angiography and Interventions, and Society of Thoracic Surgeons. J Am Coll Cardiol 2008;52(13):e1–142.
3. Ross J Jr, Braunwald E. Aortic stenosis. Circulation 1968;38(Suppl 1):61–7.
4. Dweck MR, Boon NA, Newby DE. Calcific aortic stenosis: a disease of the valve and the myocardium. J Am Coll Cardiol 2012;60(19):1854–63.
5. Cribier A, Savin T, Saoudi N, et al. Percutaneous transluminal valvuloplasty of acquired aortic stenosis in elderly patients: an alternative to valve replacement? Lancet 1986;1(8472):63–7.
6. Otto CM, Mickel MC, Kennedy JW, et al. Three-year outcome after balloon aortic valvuloplasty. Insights into prognosis of valvular aortic stenosis. Circulation 1994;89(2):642–50.
7. Bouma BJ, van Den Brink RB, van Der Meulen JH, et al. To operate or not on elderly patients with aortic

stenosis: the decision and its consequences. Heart 1999;82(2):143–8.

8. Iung B, Cachier A, Baron G, et al. Decision-making in elderly patients with severe aortic stenosis: why are so many denied surgery? Eur Heart J 2005; 26(24):2714–20.

9. Andersen HR, Knudsen LL, Hasenkam JM. Transluminal implantation of artificial heart valves. Description of a new expandable aortic valve and initial results with implantation by catheter technique in closed chest pigs. Eur Heart J 1992;13(5):704–8.

10. Bonhoeffer P, Boudjemline Y, Saliba Z, et al. Transcatheter implantation of a bovine valve in pulmonary position: a lamb study. Circulation 2000; 102(7):813–6.

11. Cribier A, Eltchaninoff H, Bash A, et al. Percutaneous transcatheter implantation of an aortic valve prosthesis for calcific aortic stenosis: first human case description. Circulation 2002;106(24):3006–8.

12. Leon MB, Smith CR, Mack M, et al. Transcatheter aortic-valve implantation for aortic stenosis in patients who cannot undergo surgery. N Engl J Med 2010;363(17):1597–607.

13. Achenbach S, Schuhback A, Min JK, et al. Determination of the aortic annulus plane in CT imaging—a step-by-step approach. JACC Cardiovasc Imaging 2013;6(2):275–8.

14. Kasel AM, Cassese S, Leber AW, et al. Fluoroscopy-guided aortic Root imaging for TAVR: "Follow the right cusp" rule. JACC Cardiovasc Imaging 2013; 6(2):274–5.

15. Lal P, Upasani P, Kanwar S, et al. First-in-man experience of percutaneous aortic valve replacement using self-expanding corevalve prosthesis. Indian Heart J 2011;63(3):241–4.

16. Grube E, Laborde JC, Gerckens U, et al. Percutaneous implantation of the CoreValve self-expanding valve prosthesis in high-risk patients with aortic valve disease: the Siegburg first-in-man study. Circulation 2006;114(15):1616–24.

17. Grube E, Schuler G, Buellesfeld L, et al. Percutaneous aortic valve replacement for severe aortic stenosis in high-risk patients using the second- and current third-generation self-expanding CoreValve prosthesis: device success and 30-day clinical outcome. J Am Coll Cardiol 2007;50(1):69–76.

18. Marcheix B, Lamarche Y, Berry C, et al. Surgical aspects of endovascular retrograde implantation of the aortic CoreValve bioprosthesis in high-risk older patients with severe symptomatic aortic stenosis. J Thorac Cardiovasc Surg 2007;134(5):1150–6.

19. Tamburino C, Capodanno D, Mule M, et al. Procedural success and 30-day clinical outcomes after percutaneous aortic valve replacement using current third-generation self-expanding Core-Valve prosthesis. J Invasive Cardiol 2009;21(3): 93–8.

20. Piazza N, Grube E, Gerckens U, et al. Procedural and 30-day outcomes following transcatheter aortic valve implantation using the third generation (18 Fr) corevalve revalving system: results from the multicentre, expanded evaluation registry 1-year following CE mark approval. EuroIntervention 2008; 4(2):242–9.

21. Moat NE, Ludman P, de Belder MA, et al. Long-term outcomes after transcatheter aortic valve implantation in high-risk patients with severe aortic stenosis: the U.K. TAVI (United Kingdom Transcatheter Aortic Valve Implantation) Registry. J Am Coll Cardiol 2011; 58(20):2130–8.

22. Linke A. 1-year outcome in real-world patients treated with TAVI: the ADVANCE study. Paris: EuroPCR; 2011. 5-21-2013.

23. Tchetche D, van der Boon RM, Dumonteil N, et al. Adverse impact of bleeding and transfusion on the outcome post-transcatheter aortic valve implantation: insights from the Pooled-RotterdAm-Milano-Toulouse in Collaboration Plus (PRAGMATIC Plus) initiative. Am Heart J 2012;164(3):402–9.

24. Smith CR, Leon MB, Mack MJ, et al. Transcatheter versus surgical aortic-valve replacement in high-risk patients. N Engl J Med 2011;364(23):2187–98.

25. Schultz CJ, Weustink A, Piazza N, et al. Geometry and degree of apposition of the CoreValve ReValving system with multislice computed tomography after implantation in patients with aortic stenosis. J Am Coll Cardiol 2009;54(10):911–8.

26. John D, Buellesfeld L, Yuecel S, et al. Correlation of Device landing zone calcification and acute procedural success in patients undergoing transcatheter aortic valve implantations with the self-expanding CoreValve prosthesis. JACC Cardiovasc Interv 2010;3(2):233–43.

27. Moussa ID. Complications of transcatheter aortic valve implantation with the CoreValve—what have we learned so far? Catheter Cardiovasc Interv 2010;76(5):767–8.

28. Piazza N, Lange R, Martucci G, et al. Patient selection for transcatheter aortic valve implantation: patient risk profile and anatomical selection criteria. Arch Cardiovasc Dis 2012;105(3):165–73.

29. van Mieghem NM, Nuis RJ, Piazza N, et al. Vascular complications with transcatheter aortic valve implantation using the 18 Fr Medtronic CoreValve System: the Rotterdam experience. EuroIntervention 2010; 5(6):673–9.

30. Piazza N, Serruys PW, Lange R. Getting safely in and out of a transcatheter aortic valve implantation procedure vascular complications according to the valvular academic research consortium criteria. JACC Cardiovasc Interv 2011;4(8):859–60.

31. Kappetein AP, Head SJ, Genereux P, et al. Updated standardized endpoint definitions for transcatheter aortic valve implantation: the Valve Academic

Research Consortium-2 consensus document. J Am Coll Cardiol 2012;60(15):1438–54.

32. Lopez-Otero D, Munoz-Garcia AJ, Avanzas P, et al. Axillary approach for transcatheter aortic valve implantation: optimization of the endovascular treatment for the aortic valve stenosis. Rev Esp Cardiol 2011;64(2):121–6.

33. Modine T, Obadia JF, Choukroun E, et al. Transcutaneous aortic valve implantation using the axillary/subclavian access: feasibility and early clinical outcomes. J Thorac Cardiovasc Surg 2011;141(2): 487–91, 491.e1.

34. Ruge H, Lange R, Bleiziffer S, et al. First successful aortic valve implantation with the CoreValve ReValving System via right subclavian artery access: a case report. Heart Surg Forum 2008;11(5):E323–4.

35. Bruschi G, Fratto P, De MF, et al. The trans-subclavian retrograde approach for transcatheter aortic valve replacement: single-center experience. J Thorac Cardiovasc Surg 2010;140(4):911–5, 915.e1–2.

36. Bruschi G, De MF, Botta L, et al. Direct transaortic CoreValve implantation through right minithoracotomy in patients with patent coronary grafts. Ann Thorac Surg 2012;93(4):1297–9.

37. Munoz-Garcia AJ, Hernandez-Garcia JM, Jimenez-Navarro MF, et al. Factors predicting and having an impact on the need for a permanent pacemaker after CoreValve prosthesis implantation using the new Accutrak delivery catheter system. JACC Cardiovasc Interv 2012;5(5):533–9.

38. Liang M, Devlin G, Pasupati S. The incidence of transcatheter aortic valve implantation-related heart block in self-expandable Medtronic CoreValve and balloon-expandable Edwards valves. J Invasive Cardiol 2012;24(4):173–6.

39. Khawaja MZ, Rajani R, Cook A, et al. Permanent pacemaker insertion after CoreValve transcatheter aortic valve implantation: incidence and contributing factors (the UK CoreValve Collaborative). Circulation 2011;123(9):951–60.

40. Jilaihawi H, Chakravarty T, Weiss RE, et al. Meta-analysis of complications in aortic valve replacement: comparison of Medtronic-Corevalve, Edwards-Sapien and surgical aortic valve replacement in 8,536 patients. Catheter Cardiovasc Interv 2012; 80(1):128–38.

41. Buellesfeld L, Stortecky S, Heg D, et al. Impact of permanent pacemaker implantation on clinical outcome among patients undergoing transcatheter aortic valve implantation. J Am Coll Cardiol 2012; 60(6):493–501.

42. Miller DC, Mack M, Svensson LG, et al. Incidence, hazards, determinants and consequences of neurologic events after TAVR and AVR in the PARTNER Trial. Vancouver (Canada): Transcatheter Valve Therapies; 2011.

43. Chieffo A, Buchanan GL, van Mieghem NM, et al. Transcatheter aortic valve implantation with the Edwards SAPIEN versus the Medtronic CoreValve Revalving system devices: a multicenter collaborative study: the PRAGMATIC Plus Initiative (Pooled-RotterdAm-Milano-Toulouse in Collaboration). J Am Coll Cardiol 2013;61(8):830–6.

44. Szeto WY, Augoustides JG, Desai ND, et al. Cerebral embolic exposure during transfemoral and transapical transcatheter aortic valve replacement. J Card Surg 2011;26(4):348–54.

45. Nietlispach F, Wijesinghe N, Gurvitch R, et al. An embolic deflection device for aortic valve interventions. JACC Cardiovasc Interv 2010;3(11): 1133–8.

46. Ghanem A, Muller A, Nahle CP, et al. Risk and fate of cerebral embolism after transfemoral aortic valve implantation: a prospective pilot study with diffusion-weighted magnetic resonance imaging. J Am Coll Cardiol 2010;55(14):1427–32.

Transcatheter Left Atrial Appendage Occlusion

Creighton W. Don, MD, PhD[a], Cindy J. Fuller, PhD[b], Mark Reisman, MD[b],*

KEYWORDS

- Transcatheter • Left atrial appendage • Occlusion • Atrial fibrillation

KEY POINTS

- Occlusion of the left atrial appendage (LAA) via surgical, epicardial, or endovascular approaches may reduce risk of stroke in patients with atrial fibrillation (AF), and does not seem to be inferior to warfarin in this regard.
- Serious periprocedural complications may negate the overall efficacy of LAA occlusion, but over the long term, as complications associated with bleeding and inconsistent anticoagulation accrue, the benefit of LAA occlusion may be more apparent.
- Adequate operator training reduces, but does not eliminate, periprocedural adverse events.
- The long-term follow-up from Percutaneous Closure of the Left Atrial Appendage Versus Warfarin Therapy for Prevention of Stroke in Patients With Atrial Fibrillation (PROTECT AF), the initial reports from Prospective Randomized Evaluation of the Watchman LAA Closure Device In Patients with Atrial Fibrillation versus Long-Term Warfarin Therapy (PREVAIL), and the small studies of the Watchman and Amplatzer Cardiac Plug devices for nonwarfarin candidates seem promising.
- Additional trials involving device and procedural refinements are in progress to ascertain whether LAA occlusion can replace anticoagulation for stroke prevention in patients with nonvalvular AF.
- The superior dosing and safety profiles of the novel oral anticoagulants raise the accepted threshold for safety and efficacy of LAA occlusion procedures, and thus underscore the need for randomized studies comparing LAA occlusion with these newer anticoagulants.

INTRODUCTION

Atrial fibrillation (AF) is the most common cardiac arrhythmia, and a major cause of stroke in the elderly.[1] An estimated 12 to 16 million Americans will have a diagnosis of AF by 2050.[2] Untreated, the annual incidence of stroke in persons with AF is 4.5%.[3] Adjusted odds ratios (ORs) for mortality in AF are 1.9 in women and 1.5 in men,[4] and 1.71

overall.[5] The risk of stroke attributable to AF increases with age from 1.5% in the 50 to 59 year age group to 23.5% at 80 to 89 years of age, with a 5-fold increase in risk for stroke over a lifetime.[6] Strokes account for 1 in 19 deaths and are a leading cause of long-term disability in the United States, costing $22.8 billion in direct medical expenses in 2009, which underestimates the total

Portions of this article were published previously in Fuller CJ, and Reisman M. Stroke prevention in atrial fibrillation: atrial appendage closure. Current Cardiology Reports 2011;13:159–166; with kind permission from Springer Science+Business Media B.V.

Funding: This publication was made possible by grant number KL2 RR025015 from the National Center for Research Resources (NCRR).

Disclosures: No conflicts of interest exist.

[a] Department of General Internal Medicine, Division of Cardiology, University of Washington Medical Center, 1959 Northeast Pacific Street, Seattle, WA 98195, USA; [b] Swedish Heart & Vascular Institute, Swedish Medical Center, University of Washington Medical Center, 1959 Northeast Pacific Street, Box 356422, Seattle, WA 98195, USA

* Corresponding author.

E-mail address: mxreisman@gmail.com

costs associated with stroke morbidity and lost productivity.[6]

Oral anticoagulation is the mainstay of medical treatment of prevention of stroke in AF (class I, level of evidence A),[7] achieving as much as a 70% reduction in the risk for nonfatal stroke per year. However, antithrombotics are associated with major and minor bleeding complications, difficulty with monitoring and compliance, drug interactions, and increased costs. Warfarin treatment requires frequent monitoring to maintain a therapeutic International Normalized Ratio (INR) and has numerous drug and dietary interactions.[8] The novel oral anticoagulants (dabigatran, apixaban, and rivaroxaban) offer more consistent anticoagulation without requiring regular monitoring, fewer drug interactions, and decreased bleeding compared with warfarin. Nevertheless, the novel anticoagulants are associated with bleeding, especially among the elderly and persons with chronic kidney disease,[9] and management of serious bleeding is significantly impeded by the inability to reverse these agents.

Alternative therapies are warranted, particularly in patients who are not candidates for anticoagulant therapy or who are at high risk of bleeding. The left atrial appendage (LAA) is a prominent source of thrombi in AF, accounting for 90% of thrombi observed in patients undergoing cardioversion.[10] In a small number of patients (3%), the LAA may also be a source of focal atrial tachycardia.[11] As a result, surgical and transcatheter techniques have been explored to reduce the risk of stroke in persons with AF by occluding the LAA. The percentage of complete closure or occlusion depends on the modality used[12,13] and appropriate anatomy. The high variability of LAA anatomy[14] does not allow for a one-device-fits-all paradigm. Several devices are under clinical evaluation or preclinical assessment. The long-term follow-up of early clinical studies has been promising, because the efficacy of LAA occlusion devices may be more apparent when compared with the long-term risk of bleeding associated with anticoagulation.

This article presents a review of the pathophysiology of LAA thrombi; discusses the role of the LAA in the cause of AF-related stroke; and examines current clinical data supporting the use of surgical, combined epicardial/endovascular, and endovascular LAA occlusion procedures compared with oral anticoagulant therapy.

STROKE RISK AND LAA THROMBI

The presence of thrombus, spontaneous echo contrast, or low velocities in the LAA that allow blood stasis are associated with increased risk of stroke.[15] Transesophageal studies show the presence of LAA thrombus in 27% of patients with chronic AF and 43% of patients with AF and clinical thromboembolism. In one report, LAA thrombus was observed on imaging or at autopsy in up to 91% of patients with stroke and AF.[16] Although cardiac sources of emboli can be associated with thrombi forming within the left ventricle, along the atrial septum, on valves, and within the left atrium, most left atrial thrombi are localized to the LAA. In a series of 1288 patients with nonrheumatic AF, 222 had left atrial thrombi, of which 91% were localized to the LAA.[16]

Among patients with nonvalvular AF, a history of prior stroke and/or transient ischemic attack (TIA) is the strongest predictor of recurrent stroke (relative risk 2.5, 95% confidence interval [CI] 1.8–3.5).[11] Patients with AF with diabetes, hypertension, renal insufficiency, and increasing age are also at increased risk for stroke. The combination of rheumatic mitral stenosis and AF is also strongly associated with embolic events. The risk for stroke seems to be similar in paroxysmal, persistent, and permanent AF. The most widely used stroke scoring systems in clinical practice are the $CHADS_2$ and $CHADS_2$ (congestive heart failure, hypertension, age $\geq$75 years, diabetes mellitus, prior stroke, TIA, or thromboembolism)-VASC (vascular disease, age 65–74 years, sex category) scores (**Box 1**), which can be used to risk stratify patients and determine optimal antithrombotic strategy.[17–19] Patients with a $CHADS_2$ score of 0 have a low stroke rate and the benefit of anticoagulation is unlikely to outweigh the bleeding risks in this group. Patients with 1 risk factor ($CHADS_2$ score = 1) should be treated with either aspirin or anticoagulation, whereas intermediate-risk patients ($CHADS_2 \geq 2$) should be anticoagulated (**Table 1**).[7]

Patients who have increased $CHADS_2$ scores with contraindications for anticoagulation should be considered for LAA occlusion. Recent data suggest that intermediate-risk and high-risk patients who are able to take anticoagulation may also benefit from LAA occlusion. Patients with a $CHADS_2$ score of greater than or equal to 1 are more likely to have left atrium or LAA thrombus or spontaneous echo contrast (SEC) than those with a $CHADS_2$ score of 0 (3.9% vs 0%, $P<.01$), and the prevalence of LAA SEC increases with increasing $CHADS_2$ score (24% with score of 0; 83% with score of 4–6, $P<.01$).[20] Obesity is also a risk factor for left atrial and LAA thrombus in AF.

LAA ANATOMY AND IMAGING
Anatomy

The LAA is derived from the embryonic left atrium.[21] It is a blind pouch lying on the anterior

Box 1
Risk model for stroke risk in AF

CHADS₂[a]

- Congestive heart failure: 1 point
- Hypertension: 1 point
- Age older than 75 years: 1 point
- Diabetes: 1 point
- History of stroke or TIA: 2 points

CHA₂DS₂-VASc[b]

- Congestive heart failure or left ventricular ejection fraction less than or equal to 40%: 1 point
- Hypertension: 1 point
- Age 75 years or older: 2 points
- Diabetes: 1 point
- Stroke/TIA/thromboembolism: 2 points
- Vascular disease (myocardial infarction, peripheral arterial disease, or aortic plaque): 1 point
- Age 65 to 74 years: 1 point
- Female sex: 1 point

[a] *Data from* Gage BF, Waterman AD, Shannon W, et al. Validation of clinical classification schemes for predicting stroke: results from the National Registry of Atrial Fibrillation. JAMA 2001;285(22):2865.
[b] *Data from* Lip GY, Nieuwlaat R, Pisters R, et al. Refining clinical risk stratification for predicting stroke and thromboembolism in atrial fibrillation using a novel risk factor-based approach: the euro heart survey on atrial fibrillation. Chest 2010;137(2):266.

surface of the heart. Normal anatomic variation in LAA morphology is shown in **Fig. 1**. An autopsy study of 500 patients showed that 54% of LAAs examined have 2 lobes, 23% have 3 lobes, 20% have only 1 lobe, and 3% have 4 lobes.[22] Four general categories of LAA anatomy have been described based on the overall appearance on computed tomography angiography (CTA): the wind sock type (1 long dominant lobe), chicken wing type (1 dominant lobe with a prominent mid bend), cactus type (dominant central lobe with secondary lobes), and cauliflower type (short length with complex internal structure). The type of LAA is associated with different risks for stroke and difficulty in performing the LAA occlusion procedure (**Table 2**).[23,24] The chicken wing and cactus shapes are most common (48.3% and 29.8% respectively).[23] The chicken wing morphology is associated with a lower rate of strokes (4%) versus the non–chicken wing types (12%; $P = .04$). The ostium of the LAA is elliptical in shape with varying long and short axes,[14,22] which may also have consequences for the design and choice of occlusion devices.[25] The inner surface of the LAA is covered with pectinate muscles that provide a trabecular structure that may promote thrombus formation.[21] In another autopsy study, casts were made of the LAA from 220 patients to evaluate LAA anatomy.[14] Ninety-two (42%) casts had an extremely bent and extremely spiral course, whereas only 16 casts (7%) had a straight course. The LAA with larger volumes and larger ostial diameters had a significantly

Table 1
Stroke events per 1000 person years by anticoagulation and CHADS₂ score

CHADS₂ Score	Warfarin	No Warfarin	Risk Ratio (95% CI)
0	0.25	0.49	0.50 (0.20–1.28)
1	0.72	1.52	0.47 (0.30–0.73)
2	1.27	2.50	0.51 (0.35–0.75)
3	2.20	5.27	0.42 (0.28–0.62)
4	2.35	6.02	0.39 (0.20–0.75)
5–6	4.60	6.88	0.67 (0.28–1.60)

Risk ratio for stroke versus all other groups.
Data from Go AS, Hylek EM, Chang Y, et al. Anticoagulation therapy for stroke prevention in atrial fibrillation: how well do randomized trials translate into clinical practice? JAMA 2003;290(20):2685–92.

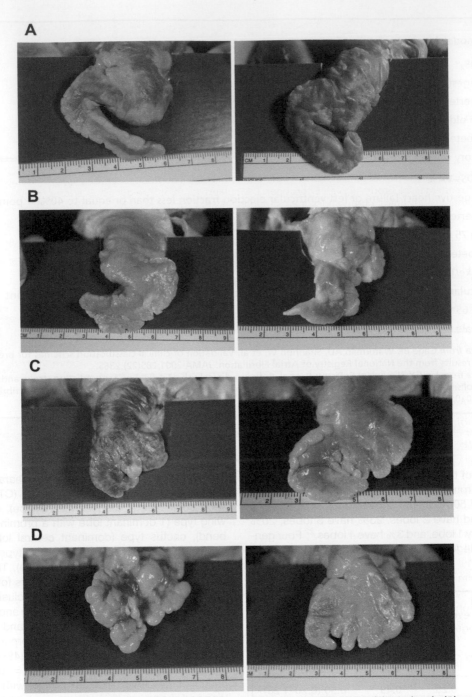

Fig. 1. Normal anatomic variation of LAA morphology: (*A*) chicken wing (*B*) cactus, (*C*) wind sock, (*D*) cauliflower. (*Courtesy of* Seattle Science Foundation, Seattle, WA; with permission.)

higher number of lobes and substructures. Patients with a history of AF had larger LAA volumes and ostial diameters (both $P<.01$) than hearts from patients who were in sinus rhythm before death.[14] The LAA volume was almost twice as large in patients with LAA thrombi ($P<.01$).[26]

Imaging

Transesophageal echocardiography (TEE), CTA, and magnetic resonance imaging (MRI) are effective modalities to assess left atrial and LAA anatomic and functional features associated with

Table 2
Anatomic and clinical features associated with different LAA types

LAA Type	Features	CHADS$_2$ ≥ 2 (%)	Prevalence (%)	Prior Stroke/ TIA (%)	OR Stroke/ TIA (95% CI)
Chicken wing	Dominant lobe with obvious bend in the mid lobe	9.1	48.3	4.4	0.2 (0.4–0.8)
Cactus	Dominant central lobe with small inferior and superior secondary lobes	18.7	29.8	12.6	1.1 (0.4–3.2)
Windsock	Single dominant lobe	15.6	19.2	10.6	2.5 (1.0–6.1)
Cauliflower	Oval ostium Complex internal characteristics Multilobed without dominant lobe	29.2	2.6	16.7	2.0 (0.2–7.2)

OR 95% CI for each group compared with the other groups combined.

Data from Di Biase L, Santangeli P, Anselmino M, et al. Does the left atrial appendage morphology correlate with the risk of stroke in patients with atrial fibrillation?: results from a multicenter study. J Am Coll Cardiol 2012;60(6):531–8.

thrombogenesis in AF[10] and feasibility of mechanical LAA occlusion. SEC on TEE, which may reflect microemboli, is increased in AF.[27] The highest amount of SEC is negatively correlated with LAA velocity.[27,28] Patients with AF and thrombus have lower LAA velocity than patients without thrombus (centimeters per second: no thrombus 32 ± 21, with thrombus 9 ± 6, P<.001).[27] Patients with AF with a history of stroke also have larger LAA depth and neck dimensions on imaging studies.[29] Increased left atrial volume index (OR 1.02; P = .018) and lower left ventricular ejection fraction (OR 1.02; P = .05) on TEE measurement can predict LAA thrombus formation. Transthoracic echocardiography (TTE) with measurement of LAA wall velocity (LAWV) was used to assess risk of recurrent stroke in patients with AF.[30] In this study, patients with TTE-LAWV less than 8.7 cm/s were more likely to experience recurrent cerebrovascular events (hazard ratio [HR] 5.05; 95% CI 2.25–11.36).[30] The combination of low LAA flow velocity, endothelial dysfunction, platelet activation, and procoagulant state may thus set up an ideal environment for thrombus formation in the LAA.

The pectinate muscles within the LAA may be mistaken for thrombi on TEE,[31] and may hinder the success of LAA ligation or occlusion. Use of real-time three-dimensional (3D) TEE can help distinguish between pectinate muscles and thrombi[32]; however, a poor two-dimensional (2D) image often predicts an inconclusive real-time 3D TEE result. In addition, 2D TEE underestimates the size of the LAA ostium relative to real-time 3D TEE,[26] which can affect the choice of device size.

CTA has become an important tool to assess LAA morphology. CTA gives an excellent 3D understanding of the location of the appendage relative to the pulmonary artery, the number of lobes, and the shape of the appendage as well as the orientation of the appendage (posterior, lateral, or anterior).[33] CTA has become essential in determining whether the LAA anatomy is favorable for successful percutaneous LAA closure.[23]

Cardiac MRI has similarly been used to define LAA and pulmonary vein anatomy for left atrial procedures,[34] but its use for planning LAA occlusion has not been described as extensively as for CTA. MRI can also provide 3D anatomy and is capable of defining tissue characteristics that can differentiate myocardium from thrombus in the LAA[35] and ventricle,[36] which CTA is unable to do consistently. However, some investigators have shown that MRI is less accurate for identifying LAA thrombus compared with TEE.[34] For both of these technologies, image quality may be compromised by patient motion and problems with gating and timing of contrast appearance in the LAA radiology protocols.

INDICATIONS FOR LAA OCCLUSION AND PATIENT SELECTION

Anticoagulation in warfarin or the new oral anticoagulants is standard of care for patients with intermediate and high risk for stroke, but for many patients consistent anticoagulation is difficult to achieve or not tolerated. Major gastrointestinal bleeding and hemorrhagic stroke are the principal adverse events with anticoagulants. Relative or absolute contraindications to anticoagulation are present in as many as 40% of patients with AF.[37] Two bleeding risk scales have been validated for patients on oral anticoagulant therapy, with the mnemonics HEMORR$_2$HAGES[38] and HAS-BLED,[39] and can help identify patients who are at high risk for significant bleeding (**Box 2**).

Patients with a high risk of bleeding are natural choices for LAA occlusion, because the long-term clinical data seem to support LAA occlusion for stroke prevention. The data for patients with contraindications to anticoagulation are also growing. A study of 150 patients with AF, CHADS$_2$ scores 2.8 ± 1.2, and contraindications to anticoagulation were treated with the Watchman device in the ASAP study. History of severe hemorrhagic syndromes was present in 93% of patients. All-cause stroke or systemic embolism occurred at a rate of 2.3% per year, which is lower than would be expected based on the patients' risk profiles.[40]

At present, there is no US Food and Drug Administration (FDA)–approved clinical indication for atrial appendage occlusion. Surgical patients undergoing a maze procedure for AF have their LAA resected or excluded using a simple surgical technique, typically performed concomitantly with a cardiac valve or bypass procedure. The Sentre-HEART LARIAT is a percutaneously delivered suture device that has 510(K) approval for use as a soft tissue ligation device, but is not specifically indicated for stroke prevention in AF. The data evaluating the safety and efficacy of the Watchman device from the Percutaneous Closure of the Left Atrial Appendage Versus Warfarin Therapy for

---

Box 2
Questionnaires for the assessment of bleeding risk in patients with AF on oral anticoagulant therapy

HEMORR$_2$HAGES[a]

Unless otherwise indicated, each item in the mnemonic receives 1 point.

- Hepatic or renal disease
- Ethanol abuse
- Malignancy
- Older age (>75 y)
- Reduced platelet count or function
- Rebleeding risk: 2 points
- Hypertension (uncontrolled)
- Anemia
- Genetic factors associated with increased bleeding propensity
- Excessive fall risk
- Stroke

HAS-BLED[b]

Unless otherwise indicated, each item in the mnemonic receives 1 point.

- Hypertension (uncontrolled, >160 mm Hg systolic)
- Abnormal renal or liver function: 1 point each, maximum 2 points
- Stroke
- Bleeding history or predisposition (anemia)
- Labile INR (<60% of time in therapeutic range)
- Elderly (age >65 y)
- Concomitant drug use (antiplatelet agents, nonsteroidal antiinflammatory drugs) or ethanol abuse: 1 point each, maximum 2 points

[a] *Data from* Lip GY, Frison L, Lane DA. Comparative validation of a novel risk score for predicting bleeding risk in anticoagulated patients with atrial fibrillation: the HAS-BLED (Hypertension, Abnormal Renal/Liver Function, Stroke, Bleeding History or Predisposition, Labile INR, Elderly, Drugs/Alcohol Concomitantly) score. J Am Coll Cardiol 2011;57(2):173–80.
[b] *Data from* Pisters R, Lane DA, Nieuwlaat R, et al. A novel user-friendly score (HAS-BLED) to assess 1-year risk of major bleeding in patients with atrial fibrillation: the Euro Heart Survey. Chest 2010;138(5):1093–100.

Prevention of Stroke in Patients With Atrial Fibrillation (PROTECT AF) and Prospective Randomized Evaluation of the Watchman LAA Closure Device In Patients with Atrial Fibrillation versus Long-Term Warfarin Therapy (PREVAIL) studies are being considered by the FDA at the time of this writing.

Until this occurs, patients with intermediate $CHADS_2$ and $CHADS_2$-VASC scores who cannot be anticoagulated can be considered for LAA occlusion using a surgical excision or percutaneous suture with a device such as the LARIAT. For patients who do not have an absolute contraindication to anticoagulation, the decision to proceed with LAA occlusion involves a complex integration of the assessed stroke, bleeding, and procedure risks with quality of life.

LAA EXCLUSION MODALITIES

Although anticoagulant therapy is recommended to reduce stroke risk in AF,[7] alternative strategies are needed for patients who have contraindications to use of anticoagulants. Hence, occlusion of the LAA has emerged as a treatment option. Three approaches have been developed to exclude the LAA. Open surgery for LAA exclusion or removal has been primarily used in combination with coronary artery bypass graft (CABG) or valve

surgery, often in conjunction with a surgical maze procedure to help reduce AF. Epicardial LAA occlusion via ligation has been used, as well as a hybrid epicardial/endovascular approach. In addition, several endovascular LAA occlusion devices are currently under evaluation (**Fig. 2**). The rates of complete occlusion are highly variable,[41,42] and periprocedural adverse event rates may depend on operator experience.[43]

Open Surgical Approaches

Surgical ligation or excision of the LAA can be performed in patients with AF deemed at high risk for stroke undergoing concurrent CABG or valve surgery. The literature consists mostly of retrospective case series or case reports.

The Left Atrial Appendage Occlusion Study (LAAOS)[12] was the first randomized, single-center study of surgical LAA occlusion in patients undergoing concurrent CABG with staples or sutures versus control. Seventy-seven patients were randomized to undergo either occlusion (n = 52) or control (no occlusion; n = 25); only 11 (14%) had a history of AF. TEE was used to test degree of occlusion at 8 postoperative weeks in 44 of 52 (85%) patients. Occlusion was successful in 29 (66%) patients, more so when stapling was used (72%) versus sutures (45%; P = .14). Two patients, both in the occlusion group, had

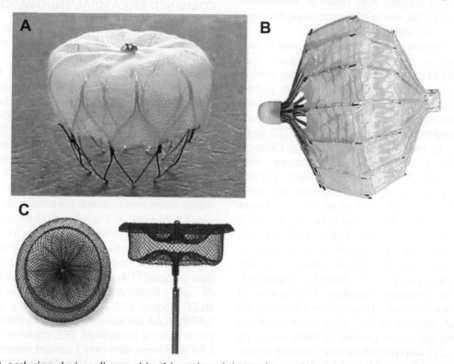

Fig. 2. LAA occlusion devices discussed in this review. (*A*) Watchman. (*B*) PLAATO. (*C*) Amplatzer Cardiac Plug. (*Courtesy of* [*A*] Atritech Division of Boston Scientific, Plymouth, MN, with permission; and [*B*] Covidien, Mansfield, MA, with permission; and [*C*] St Jude Medical, St Paul, MN; with permission.)

thromboembolic events during hospitalization. One patient with AF, patent foramen ovale, and bilateral carotid stenosis had an intraoperative stroke; the other patient had a TIA on the third postoperative day. After a follow-up period of 13 ± 7 months, no additional stroke events were reported in either occlusion or control groups.[12]

In one retrospective series,[44] 6 women with AF underwent LAA occlusion concurrently with mitral or aortic valve surgery. The LAA was occluded with running sutures, and intraoperative TEE was not performed. At follow-up TEE (23–159 postoperative days), only 1 of the patients had complete closure of the LAA ostium. All of the other 5 patients had postoperative SEC within the LAA, which was more serious than before occlusion in 2 patients. One patient with incomplete occlusion of the LAA had a stroke 4 weeks after surgery despite having an INR of 5.9.[44] The investigators concluded that intraoperative TEE was necessary to ensure complete closure of the LAA and reduce risk of postoperative stroke.

The primary issue limiting the use of surgical LAA occlusion is the variability of complete closure, ranging from 17% to 93%.[45] There is a difference between the anatomic ostium and the TEE-defined ostium of the LAA,[22] which may adversely affect occlusion regardless of the approach. Inadequate TEE visualization of the ostium during surgery may result in incomplete closure of the LAA, which allows continued formation of thrombus within the structure.

A major concern is whether incomplete occlusion is worse than no occlusion, given that reduced blood flow velocity in the LAA may enable more thrombus formation than in the fully patent situation. Kanderian and colleagues[46] performed a retrospective analysis of 137 patients who underwent surgical LAA occlusion and had TEE evaluation 8 ± 12 months following surgery. Excision resulted in a 73% successful closure rate, compared with 23% for suture exclusion and 0% for stapler exclusion (P<.01). Thrombus was visualized within the LAA in 28 of 68 (41%) patients who had unsuccessful closure following suture or stapler exclusion; however, 11% of patients who had successful closure versus 15% of patients who had unsuccessful closure suffered a stroke or TIA after surgery (P = .61). Based on these findings, the investigators identified 4 outcomes of surgical LAA closure: (1) successful closure; (2) patent LAA, defined as persistent communication of LAA with left atrium caused by dehiscence; (3) excluded LAA with persistent flow, defined as color flow jet between LAA and left atrium despite appearance of closure; and (4) remnant LAA with pouch more than 1 cm in length. The investigators

concluded that anticoagulation should not be discontinued until successful closure is confirmed by TEE evaluation.[46]

Novel epicardial devices for LAA occlusion are in development, and some new devices are beginning to be used clinically. The AtriCure (Cincinnati, OH) AtriClip system delivers a clip around the LAA with direct visualization during surgery. Its first use was described in 34 patients with AF undergoing concurrent CABG or valve replacement. The LAA was successfully occluded in all patients after 3 months as assessed by TEE.[47] Epicardial exclusion of the LAA may have other beneficial effects in AF. In a small case series (N = 10) using the AtriClip system[48] in concert with pulmonary vein isolation and off-pump coronary artery bypass, 100% of patients achieved acute electrical isolation of the LAA. The Aegis System (Vancouver, Canada), a percutaneous device, consists of a grabber with integrated electrodes to identify the LAA under fluoroscopic guidance, and a ligator (hollow suture) to cinch the LAA at the base. Ligation of the LAA was successful in 5/6 dogs in a preclinical study.[49] Necropsy after 2 to 3 months revealed an atretic remnant LAA in the animals. A silicone band delivered via a percutaneous system (Medtronic, Minneapolis, MN) resulted in complete occlusion of the LAA in 15/15 dogs.[50]

COMBINED EPICARDIAL/ENDOVASCULAR

A combination epicardial/endovascular procedure, using the LARIAT suture delivery device and magnetic-tipped guidewires with balloon-tipped endovascular catheter (SentreHEART, Palo Alto, CA), was initially tested in canines[51,52] and showed complete closure in almost all subjects and evidence for complete endothelialization at the closure site by day 7.[51] A small series of 13 patients with AF undergoing concurrent catheter AF ablation (N = 11) or mitral valve replacement (N = 2) had LAA ligation using the SentreHEART system.[53] Ten of the 11 catheter ablation and both of the mitral valve replacement patients achieved successful ligation of the LAA. Follow-up TEE performed 60 days following ligation in 6 patients revealed complete closure in 4 (67%); the remaining 2 patients had less than 2-mm jet on color flow Doppler.[53] Another series of 21 patients with AF and significantly increased average HAS-BLED scores (3.5 ± 1.0) underwent successful LARIAT LAA exclusion.[54] After 3 months, 17 of 17 patients who underwent TEE showed successful LAA exclusion, with only 1 patient showing a small amount of flow into the LAA. Three patients developed a moderate pericardial effusion, but only 1 required hospitalization and drainage.

A larger, single-center observational study consisting of 119 patients assessing the efficacy of LAA closure and procedural safety has been reported.[55] Sixteen patients were excluded by computed tomography because of orientation behind the pulmonary artery or LAA diameter larger than 40 mm. Fourteen patients were excluded because of thrombus identified during TEE or adhesions. Of the 85 patients who underwent LAA ligation with the LARIAT suture delivery device, 96% of the LAA ligations resulted in complete closure, and the remaining patient had less than a 2-mm leak by Doppler echocardiography at the 1-year follow-up. There were no device-related complications. Three access-related complications occurred in 3 patients. The adverse events included chest pain (24%), pericarditis (2.4%), late pericardial effusion (1.2%), and late thrombus formation (1.2%).[55] LAA ligation with the LARIAT suture device seems to be effective at excluding the LAA with an acceptably low access rate of complications. However, none of the epicardial procedures discussed earlier have been assessed for long-term reduction of stroke risk in humans with AF.

ENDOVASCULAR APPROACHES

Percutaneous catheter-based techniques can be performed through minimal incisions, allowing faster patient recovery and greater comfort, and have the additional advantage of using familiar techniques for the interventionist. The devices are delivered via percutaneous 9-Fr to 14-Fr catheters from the femoral vein and then through a transseptal puncture. The delivery catheters (DCs) are designed to engage the LAA. The devices are shown in **Fig. 2**. Two devices for transcatheter occlusion have been tested in large prospective clinical trials: Percutaneous Left Atrial Appendage Transcatheter Occlusion (PLAATO; ev3 Inc., Plymouth, MN; see **Fig. 2**B), which was tested in a nonrandomized trial[56]; and Watchman (Atritech division of Boston Scientific, Plymouth, MN; see **Fig. 2**A), which has been tested in 2 randomized trials against warfarin therapy.[57] Amplatzer atrial septal occluders have been used off-label to successfully close LAA,[58] and the Amplatzer Cardiac Plug (St Jude Medical, St Paul, MN; see **Fig. 2**C) is specifically designed for LAA occlusion, and is presently being evaluated in a phase 3, multicenter randomized trial. A small (N = 5) case series of the Amplatzer device has been published.[59] No periprocedural adverse events were reported, and TEE at 30 days following the index procedure showed no flow into the LAA or thrombus formation on the atrial surface of the device.

PLAATO

The first endovascular device designed specifically for LAA occlusion was deployed in patients with AF with contraindications to warfarin treatment: the PLAATO system.[60] The occluder consists of a self-expanding nitinol cage covered with polytetrafluoroethylene (see **Fig. 2**B). Three rows of anchors along the maximum circumference secure the cage within the LAA ostium. Results of the original PLAATO trial and subsequent long-term follow-up evaluations are detailed in **Table 3**. Deployment of the device was successful in the first 15 patients, with no evidence of thrombi or residual atrial shunt after septal puncture.[60] Results of the European and North American prospective feasibility studies were published in 2005.[56] Occlusion was successful in 108/111 (97%) patients, and the average duration of follow-up was 9.8 months (90.7 implant-years). There were 7 major adverse events (MAEs) in 5 patients, including 2 strokes and 4 cardiac/neurologic deaths. Three TIAs occurred. After up to 5 years of follow-up, the annualized stroke/TIA rate was 3.8%, compared with an anticipated rate of 6.6% using the CHADS$_2$ score.[61] In a single-center study of 73 patients,[62] no patients suffered a stroke in 2 years of follow-up.

The European PLAATO Study[13] included 180 patients. One-hundred and forty patients had follow-up TEE 2 months following deployment, and 126 (90%) had total occlusion. The stroke rate at 129 patient-years of follow-up was 2.3%. There were 16 MAEs in 12 patients (12.4%), 8 of which were procedure-related. The investigators pointed out in the discussion that the PLAATO device needs to be oversized by 20% to 50% relative to the LAA ostial diameter to guarantee stable placement and occlusion.[13] The manufacturer has not pursued subsequent trials of the device. Despite the noncommercialization of the PLAATO device, it showed the potential of mechanically closing the LAA for patients needing an alternative to antithrombotic treatment, both safely and what seemed to be effectively compared with historical controls. In addition, it gave many operators experience in navigating the left atrium and the LAA.

WATCHMAN

The Watchman device (see **Fig. 2**A) has incremental benefits in terms of delivery and recapture compared with the PLAATO device. Watchman is an investigational device that has a self-expanding, open-ended, nitinol cage with tines to anchor the device in place. The body of the device, specifically the aspect exposed to the left atrium,

Table 3
PLAATO Trial reports. Data are presented as mean ± standard deviation or frequency (percent)

	First Author (Year)			
	Ostermayer et al,[56] 2005	Park et al,[62] 2009	Block et al,[61] 2009	Bayard et al,[13] 2010
Number of patients/number of study sites	111/14	73/1	64/10	180/18
Age (y)	71 ± 9	73 ± 10	73 (range 43–90)	70 ± 10
No. male (%)	66 (59)	37 (51)	39 (61)	118 (62)
CHADS$_2$ score	2.5 ± 1.3	2.5 ± 1.4	2.6 ± 1.3	3.1 ± 0.8
No. of percutaneous LAA occlusion successes (%)	108 (97)	71 (97)	61 (94)	162 (90)
Duration of follow-up	9.8 mo (mean)	2 y	5 y	9.6 ± 6.9 mo
Number of strokes/Annual stroke rate (%)	2/2.2	0/0	8/3.8	3/2.3
No. of adverse events (%): device embolization	0 (0)	1 (1.4)	0 (0)	2 (1.1)
Pericardial effusion	2 (1.8)	1 (1.4)	0 (0)	5 (2.8)
Cardiac tamponade	2 (1.8)	0 (0)	1 (1.6)	6 (3.7)

From Fuller CJ, Reisman M. Stroke prevention in atrial fibrillation: atrial appendage closure. Current Cardiology Reports 2011;13:163; with permission.

is covered in a permeable polytetrafluoroethylene membrane.[63]

PROTECT AF was a prospective randomized controlled trial to assess noninferiority of the Watchman device to warfarin therapy.[57] Patients with nonvalvular AF were eligible for inclusion if they had CHADS$_2$ scores of greater than or equal to 1 and had no contraindications to warfarin treatment. There was 2:1 randomization of the Watchman to control (warfarin to achieve INR of 2.0–3.0). A total of 408 patients received a device, and 241 patients received warfarin. Intervention patients were therapeutically anticoagulated for

at least 45 days. The composite primary efficacy end point consisted of ischemic or hemorrhagic stroke, cardiovascular or unexplained death, or systemic embolism; the composite primary safety end point consisted of excessive bleeding or procedure-related complications. Mean follow-up was 18 months.

Table 4 shows the results of the PROTECT AF trial. The intention-to-treat (ITT) analysis included all randomized patients (n = 463 device, n = 244 control), whereas the successful treatment (per protocol) group included device patients who were able to discontinue warfarin following device

Table 4
Results of the PROTECT AF trial. Data are presented as rate per 100 patient-years, with 95% credible interval in parentheses. Refer to text for definitions

	Device Group	Control Group	Risk Ratio (Device/Control)
Intention-to-treat Analysis (Device n = 463, Control n = 244)			
Composite primary efficacy end point	3.0 (1.9–4.5)	4.9 (2.8–7.1)	0.62 (0.35–1.25)
Composite primary safety end point	7.4 (5.5–9.7)	4.4 (2.5–6.7)	1.69 (1.01–3.19)
Per Protocol Analysis (Device n = 389, Control n = 241)			
Composite primary efficacy end point	1.9 (1.0–3.2)	4.6 (2.6–6.8)	0.40 (0.19–0.91)
Composite primary safety end point	1.5 (0.7–2.8)	4.4 (2.5–6.7)	0.35 (0.15–0.80)

Data from Holmes DR, Reddy VY, Turi ZG, et al. Percutaneous closure of the left atrial appendage versus warfarin therapy for prevention of stroke in patients with atrial fibrillation: a randomised non-inferiority trial. Lancet 2009;374(9689):534–42.

implantation (n = 389) and control patients at the start of warfarin treatment (n = 241). The composite primary efficacy end point was noninferiority between groups in the ITT analysis (rate ratio [RR] 0.62; 95% credible interval [CrI] 0.35–1.25); however, the composite primary safety RR showed inferiority of the Watchman (1.69; 95% CrI 1.01–3.19). This was caused by 22 pericardial effusions (4.8%), 4 air emboli (0.9%), and 3 device embolizations (0.6%) in the device group, which occurred periprocedurally or shortly following implantation.

For the per protocol analysis, the composite primary efficacy and safety end points favored device implantation (efficacy RR 0.4, 95% CrI 0.19–0.91; safety RR 0.35, 95% CrI 0.15–0.80). The control group had a higher prevalence of major bleeding and hemorrhagic stroke relative to the device group (per protocol analysis: major bleeding, control 4.1% vs device 3.5%; hemorrhagic stroke, control 2.5% vs device 0.2%). The control group had INR within therapeutic range (2.0–3.0) only 66% of the time,[57] which has been seen in other studies of warfarin.[64]

Successful device implantation was achieved in 408 of 449 patients in whom implantation was attempted. Failed implantation was caused by procedural complications, unacceptable device position, size, stability, or LAA seal. Among successful implants, residual leaking was common (40.9%) and most patients had moderate (1–3-mm jet) leaks, but this decreased slightly over 12 months (32.1%), evaluated by TEE. As is the case with inadequate surgical ligation,[46] inadequate endovascular LAA occlusion may be a risk for thromboembolic events. If the leak was less than 5 mm at 45 days, patients discontinued warfarin. At 45 days after implantation, 349/408 (86%) patients in the device group discontinued warfarin per protocol, and this increased to 355/385 (92%) at 6 months. Patients remained on clopidogrel for 6 months after implantation and on aspirin permanently. There was no association between peridevice flow and adverse clinical events (stroke, peripheral embolism, or death) in the cohort regardless of continued anticoagulant therapy (P = .857).[42] The change in mental and physical quality of life measures significantly favored the Watchman group at 12 months.[65]

The results of the PROTECT AF trial need to be taken within the context of the population enrolled.[57] First, a high proportion of patients in both groups had CHADS₂ scores of 1 (device n = 157 [34%]; control n = 66 [27%]), which indicates a low-risk population that could be managed with anticoagulant or antiplatelet therapy. Many of the adverse events in the device group occurred early in the trial, which indicates an operator learning curve. Safety analysis of both PROTECT AF and the continued-access registry for the study showed significant reductions in procedure time (62 ± 34 vs 50 ± 21 min, respectively; P<.001) and in the rate of procedure-related or device-related safety events within 7 days of the procedure compared with PROTECT AF to 3.7% versus 7.7% of patients experiencing events (P = .007). The continued-access registry also had lower rates of serious pericardial effusions relative to PROTECT AF (2.2% vs 5.0%, respectively; P = .019).[43] After 1588 patient-years of follow-up (mean 2.3 years), the primary event rate was 3.0 per 100 patient-years for Watchman, which was noninferior to 4.3 for control (P = nonsignificant). However, the safety end point was worse for Watchman (5.5% vs 3.6% per year, RR 1.53, 95% CI 0.95–2.70).[66] The trend favoring LAA occlusion continued in the recently reported 4-year primary event rate of 2.3 versus 3.8 per 100 patient-years (RR 0.60, 95% CI 0.41–1.05) (Fig. 3). The data for all-cause mortality at 4 year favored the Watchman (HR 0.66, 95% CI 0.45–0.98), suggesting that, despite the early complication rate of LAA closure, the harms associated with bleeding and inconsistent anticoagulation with warfarin begin to accrue over time.

Given the early complication rate associated with the Watchman device, the FDA requested that a second randomized trial, PREVAIL (clinicaltrials.gov NCT01182441) be performed. The PREVAIL trial design is similar to PROTECT AF, but excluded patients with CHADS₂ scores equal to 1, unless they had a second high-risk characteristic (ie, woman aged greater than or equal to 75 years, left ventricular ejection fraction between 30% and 34.9%, aged 65 to 74 years with diabetes or coronary artery disease, or aged 65 years or older with documented congestive heart failure).

A total of 407 patients were randomized in a 2:1 ratio of device to medical therapy in PREVAIL. As of this writing, the study has not been published, but the preliminary data have been released.[67] Patients were older and more likely to be diabetic compared with PROTECT AF, with the baseline CHADS₂ score averaging 2.6, compared with 2.2. The adverse event rate in the first 7 days was 2.2%, less than that reported in PROTECT AF, and within the noninferiority threshold. The primary stroke/CV event/systemic emboli end point was 0.64 events per 100 patient-years in both groups, suggesting relative equivalence between the two strategies (18-month RR 1.07, 95% CrI 0.57–1.88), although this did not meet the prespecified cutoff for noninferiority. Despite the low stroke rate in the control group compared with historical controls (approximately 1.7 per 100 patient-years

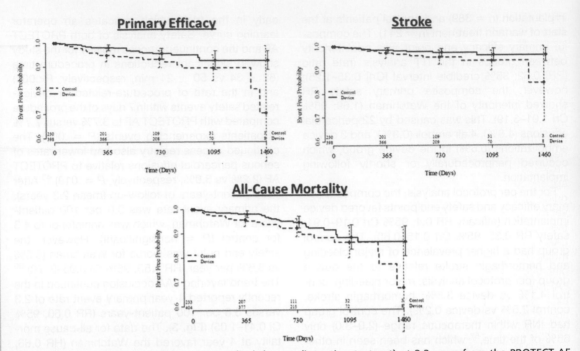

Fig. 3. Outcomes of LAA closure versus medical therapy (intention to treat) at 2.3 years from the PROTECT AF study. Primary efficacy end point of stroke, systemic embolism, and cardiovascular death. None of these comparisons were significant. Solid line, Device closure; Dotted line, Control. (*From* Reddy VY, Doshi SK, Sievert H, et al. Percutaneous left atrial appendage closure for stroke prophylaxis in patients with atrial fibrillation: 2.3-Year Follow-up of the PROTECT AF (Watchman Left Atrial Appendage System for Embolic Protection in Patients with Atrial Fibrillation) Trial. Circulation 2013;127(6):724; with permission.)

in the Randomized Evaluation of Long-Term Anticoagulation Therapy [RE-LY] study or 1.6 per 100 patient-years in the PROTECT AF study), the device seemed to perform at least as well as the controls.

AMPLATZER CARDIAC PLUG

Amplatzer devices have been used for LAA occlusion in nonrandomized trials. The first study involved off-label use of the occluder used for patent foramen ovale or atrial septal defect closure in 16 patients with AF.[58] With the exception of 1 device embolization, complete occlusion of LAA was observed in all subjects in 5 patient-years of follow-up. Several small series of patients with AF who underwent successful implantation with the Amplatzer Cardiac Plug (ACP) have been described (see **Fig. 2**C).[68,69] The ACP is specifically designed for LAA occlusion, made of a self-expanding nitinol mesh that has a flat disc and a cylindrical lobe with 2 patches of polyester sewn within the lobe and disc. The distal lobe of the device has up to 6 stabilizing wire hooks that anchor the device in the LAA. The lobe is available in sizes between 16 and 30 mm with a fixed length of 6.5 mm for all sizes. The proximal disk is 4 to 6 mm larger than the lobe. In 1 study, 86 patients

with moderate to high risk of stroke (CHADS$_2$ score 2.6 ± 1.2) underwent successful implantation with the ACP.[41] Total procedural complications were low (5.7%), and follow-up on 69 patients (25.9 patient-years) revealed no stroke or peripheral vascular thromboembolism. LAA closure was complete in 67/69 patients.[41] In a retrospective registry of 137 patients with AF who were too high risk for anticoagulation, the LAA occlusion was successful in 132 (96%) patients using the ACP.[70] Adverse events included stroke (N = 3), device embolization (N = 2), air embolism to a coronary artery (N = 2), pericardial effusion without tamponade (N = 4), or tamponade (N = 5). The 4% incidence of periprocedural tamponade was similar to that of the PROTECT AF study. A phase III clinical trial (NCT01118299) is underway randomizing 3000 warfarin-eligible patients to LAA closure using the ACP or anticoagulation. The 2 primary outcomes of the study will be safety at 45 days and ischemic stroke or peripheral embolism at 2 years. The ACP may have advantages compared with the other percutaneous devices in terms of ease of use and a more shallow design (maximum length 6.5 mm), which allows the device to occlude the ostium without being affected by the LAA length, tortuosity, or multilobed anatomy.

PROCEDURAL CONSIDERATIONS
SentreHEART LARIAT

Preprocedure considerations

The results of the 3D CTA are reviewed to assess the shape, size, and location of the appendage and determine appropriate pericardial access. If the width of the appendage is greater than 40 mm, then the device will not be able to get over the body of the appendage to ligate the neck or ostium of the appendage. The CTA also provides information as to the orientation of the appendage and thus how lateral or anterior the guide sheath needs to be to have the straightest vector to achieve launching over the distal end of the appendage and to the ostium. A superior LAA orientation behind the pulmonary artery or a multilobed LAA with the lobes oriented in different planes would be technically challenging for the LARIAT device and such patients have been excluded from the initial clinical studies. In addition, CTA helps to decide where to place the endovascular LAA wire so that the optimal orientation for capture is achieved.

A baseline TEE is performed to check for visual thrombus, pericardial thickening, or pericardial effusion. Presence of LAA thrombus is a contraindication for the procedure. The TEE views can confirm how many lobes are present. In contrast with endovascular prostheses like the Watchman, many intracardiac characteristics are not as important for the LARIAT, with the exception of defining clot, which is much better appreciated on TEE than CTA. Use of TEE in this procedure can also help delineate the extent of the pectinate muscles and the orientation of the ostium of the appendage. Pectinate muscles that appear to be proximal to the true appendage may serve as a persistent nidus of thrombus and thus a risk for stroke. After the procedure, TEE is used to assess ligation success.

Procedure

In most institutions, general anesthesia is used because of the placement of the TEE probe for extended periods of time. The patient should be off anticoagulation if clinically acceptable; antibiotic prophylaxis should be used. Once the patient is prepped and draped, the first step is to obtain access to the pericardial space. The dry tap is done with the Pajunk needle (Pajunk Medical Systems, Norcross, GA) from a subxiphoid approach, and accessed using contrast confirmation and then advancement of a 0.89-mm (0.035-inch) guidewire into the pericardium. A lateral fluoroscopic image is helpful for ensuring that the needle and wire are directed anteriorly. Once this is achieved, either over this wire or a stiffer wire, the SofTIP guide catheter is advanced and positioned in the pericardial space. TEE should be used to confirm that the catheter is not compressing the right ventricle and that there is no pericardial effusion. If an effusion does occur, drainage can be performed via a pigtail through the sheath, or a second pericardial access can be obtained.

The next step is to gain access to the left atrium using a conventional transseptal approach. The fossa should be crossed in the central position or slightly superior and posterior. The entry to the os of the LAA is anterior to the fossa and best achieved when the catheter crosses the septum to allow a straight vector toward the LAA. Leading with a soft-tipped guidewire or directly with a pigtail catheter, the LAA is accessed and an LAA angiogram can be obtained, which can be performed using the pigtail or through the transseptal catheter.

Once left atrial access is obtained, a 0.64-mm (0.025-inch) FindrWIRE with a small curve placed approximately 2 to 3 cm from the tip is back-loaded into the catheter; both are navigated to the apex of the LAA under fluoroscopic guidance. The proximal marker of the balloon should be placed just distal to the coronary sinus or circumflex artery based on TEE. The FindrWIRE should be in the distal apex of the LAA. The 0.89-mm (0.035-inch) wire is introduced through the pericardial guide cannula, directed to the endovascularly placed FindrWIRE, and connected end to end by opposite-pole magnetic tips under fluoroscopic guidance.

Once the wires have been connected, the LARIAT is placed over the wire. The LARIAT is advanced toward the LAA; the snare is reopened and advanced over the LAA. The distal snare loop of the LARIAT should align with the proximal marker of the EndoCATH balloon. The balloon is inflated with a 50:50 mixture of contrast and saline. The origin of the LAA and the epicardial surface is determined using TEE. The LARIAT snare is then closed completely. TEE and atriagram views are used to identify correct placement of the snare. If not adequate, the snare is reopened and repositioned, and then the balloon is deflated.

The 0.64-mm (0.025") FindrWIRE is retracted to the tip of the balloon while holding tension on the epicardial wire, so that the epicardial wire does not lurch forward. The EndoCATH and FindrWIRE are removed as a single unit from the LAA. Once placement is deemed satisfactory, the LARIAT suture is released and tightened until resistance is met. Two final tightenings are then performed with a suture tension force gauge, the TenSURE device.

Color duplex TEE is used to confirm adequacy of closure, and confirmed with atriagrams (30°

right anterior oblique [RAO] ± 10° cranial and 30° left anterior oblique). Once the LAA is completely excluded, the red suture release tab is cut and withdrawn from over the LAA with snare completely open. Both LARIAT and FindrWIRE are then withdrawn completely from the guide cannula, and the remnant suture tail is cut with a remote suture cutter (SureCUT).

Postprocedure care

Postprocedure care is focused on managing pericardial access issues. Often the patient does not have any drainage from the DC, and there is no effusion noted on TEE. In such cases where there is a clean entry into the pericardial space, the delivery sheath can be removed in the catheter laboratory or, for additional precautions, in the recovery area. If there is evidence of effusion or an inadvertent entry into the right ventricle, a pigtail catheter should be left in the pericardial space to drain overnight. The catheter should be removed once there is certainty that there is no reaccumulation.

Pain is common after the procedure, probably caused by irritation of the pericardial tissue. Management is typically with analgesics, often nonsteroidal antiinflammatory drugs. The pain can be debilitating and should be managed aggressively. Some operators have used direct injection of lidocaine into the pericardial space. However, the benefits of this treatment have not been studied rigorously.

Weekly follow-up by telephone is important. The patient should be asked about chest pain, dyspnea, or any changes in respiratory status. Late cases of hemothorax have been seen that may not have been recognized earlier. These cases may be related to the initial pericardial access. Although at present there is no rigorous protocol for TEE follow-up, imaging by 90 days after the procedure is highly recommended.

Watchman

Preprocedure considerations

The Watchman is an investigational device at the time of this writing. The work-up to determine whether or not the patient is a candidate is based on the eligibility criteria of the PREVAIL trial. The $CHADS_2$ score should be greater than or equal to 2 unless the patient is a woman aged 75 years or older, has a baseline left ventricular ejection fraction between 30% and 35%, or is aged 65 years or older and has diabetes, coronary artery disease, or congestive heart failure. In contrast with the LARIAT device, the Watchman work-up requires only a TEE to assess the LAA. Based on currently available device sizes, the maximal LAA

ostial diameter must be between 17 and 31 mm; therefore, careful attention should be paid to measuring the LAA ostium in several angles. LAA thrombus needs to be excluded and the usable length of the LAA to accommodate the device should be assessed. A shallow LAA, with a usable length less than the maximum diameter of the appendage may prevent the device from seating deep enough into the LAA. A multilobed cauliflower-type LAA with limited overall length poses technical challenges and may not allow adequate positioning of the Watchman. Other anatomic exclusion criteria include high-risk patent foramen ovale, implanted valve prosthesis, mitral valve stenosis, or mobile atheroma in the aortic arch or descending aorta.

Procedure

A traditional transseptal puncture is achieved to provide an orientation that optimizes access to not only the os of the LAA, but orients toward the lobe in which the operator ultimately wants to place the DC for the Watchman device. Once the transseptal puncture is performed, either directly with the Amplatz Super Stiff or using an MP catheter, the guidewire should be placed in the left upper pulmonary vein to be used as a rail. Once positioned there, the double-curve or single-curve Watchman DC (**Fig. 4**) is inserted and the Amplatz Super Stiff can be removed as the DC is positioned in the left atrial cavity. Through the catheter, a 6-Fr pigtail is advanced up the DC and placed in the LAA. Access into the LAA in most cases is via a counterclockwise or anterior rotation of the pigtail and/or DC. Once the pigtail is in the LAA, LAA images are obtained. The best working view is RAO 30° oblique and 30° caudal, which correlates with the TEE image at 135°. A simple RAO view correlates with the TEE image at 45° or 90°, whereas the cranial RAO correlates with the TEE image at 0°.

Once the pigtail catheter is in the optimal position and provides the best access, which is often the lobe that allows optimal orientation of the Watchman with relation to the os, and the length of the device is accommodated, then the DC is placed distally into the LAA over the pigtail catheter. Additional angiography is done at this point to ensure positioning and to be certain that the DC is not against the LAA wall. TEE is used continuously during the procedure to assist in positioning the catheters and to reassess LAA dimensions. It is important to be certain that the patient is euvolemic during the procedure so that true LAA measurements can be obtained. The marker bands on the DC define where the various devices will land proximally; therefore, it is critical

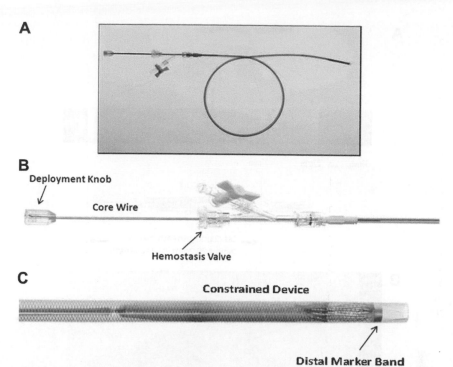

A

B
Deployment Knob
Core Wire
Hemostasis Valve

C
Constrained Device
Distal Marker Band

Fig. 4. (*A*) The Watchman DC; (*B*) proximal view of catheter; (*C*) distal view of catheter showing constrained device and marker band.

to determine which device will be placed and to make sure that the marker band corresponding with that device is located at or near the os of the LAA (**Fig. 5**).

The Watchman devices come in sizes of 21, 24, 27, 30, and 33 mm, and the appropriate device is chosen to be 2 to 4 mm greater than the maximum LAA ostium diameter (**Table 5**). For example, if the maximum LAA ostium diameter is 26 mm, a 30-mm device is selected. Once the correct size Watchman device is selected and prepared, the 6-Fr pigtail catheter is removed while keeping the DC in position with the correct sizing marker band at the os. The delivery system is inserted carefully until the distal marker band of the delivery system is lined up with the distal marker band of the DC under fluoroscopy. Once the marker bands are lined up, the delivery system is held in place and the access sheath (AS; **Fig. 6**) is retracted and snapped onto the DC (AS/DC assembly; **Fig. 7**). The DC tip position needs to be confirmed before deployment (**Fig. 8**).

The implant is slowly unsheathed within the LAA. The device is deployed by holding the deployment knob stationary while retracting the AS/DC assembly slowly to deploy the device completely. Leaving the core wire attached, the AS/DC assembly is withdrawn to a few centimeters from the device, allowing the device to align with

the LAA (**Fig. 9**). The Watchman device should meet all 4 of the device release criteria, abbreviated as PASS:

1. Position: the plane of maximum diameter of the device should be at or just distal to the LAA ostium and span it completely. The position is confirmed via TEE and fluoroscopy.
2. Anchor or stability: the AS/DC assembly is withdrawn a few centimeters from the device. Gently pull back and then release deployment knob. The device and LAA should move in unison. Stability is confirmed via TEE and fluoroscopy.
3. Size: the plane of maximum diameter of the device is measured and should be 80% to 92% of the original size measured under TEE.
4. Seal: all lobes must be distal to the device and sealed under TEE.

If any of the release criteria are not met, the device can always be recaptured. A partial recapture and redeployment can be done if the device was initially distal and did not cover all the LAA lobes. If the initial position is too proximal, a full recapture is performed. In this situation, the DC would be repositioned and deployment of a new device would be attempted. Once the operator is satisfied with placement and the device release criteria are

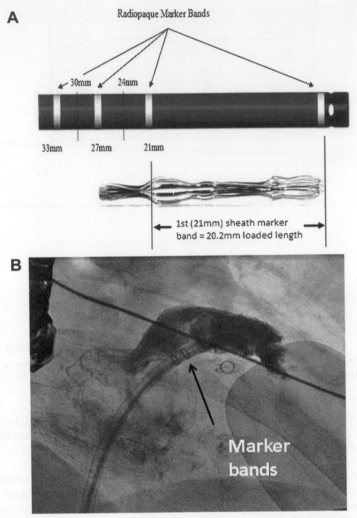

Fig. 5. (*A*) Association of radiopaque marker bands on Watchman DC with size of device; (*B*) fluoroscope shot of DC with markings at ostium of LAA.

met, the deployment knob is rotated counterclockwise 3 to 5 full turns to release device.

Postprocedure Care

Standard of care procedures should be used to control postprocedure bleeding at the access site. Patients should remain on warfarin (INR 2.0–3.0) and 81 mg aspirin for a minimum of 45 days after implantation. At 45 days, device placement should be confirmed with TEE. Cessation of warfarin at this point is at physician discretion. Patients who discontinue warfarin should begin clopidogrel 75 mg and aspirin daily through 6 months after implantation and remain on daily aspirin indefinitely. Appropriate endocarditis prophylaxis should be followed for 6 months following device implantation. Continuing endocarditis prophylaxis beyond 6 months is at physician discretion.

AMPLATZER CARDIAC PLUG
Preprocedure Considerations

At present, the ACP is an investigational device only available through a randomized multicenter clinical trial. Patients with nonvalvular AF and a CHADS2 score of greater than or equal to 2 who are eligible to take warfarin or dabigatran are included. A complete description of the inclusion and exclusion criteria is available at www.clinical-trials.gov/NCT01118299. In the study, all patients will be anticoagulated for at least 1 month before the ACP placement and put on bridge therapy leading up to the procedure. TEE measurements of the LAA ostial diameter, morphology, and length are performed for preprocedural planning and the absence of an LAA thrombus is established. The device is available in 8 diameter sizes (16, 18, 20, 22, 24, 26, 28, and 30 mm) allowing for ACP

Maximum LAA Ostium (mm)	Device Size (mm) (Uncompressed Diameter)
Watchman	
17–19	21
20–22	24
23–25	27
26–28	30
29–31	33
ACP	
12.6–14	16
15–16	18
17–18	20
19–20	22
21–22	24
23–24	26
25–26	28
27–28.5	30

Table 5
Watchman and ACP device size selection table

placement in appendages with diameters as small as 12.6 mm and as large as 28.5 mm (see **Table 5**). The size refers to the diameter of the cylindrical lobe, whereas the left atrial disc is 4 to 6 mm larger. The LAA length must be at least 10 mm to accommodate the dilator and sheath, but the device height is only 6.5 mm.

Procedure

The patient is anticoagulated to achieve an activated clotting time of longer than 250 seconds.

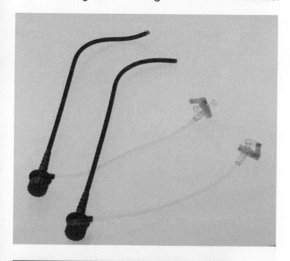

Fig. 6. The Watchman single-curve and double-curve ASs, with detail of the distal end showing the marker band.

Using a standard Mullins or similar needle/catheter, a transseptal puncture is performed and the sheath advanced to the left atrium. A pigtail catheter is advanced through this sheath and used to engage the LAA and perform angiography. Several echocardiographic and/or fluoroscopic dimensions of the LAA should be performed in multiple angles. Recommended sizing of the device is 2 to 3 cm (10%–20%) larger than the narrowest diameter of the LAA body 1 to 2 mm distal from the orifice. Once a device size is determined, the pigtail catheter is then exchanged for a TorqVue delivery sheath, which is left in the LAA. The ACP device is then prepared by screwing the ACP onto a delivery cable and advanced to the distal sheath. Using TEE guidance and fluoroscopic imaging with angiograms performed with sheath injections, the lobe of the device is deployed by retracting the sheath and positioning the lobe 1 to 2 cm distal of the LAA orifice and the left atrial disc against the LAA ostium itself. TEE should be used to verify device positioning and degree of leak, if any. Sufficient anchoring is evaluated by applying tension to the delivery cable and then releasing, the so-called wiggle test. Compression of the ACP lobe should be observed: a square lobe indicates undersizing, whereas a tapered strawberry deformation indicates oversizing or overly deep seating.[70] The device can be recaptured and repositioned by pulling it back into the sheath. Once the position is acceptable, the delivery cable can be torqued counterclockwise to release the ACP.

Postprocedure Care

Per protocol, device-treated patients receive anticoagulation for 45 days following implantation in addition to baseline aspirin therapy that is continued throughout. TEEs are performed at 45 days, 6 months, 12 months, and 24 months to assess device position and leaking, LAA closure, and thrombus formation. Based on the experience of the PROTECT AF study, clinical follow-up will include monitoring for pericardial effusions, device erosion and embolization, access site-related bleeding, and damage to other cardiac structures. If more than minimal flow of 3 mm into the LAA is seen on Doppler echocardiography assessments, then patients in the device arm should continue anticoagulation with a goal INR of 2 to 3, or be placed on dabigatran.

POTENTIAL COMPLICATIONS AND THEIR PREVENTION

The 3 major complications of the PROTECT AF trial were pericardial effusion and perforation

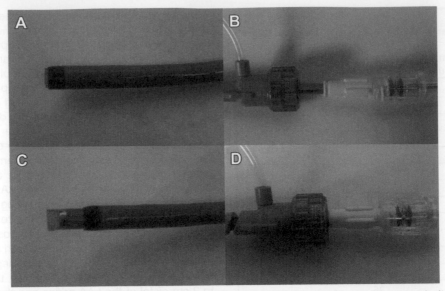

Fig. 7. The access sheath/delivery catheter assembly. (*A*) Access sheath and delivery catheter with distal markers lined up. (*B*) Position of the delivery catheter at sheath hub when distal markers are lined up. (*C*) Position of the LAA device when the access sheath is retracted and snapped into the delivery catheter. (*D*) Position of the delivery catheter at sheath hub when the access sheath is retracted and snapped into the delivery catheter.

(6.5%), intraprocedural stroke (1.1%, mostly caused by air embolism), and device embolization (0.6%).[57] Similar complications were described in the studies of the Amplatzer device. These complications were less prevalent in the PROTECT AF continuing access registry,[43] indicating the learning curve for this procedure. Using TEE to guide transseptal puncture, engaging the LAA with a pigtail or soft wire, and then advancing the delivery sheath over the pigtail may reduce the

risk of perforation and serious tamponade. Continuous TEE monitoring is essential to ensure proper device placement and to avoid puncture of the distal LAA. Catheters need to be flushed with saline to avoid air emboli. Proper anticoagulation during the case reduces thrombus formation on the catheters and devices. In addition, scrupulous attention to the echocardiographic and fluoroscopic positioning of the device and seal are needed before releasing the LAA device.

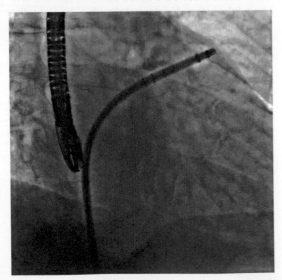

Fig. 8. Fluoroscopic confirmation of location of AS/DC assembly at the ostium of LAA.

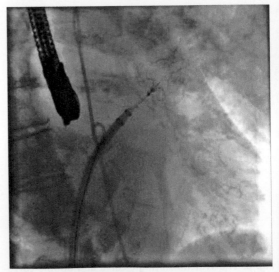

Fig. 9. Deployment of the Watchman device in the LAA before release.

The data for complications of the SentreHEART LARIAT are limited, but pericarditis, tamponade, and hemopericardium have been reported.[53] An additional patient who had pectus excavatum required thoracoscopic removal of the snare because of compression by the concave sternum.[53] A complication of this type can be avoided by thorough evaluation of the mediastinal space by 3D CTA before the procedure.

SUMMARY

Occlusion of the LAA via surgical, epicardial, or endovascular approaches may reduce the risk of stroke in patients with AF, and seems to be noninferior to warfarin in this regard. However, serious periprocedural complications may negate the overall efficacy of LAA occlusion, but, over the long term, as complications associated with bleeding and inconsistent anticoagulation accrue, the benefit of LAA occlusion may be more apparent. Adequate operator training reduces periprocedural adverse events, but does not eliminate them. The long-term follow-up from PROTECT AF, the initial reports from PREVAIL, and the small studies of the Watchman and ACP devices for nonwarfarin candidates seem promising. Nevertheless, additional trials involving device and procedural refinements are in progress to ascertain whether LAA occlusion can replace anticoagulation for stroke prevention in patients with nonvalvular AF. Furthermore, the superior dosing and safety profiles of the novel oral anticoagulants raise the accepted threshold for safety and efficacy of LAA occlusion procedures, and thus underscore the need for randomized studies comparing LAA occlusion with these newer anticoagulants.

REFERENCES

1. Wolf PA, Abbott RD, Kannel WB. Atrial fibrillation as an independent risk factor for stroke: the Framingham Study. Stroke 1991;22(8):983–8.
2. Miyasaka Y, Barnes ME, Gersh BJ, et al. Secular trends in incidence of atrial fibrillation in Olmsted County, Minnesota, 1980 to 2000, and implications on the projections for future prevalence. Circulation 2006;114(2):119–25.
3. Risk factors for stroke and efficacy of antithrombotic therapy in atrial fibrillation. Analysis of pooled data from five randomized controlled trials. Arch Intern Med 1994;154(13):1449–57.
4. Benjamin EJ, Wolf PA, D'Agostino RB, et al. Impact of atrial fibrillation on the risk of death: the Framingham Heart Study. Circulation 1998; 98(10):946–52.
5. Smith EE, Shobha N, Dai D, et al. Risk score for in-hospital ischemic stroke mortality derived and validated within the Get With the Guidelines-Stroke Program. Circulation 2010;122(15):1496–504.
6. Go AS, Mozaffarian D, Roger VL, et al. Heart disease and stroke statistics–2013 update: a report from the American Heart Association. Circulation 2013;127(1):e6–245.
7. Fuster V, Ryden LE, Cannom DS, et al. ACC/AHA/ESC 2006 guidelines for the management of patients with atrial fibrillation–executive summary: a report of the American College of Cardiology/American Heart Association Task Force on Practice Guidelines and the European Society of Cardiology Committee for Practice Guidelines (Writing Committee to Revise the 2001 Guidelines for the Management of Patients With Atrial Fibrillation). J Am Coll Cardiol 2006;48(4):854–906.
8. Holbrook AM, Pereira JA, Labiris R, et al. Systematic overview of warfarin and its drug and food interactions. Arch Intern Med 2005;165(10):1095–106.
9. Walenga JM, Adiguzel C. Drug and dietary interactions of the new and emerging oral anticoagulants. Int J Clin Pract 2010;64(7):956–67.
10. Thambidorai SK, Murray RD, Parakh K, et al. Utility of transesophageal echocardiography in identification of thrombogenic milieu in patients with atrial fibrillation (an ACUTE ancillary study). Am J Cardiol 2005;96(7):935–41.
11. Wang YL, Li XB, Quan X, et al. Focal atrial tachycardia originating from the left atrial appendage: electrocardiographic and electrophysiologic characterization and long-term outcomes of radiofrequency ablation. J Cardiovasc Electrophysiol 2007;18(5):459–64.
12. Healey JS, Crystal E, Lamy A, et al. Left Atrial Appendage Occlusion Study (LAAOS): results of a randomized controlled pilot study of left atrial appendage occlusion during coronary bypass surgery in patients at risk for stroke. Am Heart J 2005; 150(2):288–93.
13. Bayard YL, Omran H, Neuzil P, et al. PLAATO (Percutaneous Left Atrial Appendage Transcatheter Occlusion) for prevention of cardioembolic stroke in non-anticoagulation eligible atrial fibrillation patients: results from the European PLAATO study. EuroIntervention 2010;6(2):220–6.
14. Ernst G, Stollberger C, Abzieher F, et al. Morphology of the left atrial appendage. Anat Rec 1995;242(4):553–61.
15. Bernhardt P, Schmidt H, Hammerstingl C, et al. Patients with atrial fibrillation and dense spontaneous echo contrast at high risk a prospective and serial follow-up over 12 months with transesophageal echocardiography and cerebral magnetic resonance imaging. J Am Coll Cardiol 2005;45(11): 1807–12.

16. Blackshear JL, Odell JA. Appendage obliteration to reduce stroke in cardiac surgical patients with atrial fibrillation. Ann Thorac Surg 1996;61(2):755–9.

17. Gage BF, Waterman AD, Shannon W, et al. Validation of clinical classification schemes for predicting stroke: results from the National Registry of Atrial Fibrillation. JAMA 2001;285(22):2864–70.

18. Lip GY, Frison L, Halperin JL, et al. Comparative validation of a novel risk score for predicting bleeding risk in anticoagulated patients with atrial fibrillation: the HAS-BLED (Hypertension, Abnormal Renal/Liver Function, Stroke, Bleeding History or Predisposition, Labile INR, Elderly, Drugs/Alcohol Concomitantly) score. J Am Coll Cardiol 2011;57(2):173–80.

19. Go AS, Hylek EM, Chang Y, et al. Anticoagulation therapy for stroke prevention in atrial fibrillation: how well do randomized trials translate into clinical practice? JAMA 2003;290(20):2685–92.

20. Puwanant S, Varr BC, Shrestha K, et al. Role of the CHADS2 score in the evaluation of thromboembolic risk in patients with atrial fibrillation undergoing transesophageal echocardiography before pulmonary vein isolation. J Am Coll Cardiol 2009; 54(22):2032–9.

21. Al-Saady NM, Obel OA, Camm AJ. Left atrial appendage: structure, function, and role in thromboembolism. Heart 1999;82(5):547–54.

22. Veinot JP, Harrity PJ, Gentile F, et al. Anatomy of the normal left atrial appendage: a quantitative study of age-related changes in 500 autopsy hearts: implications for echocardiographic examination. Circulation 1997;96(9):3112–5.

23. Di Biase L, Santangeli P, Anselmino M, et al. Does the left atrial appendage morphology correlate with the risk of stroke in patients with atrial fibrillation? Results from a multicenter study. J Am Coll Cardiol 2012;60(6):531–8.

24. Wang Y, Di Biase L, Horton RP, et al. Left atrial appendage studied by computed tomography to help planning for appendage closure device placement. J Cardiovasc Electrophysiol 2010; 21(9):973–82.

25. Su P, McCarthy KP, Ho SY. Occluding the left atrial appendage: anatomical considerations. Heart 2008;94(9):1166–70.

26. Nucifora G, Faletra FF, Regoli F, et al. Evaluation of the left atrial appendage with real-time 3-dimensional transesophageal echocardiography: implications for catheter-based left atrial appendage closure. Circ Cardiovasc Imaging 2011;4(5):514–23.

27. Fatkin D, Kelly RP, Feneley MP. Relations between left atrial appendage blood flow velocity, spontaneous echocardiographic contrast and thromboembolic risk in vivo. J Am Coll Cardiol 1994;23(4): 961–9.

28. Handke M, Harloff A, Hetzel A, et al. Left atrial appendage flow velocity as a quantitative surrogate parameter for thromboembolic risk: determinants and relationship to spontaneous echocontrast and thrombus formation–a transesophageal echocardiographic study in 500 patients with cerebral ischemia. J Am Soc Echocardiogr 2005;18(12): 1366–72.

29. Beinart R, Heist EK, Newell JB, et al. Left atrial appendage dimensions predict the risk of stroke/TIA in patients with atrial fibrillation. J Cardiovasc Electrophysiol 2011;22(1):10–5.

30. Tamura H, Watanabe T, Nishiyama S, et al. Prognostic value of low left atrial appendage wall velocity in patients with ischemic stroke and atrial fibrillation. J Am Soc Echocardiogr 2012;25(5):576–83.

31. Willens HJ, Qin JX, Keith K, et al. Diagnosis of a bilobed left atrial appendage and pectinate muscles mimicking thrombi on real-time 3-dimensional transesophageal echocardiography. J Ultrasound Med 2010;29(6):975–80.

32. Marek D, Vindis D, Kocianova E. Real time 3-dimensional transesophageal echocardiography is more specific than 2-dimensional TEE in the assessment of left atrial appendage thrombosis. Biomed Pap Med Fac Univ Palacky Olomouc Czech Repub 2013;157(1):22–6.

33. Abbara S, Mundo-Sagardia JA, Hoffmann U, et al. Cardiac CT assessment of left atrial accessory appendages and diverticula. AJR Am J Roentgenol 2009;193(3):807–12.

34. Mohrs OK, Nowak B, Petersen SE, et al. Thrombus detection in the left atrial appendage using contrast-enhanced MRI: a pilot study. AJR Am J Roentgenol 2006;186(1):198–205.

35. Rathi VK, Reddy ST, Anreddy S, et al. Contrast-enhanced CMR is equally effective as TEE in the evaluation of left atrial appendage thrombus in patients with atrial fibrillation undergoing pulmonary vein isolation procedure. Heart Rhythm 2013; 10(7):1021–7.

36. Weinsaft JW, Kim HW, Crowley AL, et al. LV thrombus detection by routine echocardiography: insights into performance characteristics using delayed enhancement CMR. JACC Cardiovasc Imaging 2011;4(7):702–12.

37. Patel TK, Yancy CW, Knight BP. Left atrial appendage exclusion for stroke prevention in atrial fibrillation. Cardiol Res Pract 2012;2012:610827.

38. Gage BF, Yan Y, Milligan PE, et al. Clinical classification schemes for predicting hemorrhage: results from the National Registry of Atrial Fibrillation (NRAF). Am Heart J 2006;151(3):713–9.

39. Pisters R, Lane DA, Nieuwlaat R, et al. A novel user-friendly score (HAS-BLED) to assess 1-year risk of major bleeding in patients with atrial fibrillation: the Euro Heart Survey. Chest 2010;138(5):1093–100.

40. Reddy VY, Mobius-Winkler S, Miller MA, et al. Left atrial appendage closure with the Watchman

device in patients with a contraindication for oral anticoagulation: ASA Plavix Feasibility Study with Watchman Left Atrial Appendage Closure Technology (ASAP Study). J Am Coll Cardiol 2013;61(25):2551–6.

41. Guerios EE, Schmid M, Gloekler S, et al. Left atrial appendage closure with the Amplatzer Cardiac Plug in patients with atrial fibrillation. Arq Bras Cardiol 2012;98(6):528–36.

42. Viles-Gonzalez JF, Kar S, Douglas P, et al. The clinical impact of incomplete left atrial appendage closure with the Watchman Device in patients with atrial fibrillation: a PROTECT AF (Percutaneous Closure of the Left Atrial Appendage Versus Warfarin Therapy for Prevention of Stroke in Patients With Atrial Fibrillation) substudy. J Am Coll Cardiol 2012;59(10):923–9.

43. Reddy VY, Holmes D, Doshi SK, et al. Safety of percutaneous left atrial appendage closure: results from the Watchman Left Atrial Appendage System for Embolic Protection in Patients with AF (PROTECT AF) clinical trial and the Continued Access Registry. Circulation 2011;123(4):417–24.

44. Schneider B, Stollberger C, Sievers HH. Surgical closure of the left atrial appendage - a beneficial procedure? Cardiology 2005;104(3):127–32.

45. Dawson AG, Asopa S, Dunning J. Should patients undergoing cardiac surgery with atrial fibrillation have left atrial appendage exclusion? Interact Cardiovasc Thorac Surg 2010;10(2):306–11.

46. Kanderian AS, Gillinov AM, Pettersson GB, et al. Success of surgical left atrial appendage closure: assessment by transesophageal echocardiography. J Am Coll Cardiol 2008;52(11):924–9.

47. Salzberg SP, Plass A, Emmert MY, et al. Left atrial appendage clip occlusion: early clinical results. J Thorac Cardiovasc Surg 2010;139(5):1269–74.

48. Starck CT, Steffel J, Emmert MY, et al. Epicardial left atrial appendage clip occlusion also provides the electrical isolation of the left atrial appendage. Interact Cardiovasc Thorac Surg 2012;15(3):416–8.

49. Bruce CJ, Stanton CM, Asirvatham SJ, et al. Percutaneous epicardial left atrial appendage closure: intermediate-term results. J Cardiovasc Electrophysiol 2011;22(1):64–70.

50. McCarthy PM, Lee R, Foley JL, et al. Occlusion of canine atrial appendage using an expandable silicone band. J Thorac Cardiovasc Surg 2010;140(4):885–9.

51. Lee RJ, Bartus K, Yakubov SJ. Catheter-based left atrial appendage (LAA) ligation for the prevention of embolic events arising from the LAA: initial experience in a canine model. Circ Cardiovasc Interv 2010;3(3):224–9.

52. Singh SM, Dukkipati SR, d'Avila A, et al. Percutaneous left atrial appendage closure with an epicardial suture ligation approach: a prospective randomized pre-clinical feasibility study. Heart Rhythm 2010;7(3):370–6.

53. Bartus K, Bednarek J, Myc J, et al. Feasibility of closed-chest ligation of the left atrial appendage in humans. Heart Rhythm 2011;8(2):188–93.

54. Massumi A, Chelu MG, Nazeri A, et al. Initial experience with a novel percutaneous left atrial appendage exclusion device in patients with atrial fibrillation, increased stroke risk, and contraindications to anticoagulation. Am J Cardiol 2013;111(6):869–73.

55. Bartus K, Han FT, Bednarek J, et al. Percutaneous left atrial appendage suture ligation using the LARIAT device in patients with atrial fibrillation: initial clinical experience. J Am Coll Cardiol 2012;62(2):108–18.

56. Ostermayer SH, Reisman M, Kramer PH, et al. Percutaneous left atrial appendage transcatheter occlusion (PLAATO system) to prevent stroke in high-risk patients with non-rheumatic atrial fibrillation: results from the international multi-center feasibility trials. J Am Coll Cardiol 2005;46(1):9–14.

57. Holmes DR, Reddy VY, Turi ZG, et al. Percutaneous closure of the left atrial appendage versus warfarin therapy for prevention of stroke in patients with atrial fibrillation: a randomised non-inferiority trial. Lancet 2009;374(9689):534–42.

58. Meier B, Palacios I, Windecker S, et al. Transcatheter left atrial appendage occlusion with Amplatzer devices to obviate anticoagulation in patients with atrial fibrillation. Catheter Cardiovasc Interv 2003;60(3):417–22.

59. Montenegro MJ, Quintella EF, Damonte A, et al. Percutaneous occlusion of left atrial appendage with the Amplatzer Cardiac PlugTM in atrial fibrillation. Arq Bras Cardiol 2012;98(2):143–50.

60. Sievert H, Lesh MD, Trepels T, et al. Percutaneous left atrial appendage transcatheter occlusion to prevent stroke in high-risk patients with atrial fibrillation: early clinical experience. Circulation 2002;105(16):1887–9.

61. Block PC, Burstein S, Casale PN, et al. Percutaneous left atrial appendage occlusion for patients in atrial fibrillation suboptimal for warfarin therapy: 5-year results of the PLAATO (Percutaneous Left Atrial Appendage Transcatheter Occlusion) Study. JACC Cardiovasc Interv 2009;2(7):594–600.

62. Park JW, Leithauser B, Gerk U, et al. Percutaneous left atrial appendage transcatheter occlusion (PLAATO) for stroke prevention in atrial fibrillation: 2-year outcomes. J Invasive Cardiol 2009;21(9):446–50.

63. Sick PB, Schuler G, Hauptmann KE, et al. Initial worldwide experience with the WATCHMAN left atrial appendage system for stroke prevention in atrial fibrillation. J Am Coll Cardiol 2007;49(13):1490–5.

64. Hankey GJ. Replacing aspirin and warfarin for secondary stroke prevention: is it worth the costs? Curr Opin Neurol 2010;23(1):65–72.

65. Alli O, Doshi S, Kar S, et al. Quality of life assessment in the randomized PROTECT AF (Percutaneous Closure of the Left Atrial Appendage Versus Warfarin Therapy for Prevention of Stroke in Patients With Atrial Fibrillation) Trial of Patients at Risk for Stroke With Nonvalvular Atrial Fibrillation. J Am Coll Cardiol 2013;61(17):1790–8.

66. Reddy VY, Doshi SK, Sievert H, et al. Percutaneous left atrial appendage closure for stroke prophylaxis in patients with atrial fibrillation: 2.3-Year Follow-up of the PROTECT AF (Watchman Left Atrial Appendage System for Embolic Protection in Patients with Atrial Fibrillation) Trial. Circulation 2013; 127(6):720–9.

67. Boston_Scientific. PREVAIL Study: Prospective Randomized Evaluation of the WATCHMAN LAA Closure Device in Patients With Atrial Fibrillation Versus Long Term Warfarin Therapy. Available at: http://www.bostonscientific.com/watchman-eu/clinical-data/prevail-clinical-study.html. 2013. Accessed July 21, 2012.

68. Rodes-Cabau J, Champagne J, Bernier M. Transcatheter closure of the left atrial appendage: initial experience with the Amplatzer cardiac plug device. Catheter Cardiovasc Interv 2010;76(2):186–92.

69. Lam YY, Yip GW, Yu CM, et al. Left atrial appendage closure with AMPLATZER cardiac plug for stroke prevention in atrial fibrillation: initial Asia-Pacific experience. Catheter Cardiovasc Interv 2012;79(5):794–800.

70. Park JW, Bethencourt A, Sievert H, et al. Left atrial appendage closure with Amplatzer cardiac plug in atrial fibrillation: initial European experience. Catheter Cardiovasc Interv 2011;77(5): 700–6.

Atrial Septal Defect Closure

Andres F. Vasquez, MD, John M. Lasala, MD, PhD*

KEYWORDS

- Atrial septal defect • Septal closure device • Percutaneous closure • Adults

KEY POINTS

- Most secundum atrial septal defects are amenable to percutaneous closure.
- Percutaneous secundum atrial septal defect closure is safe, effective, and associated with a low complication rate.
- Appropriate patient selection is imperative to offer optimal results.
- Anatomic variations in secundum atrial septal defects may require alternative closure techniques.

INTRODUCTION

Congenital heart disease accounted for 0.3% of US admissions in 2007, with 48% related to atrial septal defects (ASDs).[1] More than one-fourth of adult congenital heart defects are ASDs, 75% of which are ostium secundum ASDs.[2] The progressive impact of volume overload on the right cardiac chambers can be halted by ASD closure. This review focuses on percutaneous ASD closure.

PUBLISHED REPORTS

Multicenter nonrandomized trials have reported closure rates of 91% to 95% and 83% to 100%, and failure or procedure adverse event rates of 7% to 8% and 16% to 24% for the device and surgical groups, respectively.[3,4] Reported closure and severe complications rates for available devices are described in **Table 1**.[3,5–11] Percutaneous closure avoids sternotomy and cardiopulmonary bypass and is associated with faster right ventricular remodeling, decreased anesthesia time, hospitalization length, and periprocedural morbidity.[3,4,12,13]

INDICATIONS FOR ASD CLOSURE AND PATIENT SELECTION

Box 1 describes indications and contraindications for ASD closure. Indications include evidence of right cardiac volume loading with or without symptoms, platypnea-orthodeoxia, and a history or high risk for paradoxic embolization.[14,15] Exercise-related cyanosis requires further evaluation before deciding on closure. Patients not meeting criteria should undergo echocardiography every 2 to 3 years. The hemodynamic impact of small ASDs may be evaluated with an exercise test with oxymetry. Closure of small ASDs (<5 mm) that do not meet criteria is controversial because it may carry a benign course untreated.[16]

Sinus venosus, coronary sinus, or primum ASDs require surgical repair. Most secundum ASDs are amenable to transcatheter closure. Surgical closure of secundum ASD is reasonable in the setting of unfavorable anatomy for percutaneous closure, after failed transcatheter closure, or when concomitant surgical repair of associated defects is required.

Bidirectional shunt and pulmonary hypertension require pulmonary vasodilator and temporary ASD balloon occlusion testing before deciding on

Disclosures: Dr J.M. Lasala is proctor and advisor for St Jude Medical. Dr A.F. Vasquez has no disclosures.
Division of Cardiology, Washington University School of Medicine, 660 South Euclid, Campus Box 8086, St Louis, MO 63110, USA
* Corresponding author.
E-mail address: jlasala@wustl.edu

Table 1
Percent closure and severe complication rates, ASD size amenable for closure, device size selection recommendations, pros and cons for Amplatzer, Buttonseal Centering on Demand, CardioSEAL, STARFlex, and Helex occluder devices

Device Type	Closure Rate (%)	Severe Complication Rate[a] (%)	ASD Size Amenable For Closure	Device Size Selection	Pros	Cons
Amplatzer	99	1.1	≤36 mm	2 mm larger than stop-flow diameter	FDA approved, self-centering, retrievable, allows repositioning, lower incidence of thrombosis	Associated with most cardiac perforation cases
Buttonseal Centering on Demand	95.6	0.9	ASD sizes 5–30 mm	1.8:1 device to stretch diameter ratio	Centering mechanism triggered by operator	Unavailable in the United States for general use
CardioSEAL/ STARFlex	93/85–98	7/2–25	<25 mm	1.6–1.7:1 device to stretch diameter ratio	Self-centering, allows 180° pivoting	Retrieval can damage device. Extracorporeal removal requires bigger sheath
Gore-Helex	90	7.1	ASD size <18–22 mm, septal thickness <9 mm	Twice stop-flow diameter	FDA approved, allows retrieval and repositioning after deployment	Not self-centering (may be an advantage in certain cases)

[a] Severe complications include need for surgery or a second device.
Data from Refs.[3,5–11]

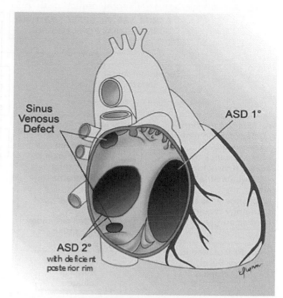

Fig. 1. ASDs are classified according to their location in the interatrial septum. Primum defects are adjacent to the atrioventricular crux, secundum defects affect the fossa ovalis region, and sinus venosus defects are observed toward the venae cavae inflow. Deficient posterior rim, as noted on this secundum defect, increases the risk of device migration when the defect diameter is more than 15 mm. (*Courtesy of* Michael C. Slack, MD, Children's National Medical Center, Washington, DC.)

closure. ASD closure in Eisenmenger syndrome responsive to pulmonary vasodilator therapy and tolerating ASD balloon occlusion test seems promising.[17,18] Fenestrated ASD device closure has been described as an alternative in borderline cases, although supporting data are lacking.

ASD ANATOMY

ASDs are classified according to location, as described in **Fig. 1**. Evaluation should include defect number, size, shape, and location. Concomitant lesions should be excluded.

Fig. 2 shows a percutaneous versus surgical closure algorithm. Favorable anatomy for percutaneous secundum ASD closure includes a stretched defect diameter 36 mm or less, septal length larger than the closure device, safe distance from the atrioventricular (AV) valves, coronary sinus, superior vena cava (SVC) and inferior vena cava (IVC), and a septal tissue rim margin greater than 5 mm in all directions.[19] The most common morphologic variation of secundum ASD involves deficient superior anterior rim (42%).[20]

Deficient and floppy rims, more peripherally located or asymmetrical secundum ASDs, ASDs between 30 and 36 mm, and multiple ASDs increase procedure complexity. Defects greater than 36 mm in diameter, without IVC rim or with extensive areas lacking rims, and those with atria smaller than the device, should be offered surgical closure.

ASD CLOSURE DEVICE OVERVIEW

Table 1 shows important characteristics of available devices.

Gore Helex Septal Occluder (HSO) (W.L. Gore, Flagstaff, AZ) (**Fig. 3**A): approved by the US Food and Drug Administration (FDA), this is a compliant, non–self-centering device that allows for retrieval and repositioning after deployment. A safety cord attached to the device protects against distal embolization and allows occluder removal even after release. It is composed of 2 circular disks made from a spiral nitinol frame attached to a polytetrafluoroethylene membrane with hydrophilic coating. It has a lower and less traumatic profile compared with the Amplatzer septal occluder (see later description). One central eyelet and 1 in each end assist with positioning. Device size ranges from 15 to 35 mm in 5-mm increments, and represents the open disk diameter. The HSO device needs to be twice the size of the measured defect, is recommended for ASD less than 18 mm in diameter and requires a 9-Fr Terumo Pinnacle introducer sheath in the absence of a guide wire or a 12-Fr Cook Check-Flo introducer sheath when using a guide wire. The sheath can be advanced across the septum in the

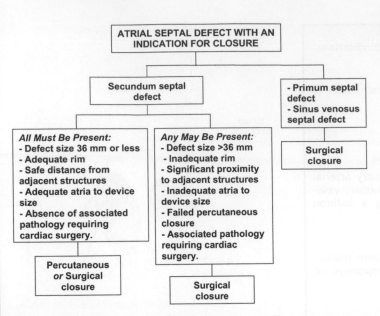

Fig. 2. Percutaneous versus surgical closure algorithm.

absence of a wire by direct manipulation using echo and fluoroscopic guidance, or by using a wire as a monorail. The device is positioned as per company specifications and cine is performed to document the locking loop across all the islets before its release. The HSO is compatible with magnetic resonance imaging (MRI) under conditions specified by the manufacturer.

Amplatzer septal occluder (ASO) (AGA Medical, Golden Valley, MN) (see **Fig. 3**B): FDA approved, this device is self-expanding, self-centering, fully retrievable, and can be repositioned. It is composed of a nitinol (nickel-titanium alloy) mesh and Dacron fabric, and consists of 2 disks linked through a central 3-mm- to 4-mm-long connecting waist, the diameter of which corresponds to the device size (ranges from 4 to 38 mm, in 2-mm increments). The 40-mm device is available in Canada but not in the United States. The left atrial disk exceeds the connecting waist diameter by

12 to 16 mm, whereas the right atrial disk exceeds the connecting waist by 8 to 10 mm. The delivery system size varies according to device size: 6 Fr for devices 4 to 10 mm, 7 Fr for devices 10 to 17 mm, 8 Fr for devices 18 to 19 mm, 9 Fr for devices 20 to 24 mm, 10 Fr for devices 26 to 30 mm, and 12 Fr for devices 32 to 38 mm. This device allows closure of small and large ASDs and is MRI compatible.

CardioSEAL and STARFlex septal occluders (CSO and SFO) (NMT Medical, Boston, MA): these discontinued devices could be partially retrieved into the long sheath, but required a 14-Fr to 16-Fr short sheath for retrieval out of the body. Retrieval could damage the device. Each device had 2 Dacron umbrellas connected through a central waist. Each umbrella had a 4-arm, cobalt-based alloy frame and 2 hinges in each arm. Available sizes (17, 23, 28, and 33 mm) represented the maximum diagonal umbrella diameter. The SFO

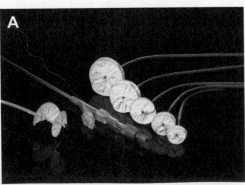

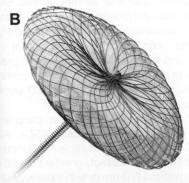

Fig. 3. (*A*) Gore HSO. (*B*) St Jude Medical Amplatzer septal occluder. (*Courtesy of* [*A*] W.L. Gore, Flagstaff, AZ, with permission; and [*B*] St Jude Medical, St Paul, MN, with permission.)

had improved pin-to-pin delivery, a smaller delivery profile, and 4 additional central nitinol rings that formed the self-centering mechanism of the device. The delivery system allowed 180° device pivoting. The SFO required a 10-Fr sheath, was MRI compatible up to 1.5 T, and was suitable for ASDs up to 25 mm.

ButtonSeal Centering on Demand (COD) device (Custom Medical Devices, Amarillo, TX): the COD has a self-centering mechanism and a circular flat left atrial umbrella composed of a Teflon-coated wire frame covered with polyurethane foam, and a counteroccluder connected by a string that is closed by radiopaque knots (buttons). It is unavailable for general use in the United States. COD requires a 10-Fr to 12-Fr sheath, and closes 5 to 30 mm ASDs. Recommended device to stretch diameter ratio is 1.8:1. Available sizes (25–60 mm in 5-mm increments) represent the occluder length.

Atrial septum defect occluder system (ASDOS) (Osypka, Rheinfelden, Germany): This device is composed of 2 self-deploying 5-arm, nitinol frame, microporous polyurethane umbrellas, requires an 11-Fr sheath and is available in sizes 25, 30, 40, 55, and 60 mm, which represent the umbrella diameter.

The Das-Angel Wings atrial septal occlusion device has been withdrawn from the market and the Guardian Angel Atrial Septal Defect Occluder (Angel Wings II) is not available for clinical use.

PATIENT PREPARATION

Contraindication to nickel, antiplatelet, anticoagulant, anesthetic, and antibiotic agents, and thrombotic and bleeding risk should be assessed. Informed consent and a cardiopulmonary, peripheral vascular, and neurologic examination should be obtained. Before the procedure, aspirin therapy should be started, and a heparin bridge may be required for oral anticoagulant clearance. Cephalosporin, clindamycin, or vancomycin is administered 30 minutes before the procedure, with a second dose at 6 to 8 hours.

CATHETERIZATION LABORATORY SETUP

Box 2 outlines additional personnel, equipment, and operator skills necessary for ASD closure by coronary catheterization teams. Transesophageal echocardiography (TEE), primarily for pediatric cases, requires an echocardiographer and general anesthesia. Intracardiac echocardiography (ICE) is performed by the operator under moderate sedation, and requires extra training, an additional 8-Fr to 10-Fr venous sheath and a disposable ultrasound catheter (AcuNav Ultrasound Catheter [Acuson, Siemens Corporation, Mountain View, CA], AcuNav catheter [Biosense Webster, Diamond Bar, CA], Ultra ICE Catheter [Boston Scientific, Natick, MA], or ViewFlex Xtra ICE Catheter [St Jude, St Paul, MN]). ICE suffers from limited depth of view, but improves visualization of the inferior-posterior atrial septum, lowers procedural and fluoroscopy times, eliminates the risks of esophageal intubation and general anesthesia, and allows same-day discharge.[21,22] Monitors should be set up for simultaneous fluoroscopic and echocardiographic visualization.

PERCUTANEOUS ASD CLOSURE
Sedation and Anesthesia

The anesthesiologist should be consulted when general anesthesia is planned (primarily for pediatric cases). Sedatives should be titrated to effect in small doses. Vital signs, pulse oxymetry, and electrocardiogram should be monitored until return to baseline.

Access

Access is obtained after local anesthesia and unfractionated heparin (75–100 units/kg) is administered, for a target activated clotting time greater than 250 seconds. A femoral approach is preferred. Hepatic vein access[23] is an alternative in the presence of infrahepatic venous interruption.

A 7-Fr short venous sheath is used for hemodynamic evaluation and accommodates most sizing balloons. Generous soft tissue predilatation is advised in preparation for a later sheath exchange. A second venous sheath (8 or 10 Fr) is needed if ICE is used. Arterial access is optional (4 Fr).

Initial Diagnostic Studies

Fluoroscopy and echocardiography guide the procedure. Defect evaluation should be performed before crossing the ASD with wires or catheters to avoid defect deformation. The diagnosis should be confirmed and associated anomalies (eg, pulmonary venous anomalies and other septal defects) should be excluded because they may make percutaneous closure inappropriate. Qp:Qs calculation estimates shunt direction and magnitude, which is related to defect size and interventricular compliance differences. In the presence of changes resulting from right-sided volume overload, a small Qp:Qs should not preclude closure.

Hemodynamic Evaluation

An end-hole catheter is used for hemodynamic assessment. Samples in heparinized syringes are obtained at room air from various sites for saturation measurement and Qp:Qs calculation.

- Qp (L/min): O_2 consumption (mL/min)/[pulmonary vein O_2 content (mL/L) – pulmonary artery O_2 content (mL/L)].
- Qs (L/min): O_2 consumption (mL/min)/[systemic arterial O_2 content (mL/L) – mixed venous O_2 content (mL/L)].

where oxygen content: [hemoglobin (g/dL) × 1.36 × O_2 saturation (%)] + [0.0031 × O_2 partial pressure (mm Hg)], and mixed venous O_2 saturation: [3(SVC) + 1(IVC)] ÷ 4.

Hypoxemia unresponsive to oxygen supplementation in presence of appropriate ventilation identifies a right to left shunt. If confirmed, pulmonary vein saturation differentiates intrapulmonary from interatrial shunt. A multipurpose or a softer Goodale-Lubin catheter is recommended. A Reuter tip deflecting wire (**Fig. 4**B) allows control of catheter tip deflection for selective pulmonary vein cannulation. A deflecting wire that is 1 size larger prevents vessel damage as a result of unintended wire exit beyond the catheter tip.

A left-to-right shunt is characterized by supranormal pulmonary arterial saturation and a step-up exceeding normal saturation variability (mean difference >7% at the atrial level and >5% at the ventricular and great vessel levels).[24] An oxymetry

run confirms the shunt location and excludes concomitant sources. An isolated step-up in the low SVC or high right atrium suggests anomalous pulmonary venous drainage associated with a sinus venosus ASD and requires surgical closure. The levophase of a pulmonary artery angiogram can confirm the diagnosis and exclude alternative anomalous pulmonary venous return (right upper lobe veins to SVC, left upper lobe veins to innominate vein, and scimitar syndrome).

Crossing the ASD and Measuring its Diameter

The septal site crossed by the catheter confirms the defect type; midseptum for secundum, high or low septum for sinus venosus, and proximal to the AV valves for primum defects. Right and left atrial pressures are commonly equal.

A multipurpose catheter is advanced across the defect and into the left upper pulmonary vein under fluoroscopy. Tactile resistance before catheter advancement beyond the fluoroscopic left mainstream bronchus and left atrial border or premature atrial contractions hints at atrial appendage position. Excessive advancement

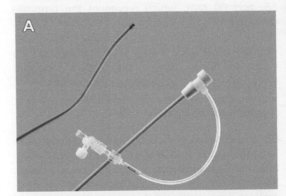

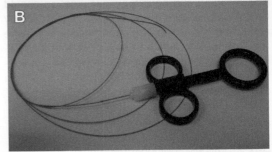

Fig. 4. (*A*) Hausdorf-lock Mullins sheath, with a 3-D curve improves perpendicular sheath alignment in relation to the septal plane. This is useful for cases with an anterior-superior atrial septal defect and absent retro-aortic rim. (*B*) Reuter tip deflecting catheter may offer guide-catheter tip control during selective pulmonary vein cannulation. Permission for use granted by Cook Medical Incorporated, Bloomington, Indiana.

into the pulmonary veins can result in vessel perforation and risks introducing air into the catheter by stimulating cough. A stiff guide wire tip is positioned in the left pulmonary vein and used as a rail for sizing balloon advancement.

Figs. 5 and **6** denote various ASD closure steps. The imaged ASD diameter guides sizing balloon selection. The balloon can be prepared in the IVC to avoid difficulties during insertion. Left anterior oblique cranial projection outlines the balloon with least foreshortening. Dynamic balloon sizing is now rarely used. It requires a Meditech sizing balloon (Boston Scientific, Watertown, MA) (available sizes: 20, 27, 33, or 40 mm), inflated in the left atrium to a diameter 5 mm greater than the imaged diameter using a 30% contrast saline mixture, then apposed onto the atrial septum to eliminate shunt by color Doppler. A steady pull is maintained during gradual balloon deflation, until it advances into the defect creating a waist. The contrast volume is then recorded, and the balloon deflated and withdrawn from the body. The balloon is again inflated using the recorded contrast volume and measured against a sizing plate. Static balloon sizing uses the highly compliant Amplatzer sizing balloon (AGA Medical Corporation), with 6-Fr to 8-Fr shaft sizes, available in 18-mm, 24-mm, and 34-mm diameters, to measure maximum defect diameters of 20, 27,

and 40 mm, respectively, or the NuMED sizing balloon (NuMED, New York) with 8-Fr to 9-Fr shaft sizes and 20-mm to 40-mm diameters. In the stop-flow method, the balloon is centered across the ASD and gradually inflated until color Doppler ceases across the ASD, identifying the stop-flow diameter at the balloon waistline. The diameter should be measured by fluoroscopy and echocardiography for agreement. Balloon inflation guided by fluoroscopy provides the stretch diameter, which is usually 30% larger than the stop-flow diameter as a result of defect stretch, and carries the risk of oversizing and septal tear. Balloon inflation provides an opportunity to search for additional septal defects (ie, additional Doppler flow other than the occluded 1° defect).

Temporary balloon occlusion of the ASD allows assessment of preload changes on cardiac output, atrial pressure, and pulmonary pressure before definitive closure, and should be performed in patients with left-to-right shunt and decreased left-sided compliance.[25] Closure should be delayed if left atrial pressure increases significantly in order to optimize afterload and preload (which may require dieresis) before attempting closure. Patients with bidirectional shunt and reduced right ventricular compliance or Eisenmenger syndrome responsive to pulmonary vasodilator therapy should also be tested before closure.

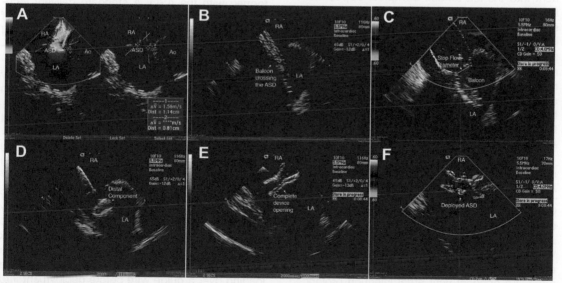

Fig. 5. (*A*) Intracardiac echocardiography images show Amplatzer septal occluder deployment steps; secundum ASD with left-to-right shunt is shown by color Doppler. (*B*) Sizing balloon is positioned across the defect. (*C*) Stop-flow diameter is obtained by balloon inflation under color Doppler guidance. (*D*) Delivery sheath across the defect exposes the self-expanding distal component. (*E*) After distal component to interatrial septum apposition, sheath is further retrieved to allow central and proximal component self-expansion. (*F*) Device is deployed. Ao, ascending aorta; ASD, secundum atrial septal defect; LA, left atrium; RA, right atrium. (*Courtesy of* Richard W. Smalling, MD, PhD, University of Texas at Houston, Houston, TX.)

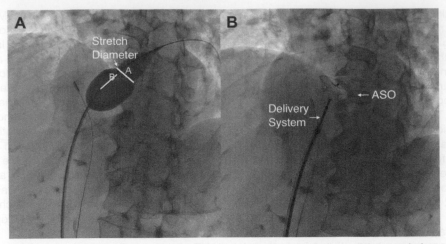

Fig. 6. (A) Fluoroscopic images show stretch diameter obtained with sizing balloon. (B) Expanded ASO is attached to the long sheath and delivery system. (*Courtesy of* Richard W. Smalling, MD, PhD, The University of Texas at Houston, Houston, TX.)

Device Insertion and Deployment

The device is advanced under fluoroscopy to the sheath tip and pulled back a short distance to document device-delivery lock before left atrial advancement. The long sheath is retracted, allowing distal component expansion. Guided by echocardiography, the distal component is gently apposed to the left atrial side of the septum. The ASO frequently prolapses the proximal component into the left atrium. Complete apposition of the distal component to the left atrial side of the septum before proximal component deployment is essential to avoid prolapse. After confirming position and absence of prolapse, further sheath retraction allows expansion of proximal component into the right atrium. Spatial relation with surrounding structures is then evaluated. A gentle tug and thrust before release confirms stability. Pericardial effusion and residual leak should be excluded by echocardiography.

Device Release, Assessment of Device Placement, and Exit of Venous Access

Cine documents release and echocardiography evaluates position, relationship with adjacent structures, residual leaks, and other defects. Vena cava, pulmonary veins, and AV valves are explored for complications such as encroachment. An optional right atrial injection prolonged into the levophase using a 7-Fr pigtail or Berman catheter evaluates for residual shunt on either direction in biplane tubes. The anteroposterior camera shows the size of the atrium and the relationship to the AV valves and systemic and pulmonary veins, whereas the lateral camera profiles

the plane of the atrial septum, confirming position. These views can be compared with follow-up chest radiographs. After ASD closure, the delivery system is removed. Sheaths are retrieved once the activated clotting time is less than 160.

SPECIAL SCENARIOS
Large Defects

Closure of defects of 30 to 36 mm can be performed with the ASO. A standard delivery technique frequently fails because of misalignment of the device to the septum (**Fig. 7**A–C). Successful techniques (**Box 3**) manipulate the device into correct position during deployment or improve alignment by changing the angle of approach or by deploying most of the device into the left atrium before approximating the septum.

A Hausdorf (Cook, Bloomington, IN), straight side-hole or Mullins sheath (Medtronic, Minneapolis, MN) reshaped (see **Fig. 4**A) or cut at the distal tip (**Fig. 8**) improves distal component to septal alignment during delivery (see **Fig. 7**D–F).[26–28] Partial deployment of the distal component into the left atrial roof or right or left upper pulmonary veins (**Fig. 9**) leads to component jump parallel to the atrial septum, which is followed by quick deployment of the proximal component before the sheath recoils out of position.[26,29] Device loading over a guide wire before deployment into a pulmonary vein may optimize positioning. A second operator can use a delivery sheath, dilator, or balloon catheter (**Fig. 10**) to hold the superior-anterior part of the distal component, preventing prolapse across the ASD, whereas the primary operator deploys the proximal component.[29,30]

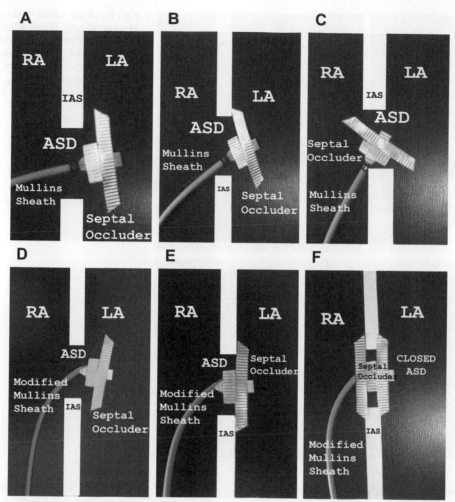

Fig. 7. Serial illustrations show occluder to ASD alignment using a standard delivery technique (*A–C*), leading to misalignment and prolapse of the distal component into the right atrium (*C*). Serial illustrations show enhanced atrial to septal alignment using a modified Mullins sheath (Cook Medical Incorporated, Bloomington, Indiana) (*D–F*), achieving good septal apposition during delivery of both components (*F*). ASD, secundum atrial septal defect; IAS, interatrial septum; LA, left atrium; RA, right atrium.

Box 3
Large ASD closure methods
• Rotation on delivery sheath
• Deployment in right upper pulmonary vein
• Deployment in left upper pulmonary vein
• Use of alternative sheaths (eg, Mullins, Hausdorf, modified Amplatzer)
• Use of right coronary catheter
• Balloon-assisted technique
• Use of dilator as buttress

Defects with Deficient Rims

When defect rim is less than 5 mm the distal component tends to prolapse across the ASD because of the orientation of the septum to the device, which may be improved by distal and partial proximal component opening into the left atrium followed by gentle tug and thrust once rim anchorage resistance is felt. A right upper pulmonary vein slide-out technique is an alternative. A jugular approach can be successful and requires crossing the ASD and mitral valve with a long sheath for stability. The distal component is slowly opened and pulled, anchoring its edge with the inferior atrial septum, to avoid slipping into the right atrium.[31] Device oversizing increases the risk of complications and should be avoided

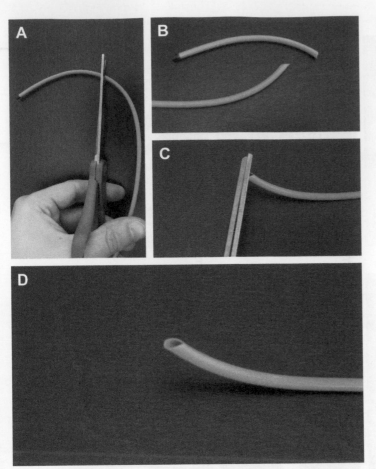

Fig. 8. (*A–D*) Serial images show a Mullins sheath (Cook Medical Incorporated, Bloomington, Indiana) being modified at the distal tip to improve distal component to septal alignment during delivery. This technique is especially useful for closure of large ASDs.

when possible, although it may be necessary in cases with aneurysmal septum.

Multiple ASD and Multifenestrated Defects

When defects are within 7 mm of each other, a single device frequently suffices. The device waist crosses the largest defect, and the large components occlude the remaining defects. Septal shift during balloon stretching or device placement frequently occludes marginal septal cribriform tissue and nearby defects with floppy septum between defects. When defects are distanced, multiple devices are necessary. The first device is deployed without release in the smaller defect, followed by deployment in the larger defect, aiming to overlap devices. The smaller device is released first, then the larger device. Fossa ovalis fenestrations may require non–self-centering devices such as the HSO or Amplatz cribriform devices.

Troubleshooting Chiari Network and Redundant Eustachian Valves

Reduction of Chiari network herniation across the ASD requires sheath retraction and repositioning.

Redundant eustachian valve interfering with deployment may be deflected with a steerable radiofrequency ablation catheter during device passage. The key component is recognition of these entities.

COMPLICATIONS AND TROUBLESHOOTING

Box 4 lists complications resulting from percutaneous ASD closure.[4,32–35] Reported severe complication rates vary from 1.1% to 7.1%[3,5–8,10] and include need for surgery or a second device.

Air embolism can be prevented by preprocedure hydration, preemptive use of positive pressure ventilation in patients with airway or pulmonary disease that is likely to produce wide negative intrathoracic pressure swings during sedation, maintenance of catheters below atrial level, delivery sheath flushing during slow withdrawal of the dilator and wire with subsequent sheath back bleeding, and prompt identification of air bubbles during fluoroscopy-assisted flushing. The right coronary artery is commonly affected because of its anterior position in a supine patient. Changes

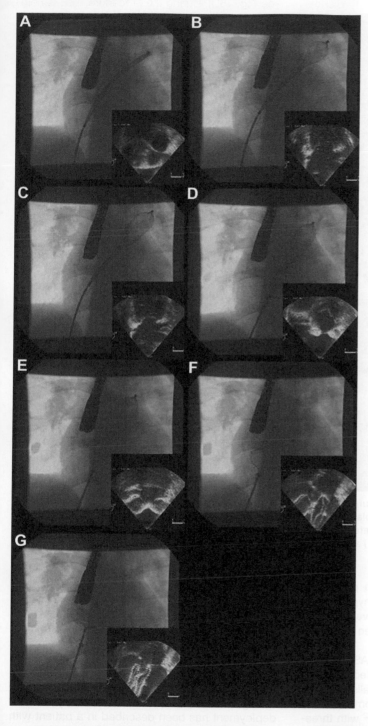

Fig. 9. (*A–G*) Fluoroscopic and echocardiographic images show serial steps involved in a left upper pulmonary vein deployment technique used for closure of a large ASD. (*B, C*) The distal component is opened into the left upper pulmonary vein, the proximal component is unsheathed as the delivery system is gently pulled. (*F*) The distal component suddenly jumps into a parallel position to the left atrial side of the interatrial septum. (*G*) This process is followed by a fast and gentle push of the proximal component against the right atrial side of the interatrial septum resulting in complete apposition.

in mentation, focal neurologic deficits, chest discomfort, ST segment changes and arrhythmias are usually transient, but can be life threatening and should be treated supportively with supplemental oxygen, analgesia, volume expansion, and standard arrhythmia therapy. Occasionally, coronary air embolism extraction may be necessary.

Nitinol is a nickel and titanium elastic alloy with enhanced shape memory properties present in ASO, SFO, HSO, ASDOS, and Angel Wings devices.[36] Metal allergy presenting as dermatitis, pericardial effusion, or severe bronchospasm has been reported with ASOs[37–39] and may require device removal if unresponsive to steroids or antihistamines.

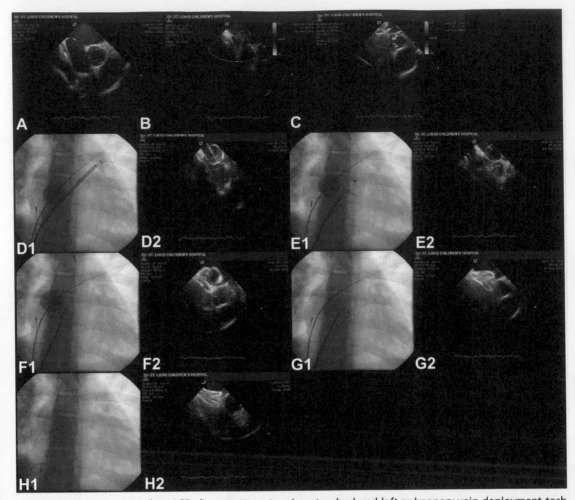

Fig. 10. (*A, B*) Large secundum ASD closure attempts using standard and left pulmonary vein deployment techniques are unsuccessful secondary to prolapse of the distal component across the retroaortic rim (*C*). A balloon-assisted technique results in successful defect closure using an ASO (AGA Medical, Golden Valley, MN). Steps are serially shown by ICE (*D1, E1, F1, G1, H1*) and fluoroscopy (*D2, E2, F2, G2*).

IVC and coronary sinus occlusion presenting with exertion dyspnea, chest pain, hypotension, presyncope, and widespread T wave inversion on electrocardiography (ECG) has been described with a 40-mm ASO.[40]

The incidence of device Amplatzer ASO erosion in the United States is 0.1%, and predominantly involves the anterosuperior atrial walls and adjacent aorta. It has been observed from 1.5 hours to 6 years after ASO deployment,[41,42] with three-fourths of cases presenting during the first week after deployment. Presentation may include pleuritic chest pain, hemopericardium, fistula formation, tamponade, and sudden death.[41,42] Rare, clinically silent cardiac erosion has been reported with CSO and SFO.[7] Defect overstretch during sizing should be avoided, because it results in diameter overestimation. Patients with deficient

anterior and superior rims or with postprocedure pericardial effusion should be closely followed.[43]

Incidence of device-associated thrombus diagnosed by TEE is 1.2% and has been primarily associated with the NMT devices. It occurs within 1 month in three-quarters of diagnosed patients,[36,44,45] with 20% developing symptoms during follow-up.[36] A presentation 1 year after deployment has been described in a patient with a poorly endothelialized HSO.[46] Thrombus can involve either atria, and seem less frequent with ASOs.[36,47] Prothrombotic disorders, postprocedure atrial fibrillation, and persistent atrial septal aneurysm are predictors for thrombus formation. Thrombus tends to resolve with heparin or warfarin and rarely requires thrombolysis or surgical removal.[36]

Box 4
Complications from ASD closure

- Allergic reactions (eg, nickel, antiplatelet agents)
- Infection, including endocarditis, which may require surgical device retrieval
- Bleeding
- Hemolysis
- Vessel trauma
- Arrhythmias
- Transient or permanent AV block and other conduction disturbances
- AV valve regurgitation
- Air embolization
- Stroke and other thromboembolic events
- Device-associated thrombus
- Cardiac or aortic erosion and perforation
- Postpericardiotomy syndrome and cardiac tamponade
- Delivery system or device failure
- Device malposition, migration, or embolization, which may require catheter or surgical removal
- Residual shunts
- Death

Device fractures are more common in larger devices and seem inconsequential, especially after device endothelialization.[6]

During ASO deployment, components rotate as they exit the sheath and return to their inherent shape. Component twist obstruction results in a cobra head malformation, which should prompt device withdrawal and redeployment. If withdrawal is unsuccessful, exchange to a larger sheath over the delivery cable ensures capture.

Device embolization can be minimized by recognizing deficient rims, confirming delivery system to device lock, avoiding device undersizing and aggressive catheter motion, retrieving and redeploying devices nonparallel to the septum, and confirming stable position with a predeployment wiggle test. After embolization, the device should be stabilized into the safest position, avoiding ventricular migration. Smaller devices may go through the heart and the distal aorta, often below the renal arteries. Position rarely allows for pulling the proximal component with a snare into correct placement. Crossing the AV valve with the device should be avoided. Retrieval with a long sheath with a beveled edge can occur within the ventricle

or after advancement across a semilunar valve. A wire, snare, or bioptome can be used for stabilization. One or 2 loop snares secure 1 of the components and pull toward the IVC, into a stiff sheath, at least 2-Fr sizes larger than the implant sheath for the ASO. SFO and CSO can be partially retrieved into the long sheath and brought back. The 14-Fr short backup sheath is then advanced into the femoral vein, and the device and long sheath are removed together. The HSO has a cord that allows for retrieval of an unlocked device with the help of a snare and the delivery sheath. Locked HSOs require snaring the distal component eyelet attached to the locking loop to unlock the device. ASO retrieval requires snaring the microscrew on the proximal component. If needed, a bioptome from an internal jugular access may better orient, elongate, and place tension from above on the distal component of the device, assisting snare retrieval toward the IVC. If retrieval into a sheath is difficult, device migration can be avoided by crossing it with a stiff wire in the infrarenal vena cava and advancing the wire tip into the SVC for stabilization. Bare vein retrieval carries high risk for vascular complications, and surgical venous cut-down is preferred and avoids intrathoracic retrieval. The ASO and HSO devices can be repositioned and redeployed. The CSO and SFO devices are damaged if pulled back into the sheath once the proximal component has been opened.

POSTPROCEDURE CARE

There is no standard regimen after device closure. Aspirin for 6 months and clopidogrel for 2 to 3 months is advised. Overnight heparin and warfarin are rarely prescribed. A second dose of prophylactic antibiotics is common. Endocarditis prophylaxis is recommended for 6 months after device closure. Predischarge hematocrit, ECG, chest radiography, and echocardiography are advised. Pericardial effusion and tamponade may occur during the following weeks after surgical repair and warrant echocardiographic examination during early visits. Frequent patient complaints include chest pain syndromes, presumably from irritation and inflammation. Nitinol reactions should be followed closely. The postprocedure incidence of atrial fibrillation is 0%.[48] Most are self-limiting.

PATIENT FOLLOW-UP

Benefits from ASD closure include improvement in exercise capacity even in asymptomatic adults, enhanced myocardial remodeling, improved ventricular function, and a decrease in pulmonary pressure.[49–58] Benefits are noted in older adults; nevertheless, the best outcome is achieved with closure before functional impairment and pulmonary arterial hypertension set in.[59] After closure, atrial arrhythmias remain prevalent compared with general population rates.[60–62] Patients undergoing surgical repair after 25 years require regular supervision for development of late cardiac failure, stroke, and atrial fibrillation.[61]

The referring physician should be informed of antiplatelet regimen, endocarditis prophylaxis, and how to identify cardiac erosion, tamponade, and device-associated thrombus. Chest pain or syncope may represent device erosion and should warrant urgent evaluation. Follow-up at 3 months, 12 months, and periodically thereafter includes ECG and echocardiography to evaluates for arrhythmias, conduction problems, chest pain, embolic events, cardiovascular and neurologic examinations, ventricular function, pericardial effusion, pulmonary pressure, device position, cardiac erosion, thrombus formation, and residual shunt. Annual follow-up is recommended when pulmonary hypertension, atrial arrhythmias, ventricular dysfunction, or coexisting cardiac lesions are present.

Isometric activity should be avoided wherever possible, especially when associated with volume depletion.[63] Pregnancy in patients with ASD and Eisenmenger syndrome is contraindicated because of excessive maternal and fetal mortality and should be strongly discouraged.

FUTURE DIRECTIONS

The biodegradable BioSTAR and BioTREK devices[64] had potential for lower atrial erosion and thrombus formation rates and allowed future transseptal access; however, the manufacturer (NMT Medical) closed operations. Gore will have a self-entering ASD system capable of closing large defects in the future. The Gore Septal Occluder (W.L. Gore, Flagstaff, AZ) is undergoing clinical trials in the United States. It offers simple deployment, superior conformability to anatomy, and easy retrieval.

SUMMARY

The progressive nature of ASDs can be dramatically altered with early identification and closure. Transcatheter closure has become the primary alternative for secundum ASD closure, with surgical closure considered for special circumstances. Device, imaging, and interventional advances coupled with operator expertise continue to improve outcomes and provide alternatives to structural heart disease therapy.

REFERENCES

1. Rodriguez FH 3rd, Moodie DS, Parekh DR, et al. Outcomes of hospitalization in adults in the United States with atrial septal defect, ventricular septal defect, and atrioventricular septal defect. Am J Cardiol 2011;108:290.
2. Lindsey JB, Hillis LD. Clinical update: atrial septal defect in adults. Lancet 2007;369:1244.
3. Du ZD, Hijazi ZM, Kleinman CS, et al. Comparison between transcatheter and surgical closure of secundum atrial septal defect in children and adults: results of a multicenter nonrandomized trial. J Am Coll Cardiol 2002;39:1836.
4. Jones TK, Latson LA, Zahn E, et al. Results of the U.S. multicenter pivotal study of the HELEX septal occluder for percutaneous closure of secundum atrial septal defects. J Am Coll Cardiol 2007;49:2215.
5. Kay JD, O'Laughlin MP, Ito K, et al. Five-year clinical and echocardiographic evaluation of the Das AngelWings atrial septal occluder. Am Heart J 2004;147:361.
6. Law MA, Josey J, Justino H, et al. Long-term follow-up of the STARFlex device for closure of secundum atrial septal defect. Catheter Cardiovasc Interv 2009;73:190.
7. Nugent AW, Britt A, Gauvreau K, et al. Device closure rates of simple atrial septal defects optimized by the STARFlex device. J Am Coll Cardiol 2006;48:538.
8. Rao PS, Berger F, Rey C, et al. Results of transvenous occlusion of secundum atrial septal defects with the fourth generation buttoned device: comparison with first, second and third generation devices. International Buttoned Device Trial Group. J Am Coll Cardiol 2000;36:583.
9. Rao PS, Sideris EB. Centering-on-demand buttoned device: its role in transcatheter occlusion of atrial septal defects. J Interv Cardiol 2001;14:81.
10. Vincent RN, Raviele AA, Diehl HJ. Single-center experience with the HELEX septal occluder for closure of atrial septal defects in children. J Interv Cardiol 2003;16:79.
11. Zamora R, Rao PS, Sideris EB. Buttoned device for atrial septal defect occlusion. Curr Interv Cardiol Rep 2000;2:167.
12. Rosas M, Zabal C, Garcia-Montes J, et al. Transcatheter versus surgical closure of secundum atrial septal defect in adults: impact of age at intervention. A concurrent matched comparative study. Congenit Heart Dis 2007;2:148.
13. Suchon E, Pieculewicz M, Tracz W, et al. Transcatheter closure as an alternative and equivalent

method to the surgical treatment of atrial septal defect in adults: comparison of early and late results. Med Sci Monit 2009;15:CR612.

14. Rigatelli G. Congenital heart diseases in aged patients: clinical features, diagnosis, and therapeutic indications based on the analysis of a twenty five-year Medline search. Cardiol Rev 2005;13:293.

15. Warnes CA, Williams RG, Bashore TM, et al. ACC/AHA 2008 guidelines for the management of adults with congenital heart disease: a report of the American College of Cardiology/American Heart Association Task Force on Practice Guidelines (Writing Committee to Develop Guidelines on the Management of Adults with Congenital Heart Disease). Developed in Collaboration with the American Society of Echocardiography, Heart Rhythm Society, International Society for Adult Congenital Heart Disease, Society for Cardiovascular Angiography and Interventions, and Society of Thoracic Surgeons. J Am Coll Cardiol 2008;52:e143.

16. Warnes CA, Williams RG, Bashore TM, et al. ACC/AHA 2008 Guidelines for the Management of Adults with Congenital Heart Disease: a report of the American College of Cardiology/American Heart Association Task Force on Practice Guidelines (Writing Committee to Develop Guidelines on the Management of Adults with Congenital Heart Disease). Circulation 2008;118:e714.

17. Dimopoulos K, Peset A, Gatzoulis MA. Evaluating operability in adults with congenital heart disease and the role of pretreatment with targeted pulmonary arterial hypertension therapy. Int J Cardiol 2008;129:163.

18. Kim YH, Yu JJ, Yun TJ, et al. Repair of atrial septal defect with Eisenmenger syndrome after long-term sildenafil therapy. Ann Thorac Surg 2010;89:1629.

19. Cooke JC, Gelman JS, Harper RW. Echocardiologists' role in the deployment of the Amplatzer atrial septal occluder device in adults. J Am Soc Echocardiogr 2001;14:588.

20. Podnar T, Martanovic P, Gavora P, et al. Morphological variations of secundum-type atrial septal defects: feasibility for percutaneous closure using Amplatzer septal occluders. Catheter Cardiovasc Interv 2001;53:386.

21. Bhindi R, Ormerod OJ. Improving procedural times during percutaneous atrial septal defect closure. J Am Coll Cardiol 2007;50:1296 [author reply: 1296].

22. Boccalandro F, Baptista E, Muench A, et al. Comparison of intracardiac echocardiography versus transesophageal echocardiography guidance for percutaneous transcatheter closure of atrial septal defect. Am J Cardiol 2004;93:437.

23. Hussain J, Strumpf R, Ghandforoush A, et al. Transhepatic approach to closure of patent foramen ovale: report of 2 cases in adults. Tex Heart Inst J 2010;37:553.

24. Antman EM, Marsh JD, Green LH, et al. Blood oxygen measurements in the assessment of intracardiac left to right shunts: a critical appraisal of methodology. Am J Cardiol 1980;46:265.

25. Tomai F, Gaspardone A, Papa M, et al. Acute left ventricular failure after transcatheter closure of a secundum atrial septal defect in a patient with coronary artery disease: a critical reappraisal. Catheter Cardiovasc Interv 2002;55:97.

26. Berger F, Ewert P, Abdul-Khaliq H, et al. Percutaneous closure of large atrial septal defects with the Amplatzer Septal Occluder: technical overkill or recommendable alternative treatment? J Interv Cardiol 2001;14:63.

27. Kannan BR, Francis E, Sivakumar K, et al. Transcatheter closure of very large (>or = 25 mm) atrial septal defects using the Amplatzer septal occluder. Catheter Cardiovasc Interv 2003;59:522.

28. Kutty S, Asnes JD, Srinath G, et al. Use of a straight, side-hole delivery sheath for improved delivery of Amplatzer ASD occluder. Catheter Cardiovasc Interv 2007;69:15.

29. Wahab HA, Bairam AR, Cao QL, et al. Novel technique to prevent prolapse of the Amplatzer septal occluder through large atrial septal defect. Catheter Cardiovasc Interv 2003;60:543.

30. Dalvi BV, Pinto RJ, Gupta A. New technique for device closure of large atrial septal defects. Catheter Cardiovasc Interv 2005;64:102.

31. Papa M, Gaspardone A, Fragasso G, et al. Feasibility and safety of transcatheter closure of atrial septal defects with deficient posterior rim. Catheter Cardiovasc Interv 2013;81(7):1180–7.

32. Kapoor MC, Singh S, Sharma S, et al. Case 6-2003: embolization of an atrial septal occluder device. J Cardiothorac Vasc Anesth 2003;17:755.

33. Peuster M, Reckers J, Fink C. Secondary embolization of a Helex occluder implanted into a secundum atrial septal defect. Catheter Cardiovasc Interv 2003;59:77.

34. Piatkowski R, Kochanowski J, Scislo P, et al. Dislocation of Amplatzer septal occluder device after closure of secundum atrial septal defect. J Am Soc Echocardiogr 2010;23:1007.e1.

35. Pratali S, Mecozzi G, Milano A, et al. Prevention of embolization of a displaced atrial septal occluder. Tex Heart Inst J 2003;30.88.

36. Krumsdorf U, Ostermayer S, Billinger K, et al. Incidence and clinical course of thrombus formation on atrial septal defect and patient foramen ovale closure devices in 1,000 consecutive patients. J Am Coll Cardiol 2004;43:302.

37. Khodaverdian RA, Jones KW. Metal allergy to Amplatzer occluder device presented as severe bronchospasm. Ann Thorac Surg 2009;88:2021.

38. Kim KH, Park JC, Yoon NS, et al. A case of allergic contact dermatitis following transcatheter closure of patent ductus arteriosus using Amplatzer ductal occluder. Int J Cardiol 2008;127:e98.

39. Lai DW, Saver JL, Araujo JA, et al. Pericarditis associated with nickel hypersensitivity to the Amplatzer occluder device: a case report. Catheter Cardiovasc Interv 2005;66:424.

40. Soo AW, Healy DG, Walsh K, et al. Inferior vena cava and coronary sinus obstruction after percutaneous atrial septal defect device closure requiring surgical revision. J Thorac Cardiovasc Surg 2006; 131:1405.

41. Divekar A, Gaamangwe T, Shaikh N, et al. Cardiac perforation after device closure of atrial septal defects with the Amplatzer septal occluder. J Am Coll Cardiol 2005;45:1213.

42. Taggart NW, Dearani JA, Hagler DJ. Late erosion of an Amplatzer septal occluder device 6 years after placement. J Thorac Cardiovasc Surg 2011;142:221.

43. Amin Z, Hijazi ZM, Bass JL, et al. Erosion of Amplatzer septal occluder device after closure of secundum atrial septal defects: review of registry of complications and recommendations to minimize future risk. Catheter Cardiovasc Interv 2004;63:496.

44. Cooke JC, Gelman JS, Menahem S, et al. Thrombus on an ASD closure device: a call for caution. Heart Lung Circ 2000;9:30.

45. Divchev D, Schaefer A, Fuchs M, et al. Thrombus formation on an atrial septal defect closure device: a case report and review of the literature. Eur J Echocardiogr 2007;8:53.

46. Zaidi AN, Cheatham JP, Galantowicz M, et al. Late thrombus formation on the Helex septal occluder after double-lung transplant. J Heart Lung Transplant 2010;29:814.

47. Anzai H, Child J, Natterson B, et al. Incidence of thrombus formation on the CardioSEAL and the Amplatzer interatrial closure devices. Am J Cardiol 2004;93:426.

48. Giardini A, Donti A, Sciarra F, et al. Long-term incidence of atrial fibrillation and flutter after transcatheter atrial septal defect closure in adults. Int J Cardiol 2009;134:47.

49. Brochu MC, Baril JF, Dore A, et al. Improvement in exercise capacity in asymptomatic and mildly symptomatic adults after atrial septal defect percutaneous closure. Circulation 2002;106:1821.

50. Giardini A, Donti A, Specchia S, et al. Recovery kinetics of oxygen uptake is prolonged in adults with an atrial septal defect and improves after transcatheter closure. Am Heart J 2004;147:910.

51. Kort HW, Balzer DT, Johnson MC. Resolution of right heart enlargement after closure of secundum atrial septal defect with transcatheter technique. J Am Coll Cardiol 2001;38:1528.

52. Patel A, Lopez K, Banerjee A, et al. Transcatheter closure of atrial septal defects in adults > or = 40 years of age: immediate and follow-up results. J Interv Cardiol 2007;20:82.

53. Salehian O, Horlick E, Schwerzmann M, et al. Improvements in cardiac form and function after transcatheter closure of secundum atrial septal defects. J Am Coll Cardiol 2005;45:499.

54. Schoen SP, Kittner T, Bohl S, et al. Transcatheter closure of atrial septal defects improves right ventricular volume, mass, function, pulmonary pressure, and functional class: a magnetic resonance imaging study. Heart 2006;92:821.

55. Schussler JM, Anwar A, Phillips SD, et al. Effect on right ventricular volume of percutaneous Amplatzer closure of atrial septal defect in adults. Am J Cardiol 2005;95:993.

56. Sun P, Wang ZB, Xu CJ, et al. Echocardiographic and morphological evaluation of the right heart after closure of atrial septal defects. Cardiol Young 2008;18:593.

57. Teo KS, Dundon BK, Molaee P, et al. Percutaneous closure of atrial septal defects leads to normalisation of atrial and ventricular volumes. J Cardiovasc Magn Reson 2008;10:55.

58. Wu ET, Akagi T, Taniguchi M, et al. Differences in right and left ventricular remodeling after transcatheter closure of atrial septal defect among adults. Catheter Cardiovasc Interv 2007;69:866.

59. Humenberger M, Rosenhek R, Gabriel H, et al. Benefit of atrial septal defect closure in adults: impact of age. Eur Heart J 2011;32:553.

60. Gatzoulis MA, Freeman MA, Siu SC, et al. Atrial arrhythmia after surgical closure of atrial septal defects in adults. N Engl J Med 1999;340:839.

61. Murphy JG, Gersh BJ, McGoon MD, et al. Long-term outcome after surgical repair of isolated atrial septal defect. Follow-up at 27 to 32 years. N Engl J Med 1990;323:1645.

62. Silversides CK, Siu SC, McLaughlin PR, et al. Symptomatic atrial arrhythmias and transcatheter closure of atrial septal defects in adult patients. Heart 2004;90:1194.

63. Santini F, Morjan M, Onorati F, et al. Life-threatening isometric-exertion related cardiac perforation 5 years after Amplatzer atrial septal defect closure: should isometric activity be limited in septal occluder holders? Ann Thorac Surg 2012;93:671.

64. Baspinar O, Kervancioglu M, Kilinc M, et al. Bioabsorbable atrial septal occluder for percutaneous closure of atrial septal defect in children. Tex Heart Inst J 2012;39:184.

Patent Foramen Ovale

Philip B. Dattilo, MD[a], Michael S. Kim, MD[b],*,
John D. Carroll, MD[c]

KEYWORDS

- Patent foramen ovale • Cryptogenic stroke • Migraine • Transcatheter closure • MIST • CLOSURE I
- RESPECT • PC Trial

KEY POINTS

- Patent foramen ovale (PFO) is a common developmental anomaly that allows for the passage of blood and other substances from the right-sided (venous) to the left (arterial) circulation.
- Presence of a PFO has been implicated as a contributing factor to cryptogenic stroke (via paradoxic embolism), migraine headaches (via absence of filtering in the pulmonary circulation of undetermined substances), and orthodeoxia-platypnea.
- Closure of PFOs to prevent strokes and migraines has been studied in 4 randomized, controlled trials evaluating 2 different types of closure devices.
- Study of PFO has been challenging, as simultaneous off-label PFO closure has been widely available concurrent with clinical trials attempting to enroll patients.
- No study has demonstrated benefit of closure using intention-to-treat analyses, although secondary and subpopulation analyses suggest that there is benefit to closure, especially in patients with atrial septal aneurysms and/or substantial degrees of right-to-left shunting.

INTRODUCTION

The patent foramen ovale (PFO), and more specifically its role in allowing deoxygenated blood, thrombi, and other unidentified substances to bypass the pulmonary circuit and directly transit from the venous to the arterial circulation, remains a subject of study and debate. Specifically, the potential role of transcatheter PFO closure in reducing clinical events and treating syndromes such as stroke, migraine headaches, and systemic hypoxemia has been, and continues to be, a "gray area" in medicine. Although there are no definitive data substantiating the benefits of PFO closure, the debate over the potential benefits of the therapy remains both healthy and lively. This article aims to describe the pertinent anatomy, available closure devices, and relevant clinical trial data, so that the reader may better understand the nuances of transcatheter PFO closure.

ATRIAL SEPTAL ANATOMY AND EMBRYOLOGY

The normal development of the interatrial septum is complex (**Fig. 1**).[1,2] Parturition results in left atrial pressure exceeding right atrial pressure, which anatomically causes the septum primum to be forced against the septum secundum.

Disclosures: Dr Carroll reports Research Support (paid to University Physicians, Inc of the University of Colorado) and consulting fees from St. Jude Medical for work relating to the RESPECT trial.
[a] Interventional Cardiology, Division of Cardiology, University of Colorado Denver, 12631 East 17th Avenue, B-132, Aurora, CO 80045, USA; [b] Structural Heart Disease Program, Division of Cardiology, University of Colorado Denver, 12401 East 17th Avenue, B-132, Aurora, CO 80045, USA; [c] Interventional Cardiology, Division of Cardiology, University of Colorado Denver, 12401 East 17th Avenue, B-132, Aurora, CO 80045, USA
* Corresponding author.
E-mail address: Michael.Kim@ucdenver.edu

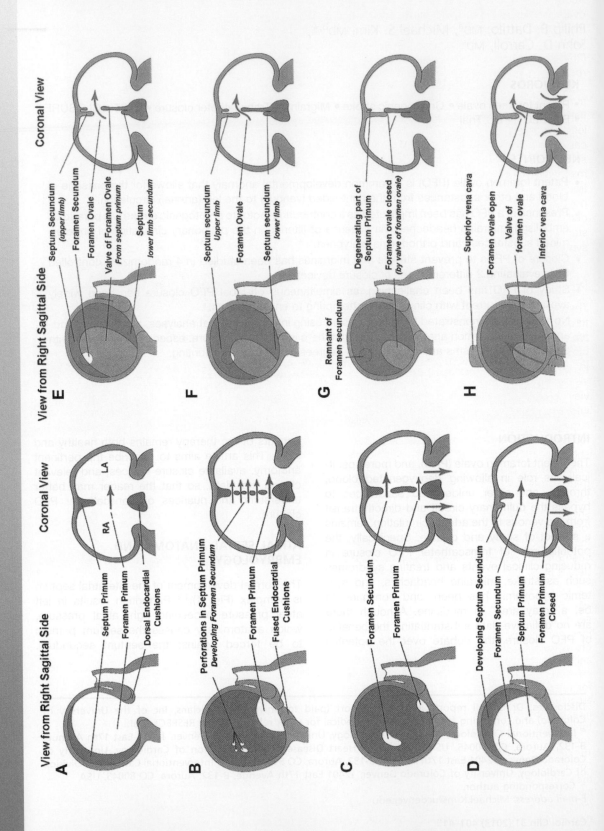

View from Right Sagittal Side   **Coronal View**

A
Septum Primum
Foramen Primum
Dorsal Endocardial Cushions

RA
LA

B
Perforations in Septum Primum
Developing Foramen Secundum
Foramen Primum
Fused Endocardial Cushions

C
Foramen Secundum
Foramen Primum

D
Developing Septum Secundum
Foramen Secundum
Septum Primum
Foramen Primum Closed

View from Right Sagittal Side   **Coronal View**

E
Septum Secundum *(upper limb)*
Foramen Secundum
Foramen Ovale
Valve of Foramen Ovale *From septum primum*
Septum *lower limb secundum*

F
Septum secundum *Upper limb*
Foramen Ovale
Septum secundum *lower limb*

G
Degenerating part of Septum Primum
Foramen ovale closed *(by valve of foramen ovale)*
Remnant of Foramen secundum

H
Superior vena cava
Foramen ovale open
Valve of foramen ovale
Inferior vena cava

Accordingly, right-to-left flow through the foramen ovale ceases. The foramen ovale fuses over time in most people, creating the anatomic structure known as the fossa ovalis. In a large minority (25%–30%), however, this fusion is incomplete, resulting in a small channel referred to as a PFO.[3]

The relationship of the septum primum to the secundum can be understood as one that results in a flap-valve mechanism. Specifically, superior and leftward aspects of the septum primum (the flap) can open into the left atrium when right atrial pressure exceeds that of the left (eg, Valsalva, cough, mechanical ventilation). This process allows for transient right-to-left interatrial shunting with the potential for transmission of paradoxic emboli, deoxygenated blood, and other unidentified substances that may play a role in various clinical syndromes.

DIAGNOSIS

There are no physical diagnosis findings specific to a PFO. When clinical suspicion warrants it, the typical screening study is a transthoracic echocardiogram (TTE) with a saline contrast study (**Fig. 2**). In addition to the standard echocardiographic views, either an apical or subcostal 4-chamber view is obtained while agitated saline is injected into the venous system (preferably through a large-bore intravenous tube in the right antecubital fossa). To improve the sensitivity of the test it should be performed at rest, with Valsalva release, and with a cough. If dynamic shunting is suspected, the echocardiogram can be done while the patient exercises as well. The sonographer should also take several dedicated views with color Doppler across the interatrial septum to assess for shunting. In cases where it is unclear if shunting seen on TTE represents a PFO or an atrial septal defect (ASD), a transesophageal echocardiogram

(TEE) is frequently obtained to further interrogate the interatrial septum (see **Fig. 2**).

Transcranial Doppler (TCD) is another imaging modality that can be useful in detecting right-to-left shunting. With this technique, agitated saline is injected into the venous system, and the TCD is used to detect saline bubbles in the intracranial circulation. This study can be done either at rest, with exercise, or with other provocative maneuvers (eg, Valsalva, cough).

In the context of an invasive study, several options are available for PFO evaluation. Intracardiac echocardiography (ICE) generally provides a highly sensitive assessment (**Fig. 3**). TEE provides an alternative to ICE although it may be less comfortable for the patient, and will generally require higher degrees of sedation or even intubation to perform. As with a TTE evaluation, during either ICE or TEE evaluation the PFO should be assessed with both color Doppler flow and agitated saline contrast injection at rest, with Valsalva release, and with a cough.

A rather straightforward technique that can be performed in the midst of an invasive assessment is the so-called wire test (see **Fig. 3**). In this evaluation, a standard 0.035-in (0.089 cm) J-wire is advanced from the femoral vein to the area of the fossa ovalis. The wire can be directed with a formed catheter such as a Judkins Right 4 or a multipurpose. Crossing of the wire into the left atrium demonstrates the presence of a PFO. With the wire across, the PFO should be partially propped open, and further imaging with ICE or TEE in combination with agitated saline injection can be performed (see **Fig. 3**).

PFO CLOSURE INDICATIONS

There are currently no specific guidelines for PFO closure. Conditions for which PFO closure has

---

Fig. 1. Embryology of the interatrial septum. The normal interatrial septum is composed of the partially overlapping septum primum and septum secundum. The septum primum originates from the roof of the atrium and grows toward the endocardial cushions (A). This process creates the initial septation of the rudimentary right and left atria. The primum grows with a concave leading edge that results in an interatrial communication referred to as the foramen primum (B). Shunting of blood from right to left through the foramen primum allows for the obligatory bypassing of the fetal pulmonary circulation. As the foramen primum closes, the superior aspect of the septum develops fenestrations. These fenestrations then coalesce to form a new interatrial communication referred to as the foramen secundum (C). Right-to-left shunting persists through the foramen secundum throughout gestation. The septum secundum forms as a result of infolding of the atria (D). It is located anterior and rightward of the septum primum. The leading edge of the septum secundum forms the foramen ovale (E). The foramen ovale lies in continuity with the foramen secundum, allowing for right-to-left shunting of blood (F). Concurrent with the growth of the septum secundum, the septum primum thins and regresses. In its mature form, the septum primum is a thin flap of tissue covering the left side of the foramen ovale (G). In a large minority of people the communication persists, resulting in a patent foramen ovale (H). LA, left atrium; RA, right atrium. (*From* Hara H, Virmani R, Ladich E, et al. Patent foramen ovale: current pathology, pathophysiology, and clinical status. J Am Coll Cardiol 2005;46(9):1769; with permission.)

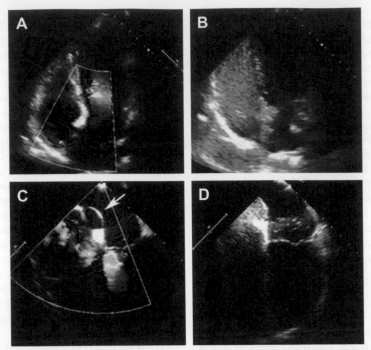

Fig. 2. Preprocedural echocardiographic imaging of the interatrial septum. Example of a transthoracic echocardiogram (TTE) evaluation of a PFO with color Doppler flow (*A*) and agitated saline contrast injection (*B*). Subsequently, a transesophageal echocardiogram (TEE) was performed with color Doppler (*C*) and agitated saline injection (*D*), demonstrating a mobile septum primum (*white arrow*) and moderate shunting across the defect.

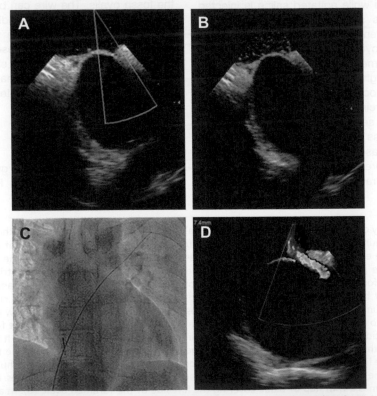

Fig. 3. The wire test using intracardiac echocardiography (ICE) guidance. Example of ICE imaging with color Doppler flow (*A*) and agitated saline contrast injection (*B*). (*C*) A fluoroscopic image with a 0.035-in (0.089 cm) stiff wire across the defect. (*D*) Color Doppler flow across the PFO being propped open by the wire.

been studied in the setting of randomized controlled trials (RCTs) include cryptogenic stroke (CLOSURE I,[4] RESPECT,[5] PC Trial,[6] and REDUCE) (**Tables 1–3**), and migraine with aura (MIST[7] and PREMIUM) (**Table 4**). Other syndromes for which PFO closure has been performed, but not specifically studied in RCTs, include orthodeoxia-platypnea,[8] high-altitude pulmonary edema,[9] decompression illness,[10] and prior to solid organ transplant. In the United States, PFO closure currently occurs either in the context of a clinical trial or in an off-label fashion using devices approved for ASD closure (eg, Amplatzer Septal Occluder [ASO], Amplatzer Cribriform Occluder, and Gore Helex Septal Occluder).

HISTORICAL PERSPECTIVE

One decade ago (early 2000s) there was significant enthusiasm for PFO closure. The excitement was based largely on observational trials and anecdotal case reports demonstrating the potential benefit of PFO closure for preventing recurrent cerebrovascular accidents (CVA).[11–17] PFO closure was believed to represent an effective therapy for a complex and very frightening condition (ie, presumed paradoxic embolism resulting in a CVA) as well as an alternative to lifelong medical therapy. Placement of closure devices was viewed as a safe and effective means of blockading the point of transit of paradoxic emboli.

With the approval of the CardioSEAL device for ventricular septal defect (VSD) closure and the Amplatzer ASO device for ASD closure, operators were able and willing to place these devices across a PFO in an off-label fashion. The Food and Drug Administration (FDA) concurrently approved implantation of the CardioSEAL and Amplatzer PFO occluder devices as part of a humanitarian device exemption pathway from 2000 to 2006. Subsequently, the Gore Helex

Septal Occluder and the Amplatzer Cribriform Septal Occluder devices were approved by the FDA for closure of secundum and fenestrated ASDs, respectively, further expanding the device options for off-label closure.[18]

As a result of the availability of these various occluders, many thousands of patients underwent transcatheter PFO closure in the early 2000s. Simultaneously, multiple clinical trials were under way investigating the effect of PFO closure on recurrent ischemic events in comparison with medical therapy (CLOSURE I, RESPECT, PC Trial, and REDUCE; see later discussion). The commonality of off-label implantation, however, arguably hindered patient enrollment, as patients deemed high-risk or uninterested in enrollment could quite easily find a provider to perform implantation of an off-label device. Whether the frequency of off-label implantation actually affected the results of these various trials is debatable. One recent study looking at the Cleveland Clinic experience, however, demonstrated that off-label closure was not only significantly more common than enrollment into a clinical trial, but that patients who underwent off-label closure had a higher risk profile than their randomized counterparts.[19]

CLOSURE DEVICES

To date, no closure device has been FDA-approved for PFO closure. PFO is known to be widely variable (eg, long vs short tunnel, presence of an atrial septal aneurysm) and difficult to assess using standard 2-dimensional imaging (**Fig. 4**).[20] Such anatomic variability often makes implantation of devices that are not specifically designed for PFO anatomy less than ideal. Although efforts are being made to better understand PFO anatomy using 3-dimensional imaging, whether such knowledge will ultimately result in more purpose-built devices to better accommodate variable anatomies is unknown. Three devices are available

Table 1				
Intention-to-treat results of the CLOSURE I trial				
End Point	Closure (N = 447)	Medical Therapy (N = 462)	Hazard Ratio (95% CI)	P Value
Composite end point[a], n (%)	23 (5.5)	29 (6.8)	0.78 (0.45–1.35)	.37
Stroke, n (%)	12 (2.9)	13 (3.1)	0.90 (0.41–1.98)	.79
TIA, n (%)	13 (3.1)	17 (4.1)	0.75 (0.36–1.55)	.44

Abbreviations: CI, confidence interval; TIA, transient ischemic attack.

[a] Defined as stroke or TIA during 2 years of follow-up, death from any cause during the first 30 days, and death from neurologic causes between 31 days and 2 years.

Data from Furlan AJ, Reisman M, Massaro J, et al. Closure or medical therapy for cryptogenic stroke with patent foramen ovale. N Engl J Med 2012;366(11):995.

Table 2
Primary and subgroup analyses of the RESPECT trial

	Hazard Ratio (95% CI)	P Value
Intention to treat	0.49 (0.22–1.11)	.08
Per protocol	0.37 (0.14–0.96)	.03
As treated	0.27 (0.10–0.75)	.007
Substantial right-to-left shunt	0.18 (0.04–0.81)	.01
Atrial septal aneurysm	0.19 (0.04–0.87)	.02

Data from Carroll JD, Saver JL, Thaler DE, et al. Closure of patent foramen ovale versus medical therapy after cryptogenic stroke. N Engl J Med 2013;368(12):1092–100.

in the United States for off-label implantation (Amplatzer Septal and Cribriform occluders and the Gore Helex device), and a fourth is undergoing FDA review (Amplatzer PFO Occluder).

Amplatzer Family of Septal Occluder Devices

The ASO device is approved for the closure of secundum-type ASDs and fenestrated Fontan closures. It is constructed of a nitinol (nickel/titanium alloy) mesh with left and right atrial discs and a central waist. In the United States, the ASO comes in sizes ranging from 4 to 38 mm (the diameter of the device waist). The left atrial disc is 12 to 16 mm wider in diameter than the waist (depending on waist size), and 4 mm wider than the right atrial disc. Because of its design, the ASO is considered a "self-centering" device.

The Amplatzer Multifenestrated Septal Occluder (also known as the Cribriform Occluder) device is approved for closure of multifenestrated secundum-type ASDs. The device is similar in design to the ASO, but differs in that the left and right atrial discs are of the same size with a small central waist. Sizing of the device is according to disc size, and comes in 18-, 25-, 30-, and 35-mm sizes. Like the ASO, the Cribriform Occluder is a self-centering device.

A device specifically designed for the closure of PFOs, the Amplatzer PFO Occluder (St Jude Medical, St Paul, MN) (**Fig. 5**) is, morphologically most similar to the Cribriform Occluder. It is constructed of nitinol mesh with left and right atrial discs joined by a short connecting waist that allows the 2 discs to move independently. The device comes in 4 sizes: the 18- and 30-mm sizes have equal disc sizes, whereas the 25- and 35-mm devices feature left atrial discs that are smaller in diameter than the right atrial discs.

Gore Helex Septal Occluder

The Gore Helex Septal Occluder (W.L. Gore & Associates, Flagstaff, AZ) (see **Fig. 5**) consists of a nitinol wire frame covered with polytetrafluoroethylene (PTFE). It is currently undergoing

Table 3
Primary and secondary outcomes of the PC Trial

	PFO Closure, N (%)	Medical Therapy, N (%)	Hazard Ratio/ Relative Risk (95% CI)	P Value
Death, stroke, TIA, or peripheral embolism	7 (3.4)	11 (5.2)	0.63 (0.24–1.62)	.34
Death	2 (1.0)	0	5.20 (0.25–107.61)	.24
Cardiovascular	0	0	Not available	
Noncardiovascular	2 (1.0)	0	5.20 (0.25–107.61)	.24
Thromboembolic event				
Stroke	1 (0.5)	5 (2.4)	0.20 (0.02–1.72)	.14
TIA	5 (2.5)	7 (3.3)	0.71 (0.23–2.24)	.56
Peripheral embolism	0	0	Not available	
Stroke, TIA, or peripheral embolism	5 (2.5)	11 (5.2)	0.45 (0.16–1.29)	.14

Data from Meier B, Kalesan B, Mattle HP, et al. Percutaneous closure of patent foramen ovale in cryptogenic embolism. N Engl J Med 2013;368(12):1087.

Table 4
Intention-to-treat results of the MIST trial

| End Point | Implant (n = 74) | | Sham Procedure (n = 73) | | Statistical Analyses | |
	Baseline	Analysis Phase	Baseline	Analysis Phase	Difference Between Implant and Sham Arms (95% CI)	P Value
Patients with no migraine attacks, n	0	3	1	3	−0.06% (−6.45–6.34)	1.0
Frequency of migraine attacks per month, mean ± SD	4.82 ± 2.44	3.23 ± 1.80	4.51 ± 2.17	3.53 ± 2.13	0.45 (−0.16–1.05)	.14
Total MIDAS score, median (range)	36 (3–108)	17 (0–270)	34 (2–189)	18 (0–240)	1 (−11–10)	.88
Headache days/3 mo (MIDAS), median (range)	27 (0–70)	18 (0–90)	30 (5–80)	21 (0–80)	1 (−5–6)	.79
HIT-6 total score, mean ± SD	67.2 ± 4.7	59.5 ± 9.3	66.2 ± 5.1	58.5 ± 8.6	0 (−3–2)	.77

Abbreviations: HIT-6, Headache Impact Test 6; MIDAS, Migraine Disability Assessment Score.

From Dowson A, Mullen MJ, Peatfield R, et al. Migraine Intervention With STARFlex Technology (MIST) trial: a prospective, multicenter, double-blind, sham-controlled trial to evaluate the effectiveness of patent foramen ovale closure with STARFlex septal repair implant to resolve refractory migraine headache. Circulation 2008;117(11):1400; with permission.

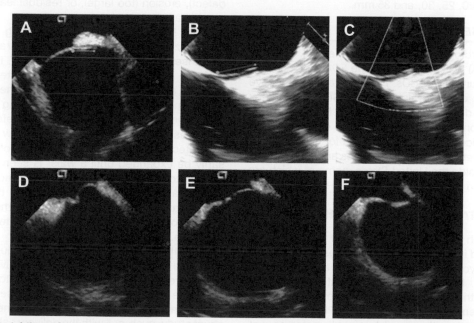

Fig. 4. Variability of PFO anatomy. (*A*) An average tunnel length (1.0 cm, denoted by the *blue bar*), with a somewhat thickened septum secundum. (*B*) A long tunnel (1.6 cm, denoted by the *blue bar*), with a thick septum secundum and mild shunting seen on color flow Doppler (*C*). (*D–F*) The PFO is shown in different phases of respiration, demonstrating an atrial septal aneurysm with more than 1 cm of excursion of the septum primum.

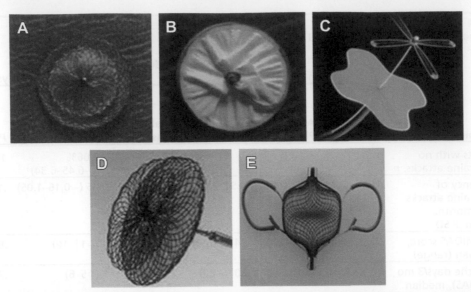

Fig. 5. Transcatheter PFO closure devices. (*A*) Amplatzer PFO Occluder (St Jude Medical, St Paul, MN). (*B*) Helex Septal Occluder (W.L. Gore and Associates, Flagstaff, AZ, USA). (*C*) Premere (St Jude Medical, St Paul, MN)*. (*D*) Occlutech PFO Occluder (Occlutech, Jena, Germany)*. (*E*) SeptRx (Secant Medical, Perkasie, PA, USA)*. *(Not currently approved for use in the United States.) *Adapted from* Steinberg D, Staubach S, Franke J, et al. Defining structural heart disease in the adult patient: current scope, inherent challenges and future directions. Eur Heart J Suppl 2010;12(Suppl E):E2–9; with permission.

investigation of PFO closure for recurrent cryptogenic stroke in the context of the REDUCE trial. It is currently approved for closure of secundum-type ASDs up to 18 mm in diameter and less than 8 mm in thickness. Available devices sizes are 15, 20, 25, 30, and 35 mm.

CardioSEAL STARFlex

The CardioSEAL device (NMT Medical, Inc, Natick, MA) was approved by the FDA for closure of secundum-type ASDs. However, after 2 negative studies of the related CardioSEAL STARFlex closure device (CLOSURE I[4] and MIST[7]) for PFO indications, the company ceased operations and the device is no longer available for clinical use.

A variety of other PFO devices are approved for use outside the United States, some of which are shown in **Fig. 5**.

PERCUTANEOUS CLOSURE TECHNIQUE

Although a detailed description of the steps involved in a transcatheter PFO closure procedure are beyond the scope of this article, several general, but important considerations regarding transcatheter PFO closure are noted here. First and foremost, clarification of the PFO anatomy at hand (both with regard to size/diameter as well as tunnel length) is of utmost importance to ensure technical success, minimize the risk of complications, and maximize the long-term benefit. Each available device has its own particular sizing recommendations and benefits/limitations with regard to particular anatomic variance. In addition, appropriate sizing should mitigate the risk of device embolization (too small for the defect), erosion (too large), or residual leak (short waist in a long tunnel defect).

Large PFOs may be measured using a compliant sizing balloon and invasive (intracardiac or transesophageal) echocardiography. Invasive balloon sizing is the most accurate sizing method available at present. Once the defect has been crossed with a wire, the sizing balloon is advanced and inflated across the defect with low pressure until Doppler color flow across the defect stops. The balloon should not necessarily be expanded until a waist is seen, as this can stretch and potentially tear the defect. However, if a waist is seen the length of the PFO tunnel can often be estimated, which may have implications on subsequent appropriate device selection.

Once the device has been placed, but before complete release from the attached delivery system, several maneuvers can be used to ensure adequate positioning and stability; these include Doppler assessment by ICE or TEE, saline bubble shunt study, push-pull with the delivery cable (specific to the Amplatzer devices), and assessment with a patient cough or Valsalva maneuver to check for stability.

POSTCLOSURE MANAGEMENT

In the authors' practice, patients are most commonly admitted for overnight monitoring and observation. Occasionally, if the patient had undergone an uncomplicated procedure completed early in the day and had been monitored during the course of the day, had an unremarkable follow-up TTE (eg, stable device, minimal to no residual shunt, no pericardial effusion) (**Fig. 6**), and patient-specific circumstances necessitated an early discharge, the patient is discharged on the same day. In general, however, the authors advocate overnight observation at a minimum, as intermediate-to-late complications (eg, hematoma, retroperitoneal hemorrhage, pericardial effusion, arrhythmia) following transcatheter PFO closure can occur and have been reported.

The authors recommend a follow-up chest radiograph after the procedure and a follow-up TTE within 24 hours of device placement. These modalities allow the operator to efficiently monitor for signs of pericardial effusion, device embolization, and residual shunting. It is worth noting that following implantation, a trivial to small residual shunt either through (Amplatzer family of devices) or around (Gore Helex) the device is a common finding, and often resolves over a period of several months following complete device endothelialization. For this reason, a TTE is generally recommended 6 months after the procedure to document either persistence or complete resolution of any residual shunting. Although no firm guidelines exist on the antiplatelet regimen following device closure of a PFO, it is the authors' practice to prescribe patients aspirin, 81 to 325 mg daily, for the first 6 months and clopidogrel, 75 mg daily, for the first 1 to 3 months after device implantation (prolonged courses reserved for larger devices).[21] It is also recommended that patients be prescribed standard bacterial endocarditis prophylaxis for invasive dental procedures for the first 6 months after implantation.

COMPLICATIONS

Potential complications noted at the time of device implantation or immediately thereafter include vascular access complications (<1%), arrhythmias (1%–5%), air embolism (<1%), pericardial effusion as a result of perforation of the atrial wall (<1%), and device embolization (1%–2%) (**Figs. 7** and **8**).[22–24]

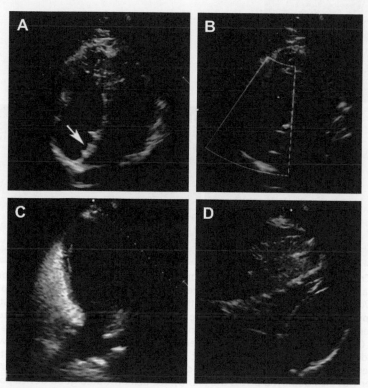

Fig. 6. Follow-up TTE. An apical 4-chamber view (*A*) shows the device (*white arrow*) in place across the interatrial septum. Color flow Doppler (*B*) demonstrates no significant shunt across the interatrial septum. A saline contrast study (*C*) documents trivial residual shunting. An alternative view of the interatrial septum (*D*) is via the subcostal approach.

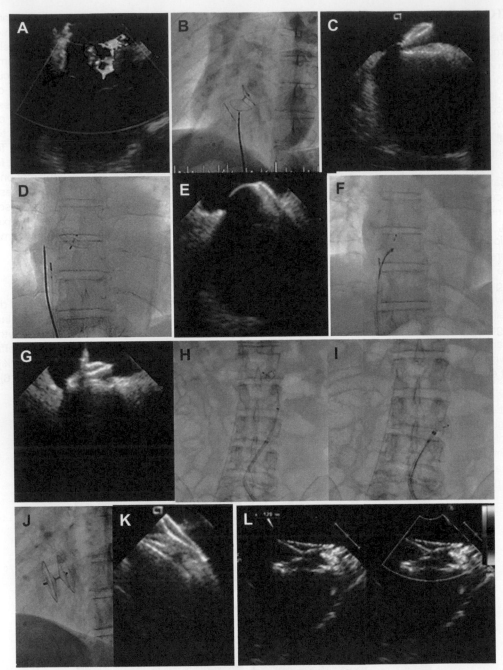

Fig. 7. Amplatzer Cribriform Occluder embolization and retrieval. Baseline ICE imaging demonstrates a large PFO with an atrial septal aneurysm (*A*). A 25-mm Amplatzer Cribriform Occluder device was deployed across the interatrial septum. With the delivery cord still attached, the push-pull test appeared to demonstrate device stability on both fluoroscopy (*B*) and ICE imaging (*C*). After release of the device (*D*), it appeared to shift. ICE imaging demonstrated absence of the typical splay of the Amplatzer device, which would indicate noncapture of the septum secundum (*E*). The decision was made to attempt retrieval with a snare (*F, G*). However, the snare did not hold and the device embolized into the systemic arterial circulation, coming to rest at the diaphragmatic aorta. Femoral arterial access was obtained, and the device was snared from below (*H, I*). A 35-mm Amplatzer Cribriform Occluder was then deployed across the PFO (*J*). ICE demonstrated good device positioning with clear capture of the septum secundum (*K*). This capture was confirmed with TEE the following day, which demonstrated absence of flow across the PFO (*L*).

As noted earlier, the authors recommend postprocedure assessment with chest radiography, TTE, and rhythm/vital sign monitoring for all patients, as these should alert the clinician to these rare but serious events.

Device embolization has been reported to occur in a delayed fashion, although it is more common for embolization to occur in the periprocedural time frame. It should be very rare for PFO closure. Other rare but potentially significant delayed adverse events include an allergic reaction either to the device[24] or to the nickel component of the device,[25,26] thrombus formation on the device (most commonly associated with the now unavailable CardioSEAL device),[27,28] and device erosion.[29] Device erosion has long been a known (albeit rare) complication of transcatheter ASD closure using the ASO, estimated to occur in approximately 0.1% of patients, but it is difficult to truly estimate the event rate because there is no mandated reporting of such events. Erosion occurs when the implanted device erodes through the atrial wall or into the aorta, and is a phenomenon most commonly associated with the ASO device.[30]

Factors associated with device erosion include device oversizing, the presence of a deficient retroaortic rim, and repetitive motion.[30] Erosion occurs suddenly and unpredictably, and can result in rapid hemodynamic collapse. Given the significant consequences of such an event, which generally necessitates emergent pericardiocentesis and/or thoracotomy, this complication has understandably garnered significant interest from the FDA. Rates of erosion after PFO closure are not

known, but have very rarely occurred outside the United States with the Amplatzer PFO Occluder. No erosions have occurred in any of the randomized PFO clinical trials.

CLINICAL TRIAL DATA

RCTs have been performed to study PFO closure for the prevention of migraine headaches and recurrent cryptogenic stroke. The prevention of recurrent cryptogenic stroke has been studied using the CardioSEAL STARFlex device in the CLOSURE I[4] study, and the Amplatzer PFO Occluder device in the RESPECT[5] and PC Trials.[6] The Gore Helex device is currently being evaluated for this indication in the REDUCE trial.

The MIST trial studied the CardioSEAL STARFlex device for migraine headache treatment[7] while the Amplatzer PFO Occluder device is currently being evaluated for this indication in the context of the PREMIUM Trial.

Cryptogenic Stroke

CLOSURE I
The Evaluation of the STARFlex Septal Closure System in Patients with a Stroke and/or Transient Ischemic Attack due to Presumed Paradoxic Embolism through a Patent Foramen Ovale (CLOSURE I) trial was a prospective, randomized, open-label trial that compared implantation of the CardioSEAL STARFlex device with medical therapy for the prevention of recurrent cryptogenic stroke. A total of 909 patients with a CVA or transient ischemic attack (TIA) within the previous 6 months, TTE evidence of a PFO with right-to-left

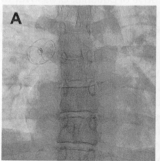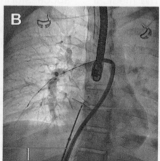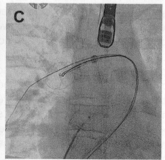

Fig. 8. Gore Helex Septal Occluder embolization. Several months following the placement of a Gore Helex device for PFO closure, a follow-up echo demonstrated absence of the device at the level of the interatrial septum. Fluoroscopy was performed (*A*), demonstrating the device in the right pulmonary artery. The patient was started on anticoagulation, then returned for an attempt at retrieval. Cineangiography demonstrated the position of the device to clearly be in a large branch of the right pulmonary artery with brisk flow past the device (*B*). A 14F Mullins sheath, supported by an Amplatzer Super stiff wire in the distal right pulmonary artery, was used to deliver a rat-tooth forceps (*C*). The forceps was cinched down with a Gooseneck snare over the jaws of the device. Despite the application of significant traction pressure, the device was clearly very adherent to the pulmonary artery. The decision was made to stop retrieval attempts. The PFO was closed with a 30-mm Amplatzer Cribriform Occluder device.

shunting, and no other obvious cause of CVA were enrolled. The results of the study were negative, with no significant difference in recurrent ischemic events noted between the two treatment arms (5.5% in the closure arm, 6.8% in the medical therapy arm, hazard ratio [HR] 0.78, 95% confidence interval [CI] 0.45–1.35, $P = .37$). The rates of vascular complications (3.2% vs 0%, $P<.001$) and atrial fibrillation (5.7% vs 0.7%, $P<.001$) associated with closure, however, were significantly higher in the device therapy arm, whereas the overall rate of adverse events were similar in both arms (16.9% vs 16.6%, $P = .90$).

RESPECT

The Randomized Evaluation of Recurrent Stroke Comparing PFO Closure to Established Current Standard of Care Treatment (RESPECT) trial was a randomized, controlled, multicenter, open-label trial conducted in the United States and Canada. The study evaluated the Amplatzer PFO Occluder for prevention of recurrent cryptogenic stroke when compared with medical therapy alone in patients who had a PFO as documented by TEE. Unlike in CLOSURE I, patients with a history of TIA or lacunar infarcts were excluded. In addition, given the length of time (8 years) required to complete study enrollment and the nature of the trial design (follow-up was continued throughout the enrollment period, and was specified to continue until the FDA made a regulatory decision), what resulted was a significantly increased number of patient-years of follow-up obtained in comparison with previously published studies.

A total of 980 patients were enrolled into RESPECT, with 499 randomized to the device group and 481 to medical therapy. The medical therapy arm of the study was divided into 1 of 5 treatment strategies: aspirin only, warfarin only, clopidogrel only, aspirin + dipyridamole, and aspirin + clopidogrel (this last group was enrolled only until 2006, when professional society guidelines changed). The choice of medication was made by the study neurologist before randomization. In the device arm, procedural success was high (>99%) and the rate of adverse events was low. Overall, 93% of patients assigned to closure underwent a procedure. There was a nonsignificant trend toward benefit with respect to the primary end point (recurrent nonfatal ischemic stroke, fatal stroke, and all-cause death within 45 days of randomization) by the intention-to-treat analysis (HR 0.49, 95% CI 0.22–1.11; $P = .08$) (see **Table 2**). In 2 other prespecified analyses, the per-protocol and as-treated cohort analyses, the device group demonstrated statistically significantly fewer events than the medical

therapy group (per-protocol; HR 0.37, 95% CI 0.14–0.96; $P = .03$; as-treated: HR 0.27, 95% CI 0.10–0.75; $P = .007$). One potential reason for this differential may be explained by the fact that 3 patients with recurrent strokes, who had been randomized to device implantation, had not yet undergone the closure procedure when the stroke events occurred. In addition, a subpopulation analysis suggested that patients with substantial right-to-left shunts and/or atrial septal aneurysms may derive the most benefit from PFO closure.

Of note, the rate of adverse events was low and did not differ between the two study groups. In particular, rates of atrial fibrillation were statistically equivalent. There was a nonsignificant trend ($P = .12$) toward higher rates of pulmonary embolism in the closure group.

PC Trial

The Clinical Trial Comparing Percutaneous Closure of Patent Foramen Ovale Using the Amplatzer PFO Occluder with Medical Treatment in Patients with Cryptogenic Embolism (PC Trial) was a randomized, multinational trial conducted in Europe, Canada, Brazil, and Australia. It compared PFO closure with the Amplatzer PFO Occluder device with medical therapy for the prevention of ischemic stroke, TIA, and peripheral thromboembolism. Patients were included if they were younger than 60 years, had had a cryptogenic stroke or peripheral thromboembolism, and had a PFO as assessed by TEE. Medical therapy was at the discretion of the treating physician.

The study enrolled 414 patients over 9 years, randomizing 204 subjects to closure and 210 subjects to medical therapy. Device implantation was successful in 96% of patients. Crossover to device implantation was noted in 28 patients randomized to medical therapy at a median of 8.8 months from enrollment. There was no difference between the two groups for the primary end point (HR for closure vs medical therapy, 0.63; 95% CI 0.24–1.62; $P = .34$). The primary end point was a composite end point including all deaths regardless of cause. The per-protocol analysis similarly demonstrated no difference (HR 0.70, 95% CI 0.27–1.85; $P = .48$). Of interest, there was only 1 stroke in the device group and 5 in the medical group, but the study was underpowered to show statistical significance of this difference. New-onset atrial fibrillation was noted in 2.9% of the closure group and in 1.0% of the medical therapy group ($P = .16$).

This trial was notable for both slow enrollment and a lower than anticipated event rate in the medical therapy group. The trial was conducted at centers where PFO closure with approved devices was possible and, thus, patient selection bias was possible. Given the overall low number of events, it was considered that there was a reasonable chance of a Type II error.

REDUCE

The Gore Helex Septal Occluder/Gore Septal Occluder and Antiplatelet Medical Management for Reduction of Recurrent Stroke or Imaging-Confirmed TIA in Patients With Patent Foramen Ovale (REDUCE) trial is a randomized trial studying the safety and efficacy of the Gore Helex Septal Occluder for PFO closure for the secondary prevention of recurrent cryptogenic stroke and imaging-confirmed shunt-related TIA in a comparison with medical therapy alone. The study enrollment criteria permit inclusion only of patients with ischemic stroke or TIA confirmed by magnetic resonance imaging and exclusion of patients with deep vein thrombosis or documented thrombi. The unique device design and lack of warfarin use in the medical therapy arm (thus comparing device closure with aspirin therapy alone) are other notable features of REDUCE. Some argue, however, that these strict entry criteria will only serve to further reduce the observed stroke rate in the study population and that the proposed 664-patient sample size will be insufficient to observe a statistically significant difference between patient cohorts.

Migraine Headache

MIST

The Migraine Intervention with STARFlex Trial (MIST) (see **Table 4**) was a prospective, randomized, double-blind, sham-controlled trial investigating the safety and efficacy of transcatheter PFO closure using the CardioSEAL STARFlex closure in comparison with best medical therapy in the treatment of migraine headaches. One hundred forty-seven patients with moderate to large right-to-left shunts were enrolled. No difference between the two groups was found in migraine cessation. The group receiving device implants demonstrated a numerically higher rate of serious adverse events, but no analysis was performed to determine the statistical significance of this finding.

PREMIUM

The Prospective Randomized Investigation to Evaluate Incidence of Headache Reduction in Subjects With Migraine and PFO Using the Amplatzer PFO Occluder Compared with Medical Management (PREMIUM) trial is actively enrolling patients to study the safety and efficacy of PFO closure using the Amplatzer PFO Occluder in the treatment of migraines. PREMIUM is a prospective, randomized, sham-controlled, double-blind,

multicenter study comparing transcatheter device closure of a PFO with medical therapy (aspirin with and without clopidogrel). The primary end point of PREMIUM is a reduction in the number of migraine attacks. Several predefined secondary end points include the change in Migraine Disability Assessment Score, reduction in use of acute or rescue migraine medications, complete defect closure, and improvement in quality of life.

Clinical Trial Challenges

As noted, clinical trials of PFO closure have been difficult to conduct and have repeatedly been hampered by slow enrollment. While widespread off-label closure within the United States and approved device availability outside the United States has arguably retarded enrollment into clinical trials in this country, the relatively low number of clinical events (ie, recurrent stroke) observed in clinical trials has also limited the ability to identify significant differences in treatment strategies. In addition, at least anecdotally, it appears that patients who are at high risk (such as those who have had a significant CVA or possess anatomy that may predispose them to recurrent events [eg, large PFO, atrial septal aneurysm]) tend to choose or be referred for off-label device placement over randomization, such that many argue that the patient population studied in clinical trials may not accurately reflect the true population at risk.

Thus, perhaps the most challenging aspect of PFO clinical trial design is selection of an appropriate study population with the ability to enroll and retain enough patients to answer the question of whether device closure adds an important additional risk reduction to recurrent strokes. To date, there seem to be reasonably clear associations between the presence of atrial septal aneurysm and high degrees of shunting with more frequent recurrent events. However, it is important that the absence of other clear causes does not necessarily make a PFO and paradoxic embolism the only potential culprit in unexplained ischemic CVA. Likewise, conditions such as migraine and systemic hypoxemia are no doubt heterogeneous in etiology, so that defining a patient subset likely to benefit from PFO closure against a background of a high rate of "bystander PFOs" is extremely challenging.

SUMMARY

Few anatomic anomalies have engendered such vigorous debate and study as the PFO. The relationship of a PFO to clinical sequelae such as paradoxic embolic stroke and migraine headaches is enigmatic, making it difficult to study. A seemingly straightforward solution, transcatheter closure, has yet to unequivocally demonstrate a positive effect on meaningful clinical outcomes. Advocates of PFO closure and its detractors are able to mount reasonable arguments for this important clinical problem that has harbored more complexity than originally anticipated. These complexities include the common occurrence of PFO that may be incidental, the difficulty of confidently assigning a specific cause to stroke, closure devices that have had substantial safety problems, and the need to demonstrate superiority versus noninferiority. Furthermore, the widespread availability of devices to perform PFO closure and the clear lack of clinical equipoise in substantial numbers of clinicians and patients has made completion of trials difficult.

To date, four randomized trials evaluating two different closure devices have provided substantial advancements in understanding this clinical problem and the identification of patient characteristics that might identify those patients most likely to benefit from device closure. The trials have had a spectrum of results, but have not definitively shown a benefit of transcatheter PFO closure for preventing recurrent cryptogenic stroke and migraine headaches. CardioSEAL-related safety and closure efficacy problems in CLOSURE and MIST made answering the central question of device benefit impossible. Whether the Amplatzer PFO Occluder or Gore Helex devices will ultimately be approved for PFO closure by the FDA remains an open question. Further evidence, potentially more definitive, will be forthcoming from the REDUCE trial, from the ongoing follow-up of more than 800 patients in the RESPECT trial, and from an upcoming pooled analysis of the RESPECT and PC Trials that used the same device.

REFERENCES

1. Anderson RH, Webb S, Brown NA. Clinical anatomy of the atrial septum with reference to its developmental components. Clin Anat 1999;12(5):362–74.
2. Anderson RH, Brown NA, Webb S. Development and structure of the atrial septum. Heart 2002; 88(1):104–10.
3. Hagen PT, Scholz DG, Edwards WD. Incidence and size of patent foramen ovale during the first 10 decades of life: an autopsy study of 965 normal hearts. Mayo Clin Proc 1984;59(1):17–20.
4. Furlan AJ, Reisman M, Massaro J, et al. Closure or medical therapy for cryptogenic stroke with patent foramen ovale. N Engl J Med 2012;366(11):991–9.
5. Carroll JD, Saver JL, Thaler DE, et al. Closure of patent foramen ovale versus medical therapy after cryptogenic stroke. N Engl J Med 2013;368(12): 1092–100.
6. Meier B, Kalesan B, Mattle HP, et al. Percutaneous closure of patent foramen ovale in cryptogenic embolism. N Engl J Med 2013;368(12):1083–91.
7. Dowson A, Mullen MJ, Peatfield R, et al. Migraine Intervention with STARFlex Technology (MIST) trial: a prospective, multicenter, double-blind, sham-controlled trial to evaluate the effectiveness of patent foramen ovale closure with STARFlex septal repair implant to resolve refractory migraine headache. Circulation 2008;117(11):1397–404.
8. Guerin P, Lambert V, Godart F, et al. Transcatheter closure of patent foramen ovale in patients with platypnea-orthodeoxia: results of a multicentric French registry. Cardiovasc Intervent Radiol 2005; 28(2):164–8.
9. Allemann Y, Hutter D, Lipp E, et al. Patent foramen ovale and high-altitude pulmonary edema. JAMA 2006;296(24):2954–8.
10. Billinger M, Zbinden R, Mordasini R, et al. Patent foramen ovale closure in recreational divers: effect on decompression illness and ischaemic brain lesions during long-term follow-up. Heart 2011; 97(23):1932–7.
11. Nendaz MR, Sarasin FP, Junod AF, et al. Preventing stroke recurrence in patients with patent foramen ovale: antithrombotic therapy, foramen closure, or therapeutic abstention? A decision analytic perspective. Am Heart J 1998;135(3):532–41.
12. Windecker S, Wahl A, Nedeltchev K, et al. Comparison of medical treatment with percutaneous closure of patent foramen ovale in patients with cryptogenic stroke. J Am Coll Cardiol 2004;44(4):750–8.
13. Khairy P, O'Donnell CP, Landzberg MJ. Transcatheter closure versus medical therapy of patent foramen ovale and presumed paradoxical thromboemboli: a systematic review. Ann Intern Med 2003;139(9):753–60.
14. Martin F, Sanchez PL, Doherty E, et al. Percutaneous transcatheter closure of patent foramen ovale in patients with paradoxical embolism. Circulation 2002; 106(9):1121–6.
15. Braun MU, Fassbender D, Schoen SP, et al. Transcatheter closure of patent foramen ovale in patients with cerebral ischemia. J Am Coll Cardiol 2002; 39(12):2019–25.
16. Hung J, Landzberg MJ, Jenkins KJ, et al. Closure of patent foramen ovale for paradoxical emboli: intermediate-term risk of recurrent neurological events following transcatheter device placement. J Am Coll Cardiol 2000;35(5):1311–6.
17. Du ZD, Cao QL, Joseph A, et al. Transcatheter closure of patent foramen ovale in patients with paradoxical embolism: intermediate-term risk of

recurrent neurological events. Catheter Cardiovasc Interv 2002;55(2):189–94.

18. Carroll JD. PFO closure in 2008: see through a glass, darkly. Catheter Cardiovasc Interv 2008; 71(3):388–9.

19. Stackhouse KA, Goel SS, Qureshi AM, et al. Off-label closure during CLOSURE study. J Invasive Cardiol 2012;24(11):608–11.

20. Carroll JD. PFO anatomy: 3D characterization and device performance. Catheter Cardiovasc Interv 2008;71(2):229–30.

21. Franke A, Kuhl HP. The role of antiplatelet agents in the management of patients receiving intracardiac closure devices. Curr Pharm Des 2006;12(10): 1287–91.

22. Du ZD, Hijazi ZM, Kleinman CS, et al. Comparison between transcatheter and surgical closure of secundum atrial septal defect in children and adults: results of a multicenter nonrandomized trial. J Am Coll Cardiol 2002;39(11):1836–44.

23. Everett AD, Jennings J, Sibinga E, et al. Community use of the Amplatzer atrial septal defect occluder: results of the multicenter MAGIC atrial septal defect study. Pediatr Cardiol 2009;30(3):240–7.

24. Jones TK, Latson LA, Zahn E, et al. Results of the U.S. multicenter pivotal study of the HELEX septal occluder for percutaneous closure of secundum atrial septal defects. J Am Coll Cardiol 2007; 49(22):2215–21.

25. Khodaverdian RA, Jones KW. Metal allergy to Amplatzer occluder device presented as severe bronchospasm. Ann Thorac Surg 2009;88(6): 2021–2.

26. Wertman B, Azarbal B, Riedl M, et al. Adverse events associated with nickel allergy in patients undergoing percutaneous atrial septal defect or patent foramen ovale closure. J Am Coll Cardiol 2006; 47(6):1226–7.

27. Krumsdorf U, Ostermayer S, Billinger K, et al. Incidence and clinical course of thrombus formation on atrial septal defect and patient foramen ovale closure devices in 1,000 consecutive patients. J Am Coll Cardiol 2004;43(2):302–9.

28. Carroll JD. Challenges in understanding rare but serious problems associated with septal occluders. Catheter Cardiovasc Interv 2012;80(3):503.

29. Carroll JD. Device erosion. Catheter Cardiovasc Interv 2009;73(7):931–2.

30. Crawford GB, Brindis RG, Krucoff MW, et al. Percutaneous atrial septal occluder devices and cardiac erosion: a review of the literature. Catheter Cardiovasc Interv 2012;80(2):157–67.

Patent Ductus Arteriosus

Mehra Anilkumar, MD

KEYWORDS

- Patent ductus arteriosus (PDA) • Congenital heart disease • Congenital defects
- Amplatzer duct occluder • Percutaneous closure

KEY POINTS

- Patent ductus arteriosus (PDA) in adults is usually is an isolated lesion with a small to moderate degree of shunt as a larger shunt become symptomatic earlier in childhood.
- Classic murmur of PDA may be the first clue to its presence, or it is detected accidently by transthoracic echocardiogram, computed tomography, or magnetic resonance angiography for an unrelated condition.
- Transthoracic echocardiogram provides complete evaluation for the diagnosis and therapeutic decisions. Transesophageal echocardiogram, diagnostic catheterization, CT, and MRI are not routinely indicated.
- All patients with PDA except silent PDA and the ones associated with Eisenmenger syndrome can be considered for closure.
- The percutaneous approach is the method of choice, with surgery in unusual cases. The percutaneous approach is very safe and effective in more than 98% of patients.
- Subacute bacterial endocarditis prophylaxis is not indicated routinely except for 6 months following the closure percutaneously or surgically.

INTRODUCTION

Ductus arteriosus (DA) is a vascular structure connecting the junction of the main and left pulmonary artery to the descending aorta just distal to the origin of left subclavian artery in fetal life and forms an important outflow conduit for right ventricular output to circumvent the high resistance pulmonary arterial circulation. After birth the duct closes functionally in 12 to 18 hours and anatomically in 2 to 3 weeks. If it remains open beyond 3 months of life in full-term infants and beyond 1 year in premature infants, it is termed persistently patent ductus arteriosus (PDA) because the incidence of spontaneous closure beyond these time limits is very low. Because of low-resistance pulmonary circulation compared with systemic circulation, in postnatal life, now it creates shunting of blood from the aorta to the pulmonary artery. The long-term effects of the extra volume of blood in the pulmonary arteries

and the left side of the heart depend on its amount and the anatomic as well as physiologic states of these structures. In isolated PDA, if the shunt volume is small to moderate, it may not be detected in childhood and may come to be diagnosed for the first time in adults. Therefore it is important for an adult cardiologist to have an understanding of its natural history, pathophysiology, and related management issues in adult patients.

Embryology/Anatomy/Histology

In fetal circulatory system development, truncus arteriosus is divided by the aorticopulmonary septum into the pulmonary trunk and ascending aorta. The truncus continues into an endothelial tube called the aortic sac or the ventral aorta from which the number of aortic arches (I, II, III, IV, VI) develop and connect it to the right-sided and left-sided dorsal aortas, which fuse together

Disclosures: The author has nothing to disclose.
Department of Cardiology, LAC-USC Medical Center, Keck School of Medicine, 1200 North State Street, Los Angeles, CA 91011, USA
E-mail address: amehra@usc.edu

Cardiol Clin 31 (2013) 417–430
http://dx.doi.org/10.1016/j.ccl.2013.05.006
0733-8651/13/$ – see front matter © 2013 Elsevier Inc. All rights reserved

below the level of the arches to form the descending thoracoabdominal aorta (**Fig. 1**).[1] The sixth aortic arch (pulmonary arch) develops around day 29. By the eight week of gestation, the ventral portions of the right and left sixth aortic arch form the proximal part of the right pulmonary artery and the proximal part of left main pulmonary artery, respectively. The dorsal portion of the right sixth arch is obliterated along with the right dorsal aorta. However, the dorsal portion of the left sixth arch persists as a vascular conduit called ductus arteriosus arising from the roof of the junction between the main and the left pulmonary arteries and joining the left dorsal aorta just distal to the left subclavian artery in normal left-sided aorta (**Fig. 2**).[2]

Anatomy

Most patients seen with isolated PDA in adults have left-sided aortic arch and the ductus arising from the left pulmonary artery forms an arch with convexity upwards and joins the anterior aspect of the descending aorta at an upper angle of approximately 30°. The length, size, and configuration of the ductus are highly variable. Krichenko and colleagues[3] classified the ductal anatomy into 5 different types (A to E) based on the angiographic appearance of PDA in the lateral angiogram (**Fig. 3**). In adults, more than 80% of ductal types are A or B, being favorable for percutaneous closure. The ductal anatomy and size have important implications in the management of PDA for both the devices used for percutaneous closure and surgical approaches for closure.

Some anatomic variations of importance in ductal origin and morphology are "reverse-oriented" PDA, ductal aneurysm, and PDA with right-sided aortic arch.

If the direction of flow in utero is from aorta to pulmonary artery due to severe right-sided obstructive lesions like tricuspid atresia or pulmonary atresia, the PDA configuration may form an arch with concavity upwards with an inferior angle less than 90° with aorta called "reverse-oriented" PDA.[4] The presence of reverse-oriented PDA especially with less than 65% inferior angle is an indication for early intervention to maintain the pulmonary blood flow in postnatal period.[5]

Ductal aneurysm without any prior intervention or infection at the site of ductus has been reported to be as high as 8% in some series.[6] The incidence is high in syndromic PDAs because of genetic abnormalities.[7] Most ductal aneurysms close spontaneously over time.[8] However, if they persist and grow large in adult life, they may cause compression on the adjacent structures like the recurrent pharyngeal nerve or trachea with associated symptoms. In rare cases, thrombosis within the aneurysm may extend to the aorta or pulmonary artery and cause embolic phenomena.[8–10]

Isolated right-sided aortic arch is an uncommon developmental abnormality, and the PDA anatomy in these patients is highly variable.[11] The variations include right-sided PDA connecting right pulmonary artery to the right descending aorta, left PDA connecting right brachiocephalic or left subclavian artery to the left pulmonary artery, or the presence of dual PDA. Sometimes in cases of left PDA arising from left subclavian artery, the subclavian artery arises from the right descending aorta and runs behind the trachea and esophagus, forming a vascular ring around them by the right aortic arch anteriorly, and to the right, the left subclavian artery at the back and the PDA to the left. The patients may present with compressive symptoms related to the trachea and/or the esophagus.[12]

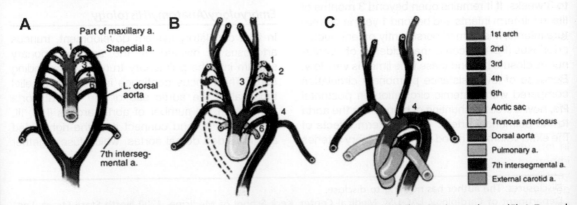

Fig. 1. Embryologic development of the aortic arches and ductus arteriosus. (A) A 29-day embryo. (B) A 7-week embryo. (C) An 8-week embryo. a, artery; L, left. (*From* Groshong SD, Tomashefski JF, Cool CD. Pulmonary vascular disease. In: Tomashefski JF, ed. Dail and Hammar's pulmonary pathology, 3rd edition, vol. 1. New York: Springer Science+Business Media, 2008; with permission.)

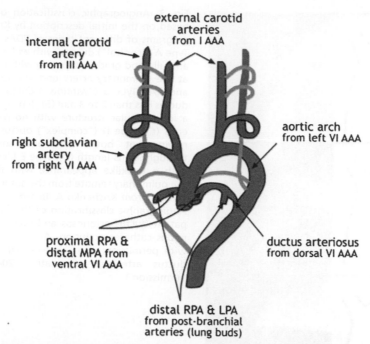

internal carotid
artery
from III AAA

external carotid
arteries
from I AAA

aortic arch
from left VI AAA

right subclavian
artery
from right VI AAA

proximal RPA &
distal MPA from
ventral VI AAA

ductus arteriosus
from dorsal VI AAA

distal RPA & LPA
from post-branchial
arteries (lung buds)

Fig. 2. Degenerated aortic arch arteries (AAA) and final great vessels as well as ductal anatomy. LPA, left pulmonary artery; MPA, main pulmonary artery; RPA, right pulmonary artery. (*From* Abdulla R, Blew GA, Holterman MJ. Cardiac embryology. Pediatr Cardiol 2004;25:199; with permission.)

Histology

Histologically ductal tissue goes through significant maturational changes throughout the fetal life (**Fig. 4**).[13,14] Fully matured ductal tissue at term has an arterial configuration with medial muscle fibers arranged in longitudinally and spirally in contrast to the adjacent aorta and pulmonary artery, which aid in the closure process with the constriction.[14–16] Maturity of ductal tissue also determines the responsiveness to oxygen tension in the blood and the prostaglandins.[17,18] In addition, the response of the muscle fiber to oxygen tension is also different compared with pulmonary artery. Low oxygen tension causes vasoconstriction of the pulmonary vasculature but causes relaxation of the ductal muscle cells.

Physiology of Fetal Circulation and Postnatal Period

In intrauterine circulation, patency of DA is very important because almost 60% of the combined ventricular output crosses across the DA into the descending aorta and only 7% enters the pulmonary circulation as the unexpanded lungs and the pulmonary arteries offer significantly high vascular resistance, compared with the ductus and the descending aorta.[19,20] The size of the ductus as large

as the aorta poses no resistance and the systemic resistance is low because of placental circulation. The patency is maintained because of the vasodilatory response of the muscles to low blood oxygen tension, circulating and locally produced prostaglandins, and the nitric oxide derived from the ductal endothelium.[16] The prostaglandins (PG E_2, and PGI_2) concentrations are high in fetal life because of increased production by the placental tissue coupled with decreased clearance by the lung tissue. They act via specific G-protein-coupled receptors on the muscle cells and cause muscle relaxation.[21] PGE_2 is considered to be the most important endogenous prostaglandin involved in the regulation of DA patency. Immature duct is more responsive to the vasodilatory effects of prostaglandins and is less responsive to oxygen tension, whereas mature duct is more sensitive to changes in oxygen tension and less responsive to PGE_2.[22]

In full-term infants, initial "functional" closure of the ductus occurs within 10 to 15 hours of birth and is followed by a permanent "anatomic" occlusion with replacement by a fibrous ligament (ligamentum arteriosum) over the following 2 to 3 weeks. The functional closure is related to multiple mechanisms, the most important being high arterial Po_2. The full expansion of the lung tissue

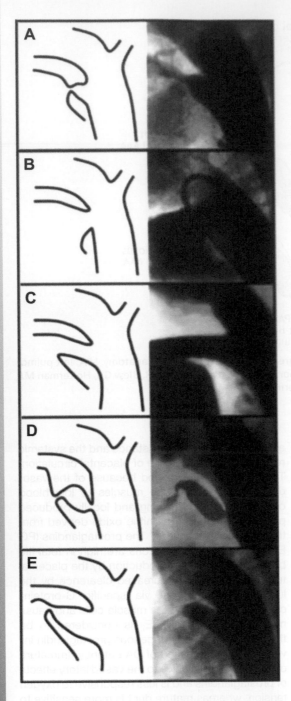

Fig. 3. Angiographic classification of ductal anatomy based on the initial description by Krichencko. Left angiograms of different types of PDAs with the sketches. Type A ("conical") ductus, with wider diameter of aortic ampulla and gradual tapering with narrowest diameter at the pulmonary artery end, giving a conical appearance (A). Type B ("window") ductus, with a length of ductus less than 2 to 3 mm (B). Type C ("tubular") ductus, a long tubular structure with no narrowing at either ends (C). Type D ("complex") ductus, ductus with narrowings at both ends and sometimes multiple throughout its length (D). Type E ("elongated") ductus, with a beaklike appearance with the constriction at the pulmonary remote from the anterior edge of the trachea." (*From* Krichenko A, Benson LN, Burrows P, et al. Angiographic classification of the isolated, persistently patent ductus arteriosus and implications for percutaneous catheter occlusion. Am J Cardiol 1989;63:877–9, with permission; and Schneider DJ, Moore JW. Patent ductus arteriosus. Circulation 2006;114:1875, with permission.)

and oxygenation of blood leads to a significant rise in arterial P_{O_2}. The oxygen inhibits muscle voltage-dependent potassium channels in the ductal smooth muscle cells, which leads to an influx and overload of calcium inside the cells and vasoconstriction.[23,24] The loss of placenta and functioning lung tissue with increased pulmonary blood flow leads to a marked reduction in the levels of circulating PGE_2 and the loss of opposing vasodilatory response. Hemodynamic changes with a drop in blood pressure within the lumen of the ductus further contribute to its functional closure.

After this constriction, the ductal endothelial cells detach; the subendothelial region swells, and smooth muscle cells migrate into the region. The innermost layer of smooth muscle cells and the endothelium suffer a significant hypoxic injury and release growth factors in response. The

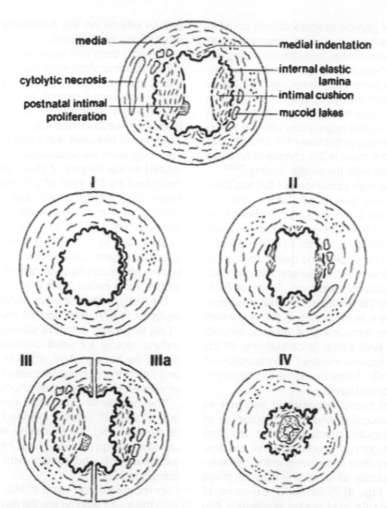

Fig. 4. Schematic presentation of the 4 maturational stages. Stage I, immature; Stage IIIa, patent ductal histology. (*From* Gittenberger-De Groot AC, Van Ertbruggen I, Moulaert AJ, et al. The ductus arteriosus in the preterm infant: histologic and clinical observations. J Pediatr 1980;96:89; with permission.)

growth factors stimulate endothelial proliferation, leading to extensive neointimal thickening and infolding followed by gradual cellular death and replacement by fibrous tissue.[25]

The duct will remain open if the normal response at birth is interrupted because of the developmental changes in the histopathologic architecture of the ductal tissue or changes in the oxygen tension at birth. However, the exact mechanisms as to why the duct will not close in some full-term infants remain unknown.

Epidemiology

Incidence

In normal term infants, the spontaneous closure of DA may be delayed until 3 months of life, after which the closure rate is less than 0.6% per year.[26] The duct may remain patent but very small to be clinically detected by murmur for the rest of life unless detected incidentally by echocardiography (silent PDA).[27] Therefore, the reported incidence of persistently patent PDA is variable and is estimated to be 1 in 2000 births, accounting for 5% to 10% of children born with congenital heart disease. The incidence will be more common (1 in 500), if the estimates of silent PDAs are included.[28,29] It is more common in female patients (F:M ratio ~2:1).

In contrast to term infants, in premature infants due to development immaturity of ductal tissue, closure during the postnatal period may be delayed up to 1 year and the incidence of PDA after 1 year may remain high.

Etiologic factors

PDAs in term infants are mostly sporadic in nature. Most cases are thought to be multifactorial with a combination of genetic predispositions coupled with critically timed environmental exposure, such as low oxygen tension due to asphyxia during delivery, rubella infection during pregnancy, or unknown viral infections and chemicals.[30,31] These findings are based on the epidemiologic studies of multifactorial mode of inheritance for the conditions that show familial aggregates with the recurrence rate in a sibling of between 1% and 5%. For a patient with PDA, there is 3% chance of finding a parent or a sibling with the similar finding.[30,32]

In addition, the high incidence of PDA has been observed in several genetic syndromes with defined abnormalities like chromosomal aberrations (such as trisomy 21), single-gene mutations (such as Holt-Oram syndrome), and some X-linked mutations, but to date no single gene defect specific for PDA has been identified.[32] Genetic research has identified the cause of syndromic forms of PDA, such as the TFAP2B mutations in Char syndrome with abnormalities in transcription factors, which interfere with the remodeling of vascular smooth muscle cells.[33] With better understanding of the genes and the factors involved in maturation of ductal muscle cells, future therapies can be developed to target ductal patency.

The most well-known association between an environmental exposure and a high incidence of PDA is the Rubella infection during the first trimester of pregnancy, particularly in the first 4 weeks,[34,35] resulting in an arrest in the development of the ductus at a very immature stage (stage 1) (see **Fig. 4**).[13] Similarly, exposure of the fetus to valporic acid during pregnancy has been associated with fetal valporate syndrome, which has a high incidence of PDA as a component.[36,37] The children born at high altitude and suffering asphyxia during delivery may carry a higher risk of PDA due to exposure to low oxygen tension.[38,39]

Natural history and pathophysiology

After birth, the ductal tissue constricts; the systemic resistance increases markedly as the placenta is disconnected from the systemic circulation, and the pulmonary vascular resistance decreases significantly over time.[40] Therefore, in patients with whom ductus remain persistently patent, the direction of flow is left to right and the amount of shunt is determined by the difference in systemic and pulmonary vascular resistance, but importantly, by the resistance to blood flow offered by residual diameter, geometry, and distensibility of the ductus.[41] In patients with PDA without any associated congenital heart defects the natural history and clinical manifestations are mainly related to the amount of shunted blood

and its effects on the pulmonary circulation and the left side of the heart.

In infants born with large unrestricted PDAs, the immediate and short-term mortalities are high and such patients are unlikely to be encountered by an adult cardiologist except for the survivors with Eisenmenger syndrome.[42] In most infants, the ductus is restrictive and a significant pressure gradient exists between aorta and pulmonary artery. The long-term hemodynamic consequences are related to the degree of shunt and the PDAs are described by the ratio of pulmonary (QP) to systemic (QS) arterial blood flow: small PDA with QP:QS <1.5 to 1, moderate PDA with QP:QS between 1.5 and 2.2 to 1, and large PDA being QP:QS >2.2 to 1.[43] A very small PDA where the shunt is minimal and there is no audible murmur, but the shunt can be detected on routine echocardiography is called silent PDA.[27]

Currently, with routine availability of echocardiography, early detection of moderate to large PDAs with early definitive closure has altered the natural history for adult cardiologists, who may encounter largely silent, small or moderate PDAs and rarely the occasional missed large PDAs with or without Eisenmenger syndrome.

The degree of pulmonary overcirculation and left ventricular volume overload in a small PDA is minimal and therefore the natural history is usually benign unless it is interrupted by an incidence of endarteritis with its associated complications.

In moderate and large PDAs, risks associated with the shunt volume are the development of progressive arterial changes in the pulmonary arteries with development of pulmonary hypertension and dilatation of the left atrium as well as left ventricle with eventual development of congestive heart failure.[44-46] The time course of these changes and onset of clinical symptoms are highly variable but patients may present usually with symptoms if detected for the first time in the third decade.[26] If pulmonary overcirculation remains uncorrected, the arteriolar medial hypertrophy, intimal proliferation, and eventual obliteration of pulmonary arterioles and capillaries will lead to an irreversible marked increase in pulmonary arterial pressure. When pulmonary vascular resistance exceeds the systemic vascular resistance, ductal shunting is reversed and becomes right to left (Eisenmenger syndrome).[42,46]

Clinical Manifestations

The clinical manifestations are largely dependent on the amount of extra blood recirculating in the pulmonary artery, capillaries, pulmonary veins, left atrium, left ventricle, ascending aorta, and the length of time the situation continues.

In large PDAs, the large volume of blood leads to the very early development of pulmonary congestion, decreased lung compliance, and failure of the left ventricle, often presenting within weeks after birth with failure to thrive, recurrent pulmonary infections, and even death. If patients survive, most of the cases will develop progressively severe pulmonary hypertension. Eisenmenger syndrome will present to the adult cardiologist with right-sided failure, exercise intolerance, and the lower extremity blueness.

Most patients with moderate left-to-right shunt compensate well throughout childhood and may remain completely asymptomatic in early adulthood but will eventually present with exercise intolerance and symptoms related to left ventricular failure, usually starting in the third decade.

Patients with a small PDA are usually asymptomatic throughout life and are brought to the attention of an adult cardiologist only during an echocardiographic evaluation of a heart murmur found during routine cardiac examination or diagnosed by echocardiography, computed tomography (CT), or magnetic resonance imaging (MRI) of the chest for an unrelated condition.[47]

Physical Examination

In patients with a small PDA, murmur is usually the only abnormal finding. Typically the description in an adult patient is a grade 2 to 3 continuous murmur, referred to as a machinery murmur with peaks around the second heart sound, heard best in the left infraclavicular area with radiation to the left sternal border and left interscapular area. The presence of a palpable thrill in the same region along with louder audible murmur indicates a moderate to large PDA. Larger blood flow from the left atrium to the left ventricle in diastole may give rise to a third heart sound with apical diastolic rumble. With a progressive increase in pulmonary vascular resistance, the diastolic component will gradually disappear and in patients with Eisenmenger syndrome no murmur is detected during systole or diastole because shunting is minimal and right to left with equal pressures in the pulmonary artery and aorta. However, due to pulmonary hypertension and right ventricular failure, pulmonary regurgitation and/or tricuspid regurgitation murmur may be detected.

The first heart sound in patients with PDA is normal and, depending on the degree of pulmonary hypertension, S2 may be split with an accentuated P2 component. The presence of a third heart sound indicates significant shunt volume.

Similarly, a wide pulse pressure with bounding pulses and displaced hyperdynamic apical impulse indicates significant left-to-right shunting seen in moderate to large PDA.

Patients presenting with Eisenmenger syndrome will have differential cyanosis more marked with exertion and clubbing characteristically in lower extremities and not in upper extremities due right to left shunting entering the descending aorta distal to the left subclavian artery in a typical case of isolated PDA.

Electrocardiogram

The electrocardiographic findings are nonspecific, usually normal in small PDA, and not useful in making the diagnosis of PDA. However, the presence of electrocardiographic findings of the left ventricular hypertrophy and left atrial enlargement indicate moderate or large PDA. The signs of right ventricular hypertrophy and right atrial enlargement indicate an advanced stage of severe irreversible pulmonary hypertension.

Chest Radiograph

In an adult patient with a small PDA, the chest radiograph will be normal. If the shunt volume is moderate to large, the chest radiograph shows increased pulmonary vascular markings with prominent ascending aorta, and enlarged cardiac silhouette with prominence of the left atrium, left ventricle. Peripheral pruning of vascular markings with large pulmonary arterial shadow and right pulmonary artery indicates severe pulmonary hypertension. In some older adult patients calcification of the ductus, especially in lateral chest radiograph, may be detected.

Echocardiogram

The diagnosis of PDA is suspected by clinical examination but transthoracic echocardiogram (TTE) is the procedure of choice to confirm the diagnosis and in some patients with no audible murmur (silent PDA) the only tool to detect the presence of PDA. Transesophageal echocardiogram is generally not necessary in most cases except sometimes to evaluate associated lesions.

TTE allows the assessment of ductal size, geometry, the degree of shunt, and pulmonary artery pressures.[48,49]

Most commonly, ductus can be detected in high parasternal short-axis view or suprasternal notch view by 2-dimensional imaging with superimposed color flow. Color flow Doppler is a very sensitive technique to detect even tiny ductus showing retrograde high-velocity flow entering the pulmonary artery trunk near the origin of the left pulmonary artery in a high left parasternal view. It is important to show the origin of the retrograde flow to aorta to differentiate it from other shunts like coronary to pulmonary fistulae. In addition, color flow imaging in the same views helps measure the diameter of the ductus and assess the geometry (**Fig. 5**).

The degree of shunt is indirectly estimated by the presence or absence of an enlarged left atrium or left ventricle and is used as a guide in the management of the patients (**Fig. 6**). In patients with small PDA with a shunt ratio less than 1.5, the left ventricular and left atrial size assessed by M-mode or 2-dimensional echocardiography will be normal and suggests a benign long-term outcome. In contrast, the mere presence of left atrial and left ventricular enlargement indicates significant shunt volume and dictates definitive therapy for the closure of PDA before the development of irreversible pulmonary hypertension. A left atrium/aorta ratio greater than 1.3/1 is considered to be a reliable marker of a hemodynamically significant ductal shunt.

Shunt ratio can also be calculated by measuring the right ventricular outflow area multiplied by the pulse Doppler-measured Time-Velocity Integral (TVI) at the site giving the systemic flow before shunting in the pulmonary artery and left ventricular outflow tract area and TVI giving the pulmonary blood flow.[50] However, because of errors in measurements in the areas, these calculations of shunt ratios have been found to be unreliable compared with direct measurements by cardiac catheterization.

Doppler echocardiography is helpful in the assessment of the pulmonary artery pressures and the degree of left-to-right shunt. In the absence of any detectable tricuspid regurgitation to measure right ventricular systolic pressure, the velocity of flow measured by continuous wave Doppler across the ductus gives the direct measurement of pulmonary artery systolic and diastolic pressures by subtracting the peak gradients from the simultaneously recorded aortic systolic and diastolic cuff pressures (**Fig. 7**). Geometry of ductus (longer and tortuous vessel) along with an incorrect angle of interrogation to the ductal flow will make the measurements less reliable and caution should be exercised in the interpretation.

Color Doppler shows the turbulence in both systole and diastole. The presence of bidirectional or pure right-to-left flow indicates elevated pulmonary artery pressures. In Eisenmenger patients, the PDA may be difficult to visualize, even if it is large due to a lack of significant flow across it with equalized pressures in the aorta and pulmonary artery. Echocardiographic features of enlargement of the right cardiac chambers, septal flattening, right ventricular hypertrophy, or high-velocity tricuspid and/or pulmonary regurgitation should be a prompt to look for a PDA.

CT and MRI

When questions exist after TTE, CT or MRI can be used in adult patients with PDA in whom surgical or percutaneous closure is planned to ascertain the size, geometry, and degree of calcification.[51,52] Routine evaluation by CT or MRI is not necessary. CT to detect calcification of the ductus in older individuals presenting with a large PDA is very useful in planning the type of surgical approach.[53–55]

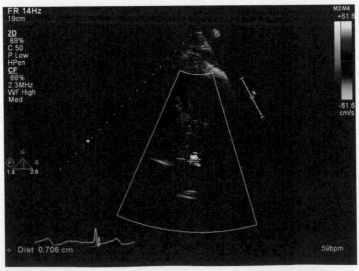

Fig. 5. High parasternal view with color flow imaging showing the size of the PDA.

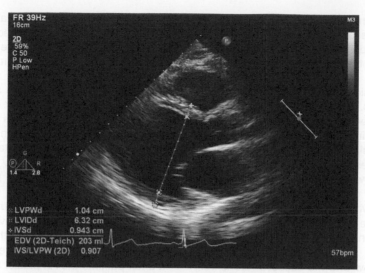

Fig. 6. Parasternal long-axis view showing increased left ventricular size in diastole.

Cardiac Catheterization

Diagnostic cardiac catheterization is not indicated for uncomplicated PDA with adequate noninvasive imaging (class III-B).[56] Cardiac catheterization in an adult patient with PDA is performed at the time of planned percutaneous closure in patients meeting the criteria after initial evaluation by TTE. Therefore patients with small or silent PDA do not need a catheterization. In patients with pulmonary hypertension detected by echocardiography or other clinical evaluations, catheterization is recommended to assess the degree of left-to-right shunt, pulmonary vascular resistance, and the reactivity to vasodilators or balloon occlusion of PDA before considerations for closure of the PDA.[57]

Management

The first decision in the management of an adult patient with PDA is whether to close the ductus or follow the patient with repeat assessments.

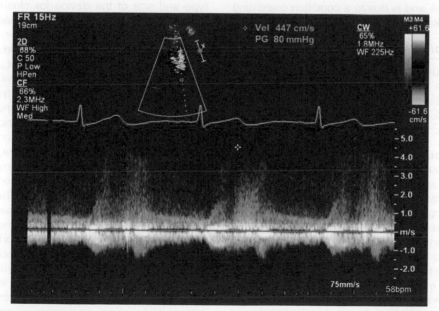

Fig. 7. Continuous wave Doppler along the axis of the PDA flow in both systole and diastole and the peak gradient of 80 mm Hg (by simplified Bernoulli equation, $4v^2$). This gradient is subtracted from the systolic cuff pressure to yield systolic PA pressure. High velocities by Doppler through ductus mean low pulmonary artery pressures.

The current American College of Cardiology/ American Heart Association and European Society of Cardiology guidelines suggest to close almost all PDAs except the small, silent ducti with no audible murmurs and patients with pulmonary arterial hypertension (PAH) with net right-to-left shunting (class III).[56,57] The class I indications are (1) shunt associated with evidence of volume overload on the left atrium or left ventricle (left atrium or left ventricular enlargement); (2) development of PAH but the pressure and the resistance still remain less than two-thirds of the systemic levels; (3) prior history of endarteritis.

Small PDAs with normal PA pressures and normal heart size with a shunt ratio less than 1.5/1 can be considered for closure (class IIa) because the risk associated with percutaneous closure is very low and the success rate is very high or can be followed with repeat evaluations every 3 to 5 years. The dilemma exists regarding the risks associated in patients with severe PAH with pulmonary pressures more than two-thirds of the systemic levels or even equal to systemic pressures. In such cases ductus can be closed with caution if the net shunt still remains left to right with QP/QS ratio greater than 1.5/1 or one can demonstrate reduction in PA pressures with vasodilator therapy (NO vascular reactivity) or by balloon occlusion at the time of cardiac catheterization (Class IIa). Small studies have shown that over time the pulmonary arterial pressures will regress but concern still remains if PAH is unrelated to PDA and is due to a condition coexisting with PDA like primary PAH.[58,59]

Methods of PDA Closure

The adult ductal tissue has no response to COX inhibitors like indomethacin in adult PDA patients unlike in infants. Therefore, the 2 primary modes of closure for PDA remain percutaneous or surgical approaches.

Percutaneous Methods

Percutaneous closure of the PDA is the preferred method in adult patients (class I)[56,57] as surgery in adults carries an increased perioperative risk due to ductal friability, calcification, and associated comorbid conditions like coronary artery disease or aortic atherosclerosis. Device closure is the method of choice, even if cardiac surgeries are needed for other associated cardiac lesions.

The first experience of transcatheter closure of the PDA was reported by Portsmann and co-workers in 1967,[60] followed by Rashkind and Cuaso[61] in 1979 with the use of a double-umbrella device. After US Food and Drug Administration approval of the Amplatzer duct occluder

device in 2003 based on data from multicenter registry,[62] the 2 commonly used devices to close PDAs in the United States are the coils in PDA less than 3 mm size and Amplatzer duct occluders for PDAs between 3 and 12 mm (see Fig. 9).[63] In type B PDAs with a length less than 3 mm, closure with Amplatzer (St. Jude Medical Inc, MN) septal occluder has been reported.[64] Additional sizes up to 16 mm are available for countries outside the United States. As ductal geometry and size are extremely variable, the new devices, like ADO II (St. Jude Medical Inc, MN), are undergoing trials.

The basic technique for percutaneous closure of PDA is to cross it with a delivery catheter from either the pulmonary artery or the aorta and place the coils or the occluder devices along its length. In adult patients the Amplatzer duct occluder has become the device of choice for moderate to large-sized PDA. The procedure is performed under conscious sedation and local anesthesia with a 7-Fr sheath placed in the femoral vein and 5- to 6-F sheath in the femoral artery. Initially the pressure measurements and oxygen saturations are obtained from the right and left sides of the heart to calculate the pulmonary and systemic blood flows to determine the pulmonary as well as systemic vascular resistances. Subsequently, an aortic angiogram is performed in a 90° lateral projection with a pigtail catheter in the proximal descending aorta (Fig. 8) to ascertain the size and shape of the PDA to select the appropriate type and size of the device for closure. For the most common type A PDA, the measurements obtained are the narrowest diameter, the length from pulmonary end to aortic end and the vertical length of the ampulla. The size of the device selected is usually 2 mm larger at the pulmonary end than the narrowest diameter of the PDA.

Using a multipurpose catheter and the wire, PDA is crossed across from the pulmonary artery and the catheter is advanced into the distal descending aorta. Using a stiff guide wire, PDA delivery sheath is exchanged for the multipurpose catheter. The selected device attached to the delivery cable is slowly advanced to the tip of the sheath and the retention disc is exposed by pulling back on the sheath. The sheath and the device are now pulled back together into the aortic ampulla. With the retention disc firmly secured in the ampulla, the sheath is retracted to place the remaining part of the device along the length of the PDA. After 10 minutes, with the delivery cable still attached, an aortic angiogram is performed to confirm the device position as well as the residual shunt (Fig. 9). If the results are satisfactory, the device is released and the cable is pulled back into

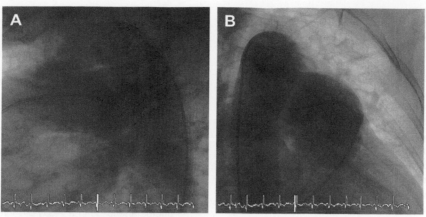

Fig. 8. An aortic angiogram showing the type A PDA in (*A*) 90° lateral projection. (*B*) Simultaneous RAO 32° projection.

the delivery sheath and the delivery system is removed. A repeat aortogram 10 to 15 minutes after the release may be optional to reaffirm immediate device stability.

The patient is usually observed overnight and discharged the following day after confirming the device position by chest radiograph and TTE. Along with periodic clinical follow-up, at 6 months after the procedure, a TTE is performed to document complete closure of the PDA. If any residual shunt is still detectable by echocardiography, it should be repeated at 1 year. Subacute bacterial endocarditis prophylaxis is recommended for a minimum of 6 months and it is advisable to be continued until complete closure is documented.

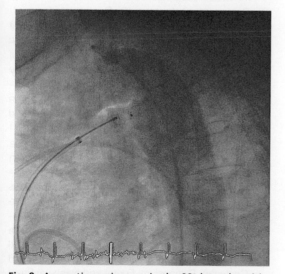

Fig. 9. An aortic angiogram in the 90° lateral position showing delivery cable still attached, PDA device well secured, and minimal residual shunt.

The evidence on the efficacy of percutaneous closure devices for PDA primarily consists of a clinical series and a small number of nonrandomized comparative studies.[62,65,66] Overall the implantation success rate of ADO is 99% with immediate closure at the time of implantation of 76%, at day 1 of 89%, and at 6 to 12 months of 99% by echocardiography. Major complications are extremely uncommon with mortality in 1 out of 439 cases. In the pivotal registry the major events were reported in 2.3% (10/439) of patients with device embolization in 2/439 patients. Most of the patients are discharged home within 24 hours.[62]

Given the variations in PDA configurations and sizes, Amplatzer duct occluder is not the optimal device for closure of all PDAs. However, the modifications in the Amplatzer device currently being tested and other new devices being developed will certainly allow for the percutaneous management of PDAs in most patients.

Surgical approaches

Surgical ligation had been the gold standard for PDA treatment since it was introduced in 1939 by Gross and Hubbard.[67] However, with the availability of safer catheter-based therapy, surgery is reserved for rare cases of very large PDA, unusual ductal anatomy like ductal aneurysm, or significant endarteritis/abscess at the site of PDA, making them unsuitable for percutaneous closure.[56] The approaches can be via lateral thoracotomy, median sternotomy, or video-assisted thoracoscopic ligation.[68–71] Successful closure rate is almost 100% but the morbidity of surgery is higher and the length of stay is longer compared with percutaneous closure.[70] Complications of surgery include injury to recurrent laryngeal nerve or phrenic nerve.

Long-term Management

In patients with silent PDA, no routine follow-up evaluation or endocarditis prophylaxis is indicated.[71]

In patients with small PDA with a shunt ratio less than 1.5 to 1 without evidence of left atrial or ventricular enlargement by TTE, it is reasonable to follow them without closure at 3- to 5-year intervals with repeat TTE evaluation.[56] Patients who undergo percutaneous closure with no residual shunt after 6 months do not need any further regular follow-up.

Patients with moderate-to-large PDAs who are treated for signs of congestive heart failure and/or left-sided volume overload may remodel left ventricularsize; however, these patients may require repeat evaluation and management of left ventriculardysfunction even after successful percutaneous or surgical closure. Similarly, patients presenting with pulmonary hypertension may not regress the pulmonary arterial changes and should be followed in specialized adult congenital clinics with pulmonary hypertension specialists at regular intervals with current pulmonary hypertension management strategies as required. Patients with Eisenmenger syndrome must be followed by adult congenital heart disease specialists.

Current guidelines do not recommend antibiotic prophylaxis for uncorrected PDA. However, antibiotic prophylaxis is recommended for both surgical closure and percutaneous closure for 6 months after the procedure if the complete closure is documented by TTE at 6 months. Patients with residual shunt detected by TTE will continue to require future subacute bacterial endocarditis prophylaxis.[72]

REFERENCES

1. Groshong SD, Tomashefski JF, Cool CD. Pulmonary vascular disease. In: Tomashefski JF Jr, editor. Dail and Hammar's pulmonary Pathology, 3rd edition, vol. 1. 2008. p. 1033.
2. Abdulla R, Blew GA, Holterman MJ. Cardiac embryology. Pediatr Cardiol 2004;25:191–200.
3. Krichenko A, Benson LN, Burrows P, et al. Angiographic classification of the isolated, persistently patent ductus arteriosus and implications for percutaneous catheter occlusion. Am J Cardiol 1989;63:877–9.
4. Berning RA, Silverman NH, Villegas M, et al. Reversed shunting across the ductus arteriosus or atrial septum in utero heralds severe congenital heart disease. J Am Coll Cardiol 1996;27:481–6.
5. Hinton R, Michelfelder E. Significance of reverse orientation of the ductus arteriosus in neonates with pulmonary outflow tract obstruction for early intervention. Am J Cardiol 2006;97:716–9.
6. Jan SL, Whang B, Fu JW, et al. Isolated neonatal ductus arteriosus aneurysm. J Am Coll Cardiol 2002;39:342–8.
7. Dyamenahalli U, Smallhorn JF, Geva T, et al. Isolated ductus arteriosus aneurysm in the fetus and infant: a multi-institutional experience. J Am Coll Cardiol 2000;36:262–9.
8. Rutishauser M, Ronen G, Wyler F. Aneurysm of the nonpatent ductus arteriosus in the newborn. Acta Paediatr Scand 1977;66:649–51.
9. Berger M, Ferguson C, Hendry J. Paralysis of the left diaphragm, left vocal cord, and aneurysm of the ductus arteriosus in a 7-day-old infant. J Paediatr 1960;56:800–2.
10. Roughneen PT, Parikh P, Stark J. Bronchial obstruction secondary to aneurysm of a persistent ductus arteriosus. Eur J Cardiothorac Surg 1996; 10:146–7.
11. Achiron R, Rotstein Z, Heggesh J, et al. Anomalies of the fetal aortic arch: a novel sonographic approach to in-utero diagnosis. Ultrasound Obstet Gynecol 2002;20(6):553–7.
12. Backer CL, Ilbawi MN, Idriss FS, et al. Vascular anomalies causing tracheoesophageal compression. Review of experience in children. J Thorac Cardiovasc Surg 1989;97(5):725–31.
13. Gittenberger-de Groot AC, Moulaert AJ, Hitchcock JF. Histology of the persistent ductus arteriosus in cases of congenital rubella. Circulation 1980;62:183–6.
14. Gittenberger-De Groot AC, Van Ertbruggen I, Moulaert AJ, et al. The ductus arteriosus in the preterm infant: histologic and clinical observations. J Pediatr 1980;96:88–93.
15. Desligneres S, Larroch JC. Ductus arteriosus, 1: anatomical and histologic study of its development during the second half of gestation and its closure after birth; 2: histological study of a few cases of patent ductus arteriosus in infancy. Biol Neonate 1970;16:278–96.
16. Silver MM. The morphology of the human newborn ductus arteriosus: a reappraisal of its structure and closure with special reference to prostaglandin E1 therapy. Hum Pathol 1981;12:1123–36.
17. Heymann MA, Rudolf AM. Control of the ductus arteriosus. Physiol Rev 1975;55:62–78.
18. Coceani F, Olley PM. The response of the ductus arteriosus to prostaglandins. Can J Physiol Pharmacol 1973;51:220–5.
19. Heymann MA, Creasy RK, Rudolph AM. Quantitation of blood flow patterns in the foetal lamb in utero. In: Proceedings of the Sir Joseph Barcroft Centenary Symposium: Foetal and Neonatal Physiology. Cambridge (United Kingdom): Cambridge University Press; 1973. p. 129–35.

20. Reed KL, Meijboom EJ, Sahn DJ, et al. Cardiac Doppler flow velocities in human fetuses. Circulation 1986;73:41–6.

21. Leonhardt A, Glaser A, Wegmann M, et al. Expression of prostanoid receptors in human ductus arteriosus. Br J Pharmacol 2003;138:655–9.

22. Bhattacharya M, Asselin P, Hardy P, et al. Developmental changes in prostaglandin E(2) receptor subtypes in porcine ductus arteriosus. Possible contribution in altered responsiveness to prostaglandin E(2). Circulation 1999;100:1751–6.

23. Michelakis E, Rebeyka I, Bateson J, et al. Voltage-gated potassium channels in human ductus arteriosus. Lancet 2000;356:134–7.

24. Fay FS. Guinea pig ductus arteriosus. I. Cellular and metabolic basis for oxygen sensitivity. Am J Physiol 1971;221:470–9.

25. Fay FS, Kooke PH. Guinea pig ductus arteriosus, II: irreversible closure after birth. Am J Physiol 1972; 222:841–9.

26. Campbell M. Natural history of persistent ductus arteriosus. Br Heart J 1968;30:4–13.

27. Hammerman C, Strates E, Valaitis S. The silent ductus: its precursors and its aftermath. Pediatr Cardiol 1986;7(3):121–7.

28. Mitchell SC, Korones SB, Berendes HW. Congenital heart disease in 56,109 births: incidence and natural history. Circulation 1971;43:323–32.

29. Hoffman JI, Kaplan S. The incidence of congenital heart disease. J Am Coll Cardiol 2002;39:1890–900.

30. Nora JJ. Multifactorial inheritance hypothesis for the etiology of congenital heart diseases: the genetic-environmental interaction. Circulation 1968;38:604–17.

31. Mani A, Meraji S, Houshyar R, et al. Finding genetic contributions to sporadic disease: a recessive locus at 12q24 commonly contributes to patent ductus arteriosus. Proc Natl Acad Sci U S A 2002;99:15054–9.

32. Schneider DJ, Moore JW. Patent ductus arteriosus. Circulation 2006;114:1873–82.

33. Satoda M, Zhao F, Diaz GA, et al. Mutations in TFAP2B cause Char syndrome, a familial form of patent ductus arteriosus. Nat Genet 2000;25: 42–6.

34. Swan C, Tostevin AL, Black GH. Final observations on congenital defects in infants following infectious disease during pregnancy with special reference to rubella. Med J Aust 1946;2:889–908.

35. Gibson S, Lewis K. Congenital heart disease following maternal rubella during pregnancy. Am J Dis Child 1952;83:117–9.

36. Anoop P, Sasidharan CK. Patent ductus arteriosus in fetal valproate syndrome. Indian J Pediatr 2003; 70:681–2.

37. Kini U. Fetal valproate syndrome: a review. Paediatr Perinat Drug Ther 2006;7(3):123–30.

38. Alzamora-Castro V, Battilana G, Abugattas R, et al. Patent ductus arteriosus and high altitude. Am J Cardiol 1960;5:761–3.

39. Olley PM. The ductus arteriosus, its persistence and its patency. In: Anderson RH, Shinebourne EA, Macartney FJ, et al, editors. Paediatric Cardiology. Edinburgh (United Kingdom): Churchill Livingstone; 1987. p. 931–58.

40. Evans NJ, Archer LN. Postnatal circulatory adaptation in healthy term and preterm neonates. Arch Dis Child 1990;65(1):24–6.

41. Tomita H, Fuse S, Hatakeyama K, et al. Epinephrine-induced constriction of the persistent ductus arteriosus and its relation to distensibility. Jpn Circ J 1998;62:913–4.

42. Blount SG, Vogel JH. Pulmonary hypertension. In: Moss AJ, Adams FH, editors. Heart disease in infants, children and Adolescents. Baltimore (MD): Williams and Wilkins; 1968. p. 947.

43. Braunwald E, editor. Braunwald's heart disease. Philadelphia: Saunders Elsevier; 2008. p. 1585–6.

44. Marquis RM, Miller HD, McCormack RJ, et al. Persistence of ductus arteriosus with left to right shunt in the older patient. Br Heart J 1982;48: 469–84.

45. Espino-Vela J, Cardenas N, Cruz R. Patent ductus arteriosus with special reference to patients with pulmonary hypertension. Circulation 1968;38(Suppl V): V45–60.

46. Bessinger FB Jr, Blieden LC, Edwards JE. Hypertensive pulmonary vascular disease associated with patent ductus arteriosus: primary or secondary? Circulation 1975;52:157–61.

47. Goitein O, Fuhrman CR, Lacomis JM. Incidental finding on MDCT of patent ductus arteriosus: use of CT and MRI to assess clinical importance. Am J Roentgenol 2005;184(6):1924–31.

48. Becker TE, Ensing GJ, Darragh RK, et al. Doppler derivation of complete pulmonary artery pressure curves in patent ductus arteriosus. Am J Cardiol 1996;78:1066–9.

49. Silverman NH. Pediatric echocardiography. Baltimore (MD): Williams & Wilkins; 1993. p. 173.

50. Hiraishi S, Horiguchi Y, Misawa H, et al. Noninvasive Doppler echocardiographic evaluation of shunt flow dynamics of the ductus arteriosus. Circulation 1987;75(6):1146–53.

51. Morgan-Jughes GJ, Marshall AJ, Roobottome C. Morphologic assessment of patent ductus arteriosus in adults using retrospectively ECG-gated multidetector CT. Am J Roentgenol 2003;181: 749–54.

52. Brenner LD, Caputo GR, Mostbeck G, et al. Quantification of left to right atrial shunts with velocity-encoded cine nuclear magnetic resonance imaging. J Am Coll Cardiol 1992;20: 1246–50.

53. John S, Muralidharan S, Jairaj PS, et al. The adult ductus: review of surgical experience with 131 patients. J Thorac Cardiovasc Surg 1981;82:314–9.

54. Fisher RG, Moodie DS, Sterba R, et al. Patent ductus arteriosus in adults–long-term follow-up: nonsurgical versus surgical treatment. J Am Coll Cardiol 1986;8:280–4.

55. Ng AS, Vlietstra RE, Danielson GK, et al. Patent ductus arteriosus in patients more than 50 years old. Int J Cardiol 1986;11:277–85.

56. Warnes CA, Williams RG, Bashore TM, et al. ACC/AHA 2008 guidelines for the management of adults with congenital heart disease. Circulation 2008; 118:e714–833.

57. Baumgartner H, Bonhoeffer P, et al. ESC Guidelines for the management of grown-up congenital heart disease (new version 2010). Eur Heart J 2010;31:2915–57.

58. Bhalgat PS, Pinto R, Dalvi BV. Transcatheter closure of large patent ductus arteriosus with severe pulmonary arterial hypertension: short and intermediate term results. Ann Pediatr Cardiol 2012;5(2):135–40.

59. Zhang CJ, Huang YG, Huang XS, et al. Transcatheter closure of large patent ductus arteriosus with severe pulmonary arterial hypertension in adults: immediate and two-year follow-up results. Chin Med J (Engl) 2012;125(21):3844–50.

60. Portsmann W, Wierny L, Warnke H. Closure of persistent ductus arteriosus without thoracotomy. Ger Med Mon 1967;12:259–61.

61. Rashkind WJ, Cuaso CC. Transcatheter closure of a patent ductus arteriosus: successful use in a 3.5-kg infant. Pediatr Cardiol 1979;1:3–7.

62. Pass RH, Hijazi Z, Hsu DT, et al. Multicenter USA Amplatzer patent ductus arteriosus occlusion device trial: initial and one-year results. J Am Coll Cardiol 2004;44:513–9.

63. Wang JK, Hwang JJ, Chiang FT, et al. A strategic approach to transcatheter closure of patent ductus: Gianturco coils for small-to-moderate ductus

and Amplatzer duct occluder for large ductus. Int J Cardiol 2006;106(1):10–5.

64. Fatema NN. Closure of large patent ductus arteriosus in a Patient with Severe Pulmonary Hypertention by Amplatzer Septal Occluder (ASO) - A Case Report. J Armed Forces Med Coll, Bangladesh 2009;5(1). p. 46–48.

65. Wang JK, Wu MH, Hwang JJ, et al. Transcatheter closure of moderate to large patent ductus arteriosus with the Amplatzer duct occluder. Catheter Cardiovasc Interv 2007;69(4):572–8.

66. Chen ZY, Wu LM, Luo YK, et al. Comparison of long-term clinical outcome between transcatheter Amplatzer occlusion and surgical closure of isolated patent ductus arteriosus. Chin Med J (Engl) 2009;122(10):1123–7.

67. Gross RE, Hubbard JP. Surgical Ligation of a Patent Ductus Arteriosus: Report of First Successful Case. JAMA 1939;112(8):729–31.

68. Chen H, Weng G, Chen Z, et al. Comparison of long-term clinical outcomes and costs between video-assisted thoracoscopic surgery and transcatheter amplatzer occlusion of the patent ductus arteriosus. Pediatr Cardiol 2012;33(2):316–21.

69. Hongxin L, Wenbin G, Zhu M, et al. New minimally invasive technique of perpulmonary device closure of patent ductus arteriosus through a parasternal approach. Ann Thorac Surg 2012;93(3): 862–8.

70. Toda R, Moriyama Y, Yamashita M, et al. Operation for adult patent ductus arteriosus using cardiopulmonary bypass. Ann Thorac Surg 2000;70(6): 1935–7.

71. Mavroudis C, Backer CL, Gevitz M. Forty-six years of patient ductus arteriosus division at Children's Memorial Hospital of Chicago. Standards for comparison. Ann Surg 1994;220(3):402–9.

72. Nishimura RA, Carabello BA, Faxon DP, et al. ACC/AHA 2008 guideline update on valvular heart disease: focused update on infective endocarditis. Circulation 2008;118:887–96.

Percutaneous Paravalvular Leak Closure

Robert Kumar, MD, Vladimir Jelnin, MD, Chad Kliger, MD,
Carlos E. Ruiz, MD, PhD*

KEYWORDS

- Percutaneous closure • Prosthetic valve • Paravalvular regurgitation • Congestive heart failure
- Hemolytic anemia

KEY POINTS

- Percutaneous closure of paravalvular leaks in symptomatic patients offers a less-invasive option than surgical reoperation, with lower procedural morbidity.
- Preprocedural planning and intraprocedural guidance with multimodality imaging techniques, including 3-dimensional (3D) transesophageal echocardiography and 3D/4D computed tomography angiography are keys to procedural success.
- Technical success is facilitated by operator experience and comfort with antegrade transseptal, retrograde aortic, and transapical access.
- Familiarity with the full range of available closure devices allows optimal devices selection for patient-specific anatomy.
- Complication rates are low at experienced centers, but prompt recognition and management of potential complications are important when performing percutaneous paravalvular leak closure.

INTRODUCTION

Prosthetic paravalvular leaks (PVLs) are a known complication of surgical valve replacement that may present as anywhere from an incidental imaging finding to severely symptomatic paravalvular regurgitation requiring urgent treatment. PVLs may occur in up to 12% of patients after valve replacement. They are the primary reason for reoperation in 5% to 9% of patients, and are second only to valve degeneration as a cause for reoperation.[1,2] As an alternative to surgical reoperation for PVLs, percutaneous closure of PVLs has emerged as a less-invasive technique that is being performed with increasing frequency worldwide, and may offer comparable rates of success with lower procedural morbidity.[3–6] This article reviews PVLs as a complication of surgical valve replacement, and the most recent developments in transcatheter techniques for PVL closure.

PATHOGENESIS OF SURGICAL PVLS

PVLs occur because of a separation of the prosthetic valve or ring from the adjacent tissue of the mitral or aortic annulus, and may develop during the immediate postoperative period and up to several years after valve implantation. PVLs may result early after valve implantation from factors such as local calcification or technical difficulties during surgery, or later from endocarditis, gradual resorption of calcified tissue, and dynamic forces exerted on the prosthesis during the cardiac cycle.[7,8] PVLs occur with similar frequency with both mitral and aortic prostheses, and up to 74% occur within the first year of valve implantation.[9]

Disclosures: The authors have nothing to disclose.
Department of Structural and Congenital Heart Disease, Lenox Hill Heart and Vascular Institute, North Shore/LIJ Health System, 130 East 77th Street, 9th Floor Black Hall, New York, NY 10021-10075, USA
* Corresponding author.
E-mail address: cruiz@nshs.edu

cardiology.theclinics.com

CLINICAL PRESENTATION AND DIAGNOSIS

Many PVLs are asymptomatic, but some patients may present with heart failure, hemolysis, or a combination of both. On physical examination, a regurgitation murmur may be present, with location, pitch, and intensity varying with the position and trajectory of the regurgitant jet. Mitral PVLs can be heard as a holosystolic murmur, usually at the left sternal border or in the midaxillary line. Aortic PVLs may be heard as a diastolic decrescendo murmur along the left sternal border. If a PVL is suspected based on symptoms or physical examination, additional laboratory and imaging studies may confirm the diagnosis. In patients with heart failure, brain natriuretic peptide levels may be elevated, and a chest radiograph may show pulmonary congestion or pleural effusion. In patients with hemolysis, l-lactate dehydrogenase (LDH) levels are elevated (>460 U/L); levels greater than 1000 U/L may be present with severe hemolysis.[10] Peripheral blood smear may show schistocytes because of red blood cell fragmentation through a high-velocity paravalvular regurgitant jet. New renal failure may be present with significant hemolysis caused by hemosiderin deposits in renal glomeruli, and may be reversible with resolution of the hemolysis.[11,12]

RATIONALE FOR PERCUTANEOUS PVL CLOSURE

When PVLs are symptomatic, medical therapy consisting of diuretics and afterload reduction can be used to treat heart failure. Hemolysis may be treated with a combination of iron, folate, and vitamin B_{12} supplements; erythropoietin injection; and packed-red blood cell transfusions in severe cases.[13] However, these measures may not completely relieve symptoms, and patients may experience progressive heart failure and/or continued hemolysis. The goal of percutaneous closure, therefore, is to reduce or eliminate paravalvular regurgitation to alleviate heart failure and hemolysis and avoid progressive ventricular dysfunction.

DIAGNOSTIC IMAGING

Echocardiography, including transthoracic echocardiography (TTE) and transesophageal echocardiography (TEE), and cardiac computed tomographic angiography (CTA) are the major imaging modalities used to diagnose and characterize PVLs and aid in procedural guidance at most centers. Cineangiography may provide additional diagnostic information and procedural guidance in the catheterization laboratory. To describe the location of the PVL on imaging

studies and in the catheterization laboratory, the authors' center uses a clock-face approach. In this scheme, the 12 o'clock position is at the mitral-aortic continuity, such that the 12 o'clock positions of the mitral and aortic valves are adjacent. The hours are numbered according to a surgical view of the valves, as shown in **Fig. 1**. For the aortic valve, the left coronary cusp extends from 12 to 4 o'clock, the right coronary cusp extends from 4 to 8 o'clock, and the noncoronary cusp extends from 8 to 12 o'clock, approximately. For the mitral valve, the left atrial appendage corresponds to the 9 o'clock position, the mitral-aortic continuity is at 12 o'clock, and the interatrial septum is adjacent to the 3 o'clock position. A scheme such as this facilitates accurate communication between all physicians involved in the procedure, and other schemes may be used by other centers, depending on preference.

ECHOCARDIOGRAPHY

TTE is often the initial imaging study during PVL assessment. Two-dimensional (2D) TTE with color Doppler imaging can identify the leak location and the possible presence of multiple leaks, assess chamber size and ventricular function, and evaluate the function of the prosthetic valve. In some cases, acoustic shadowing from the prosthetic valve may interfere with TTE assessment of the PVL, and TEE may provide superior characterization of the leak. The use of 3D TEE can further characterize the leak location, size, and severity (**Fig. 2**). Both qualitative and quantitative echocardiographic methods can be used to characterize PVLs. Because of the variable size, shape, and trajectory of PVLs, a single parameter may underestimate or overestimate the severity of regurgitation, and the use of multiple parameters in conjunction with the patient's clinical condition are important to correctly identify the severity and clinical importance of the leak. For aortic PVLs, the width and density of the regurgitant jet and jet deceleration time may provide semiquantitative evaluation of PVL severity, although eccentric jets may be difficult to assess because of off-axis measurement. If a proximal isovelocity surface area (PISA) shell is identifiable, regurgitant volume may be calculated to provide a quantitative measurement of PVL severity. Diastolic flow reversal in the descending aorta assessed by Doppler echocardiography may indicate severe paravalvular regurgitation, if present.[14] For mitral PVLs, the area of the regurgitant jet on 2D color Doppler imaging may estimate the severity of regurgitation. Measurement of the vena contracta

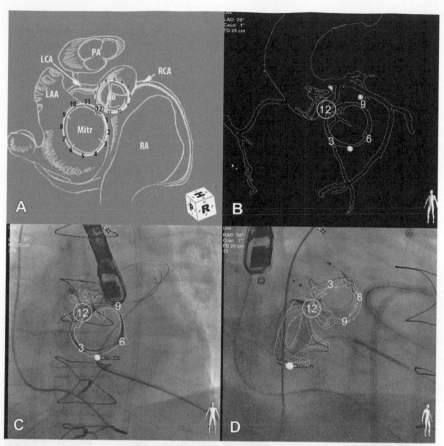

Fig. 1. Clock-face approach to PVL location. (*A*) Diagram of a surgical view of the exposed left atrium, showing the clock-face positions of the mitral and aortic valves. The mitral-aortic continuity is identified at the 12 o'clock position for the mitral and aortic valves. (*B*) Diagram of aortic and mitral prosthetic valves, aorta, and coronary arteries in a patient with a mitral PVL at the 4 o'clock position, as seen from a 29° left anterior oblique (LAO) view. (*C, D*) Fluoroscopic views of the same patient in Fig. 1B, in the anteroposterior (AP) and 50° right anterior oblique (RAO) views, respectively. The mitral (*C*) and aortic (*D*) clock-face positions are labeled. Ao, aorta; LAA, left atrial appendage; LCA, left coronary artery; Mitr, mitral valve; PA, pulmonary artery; RA, right atrium; RCA, right coronary artery.

width and calculation of the regurgitant volume can provide quantitative assessment of the severity of regurgitation.[15] A large PISA shell may correlate with the size of the PVL, although quantitative methods of assessing regurgitation have not been well validated for PVLs. Pulmonary vein flow reversal may be present with severe regurgitation.[14]

CTA AND COMPUTED TOMOGRAPHY–FLUOROSCOPY FUSION IMAGING

Cardiac CTA with 3D and 4D reconstruction provides excellent anatomic evaluation of PVLs. CTA can identify the leak location and size, assess for significant calcification within the track and in adjacent annular tissue, and assist in choosing the appropriate access route for closure (**Fig. 3**). The

recent development of computed tomography (CT)–fluoroscopy fusion imaging has allowed CT imaging to provide a valuable tool for guidance during percutaneous PVL closure.[5,16] With CT-fluoroscopy fusion, single-phase CT data are reconstructed into 3D images and are then segmented into the individual components of the cardiac and thoracic anatomy. The CT data are coregistered to fluoroscopy and the relevant structures, such as the cardiac chambers, valves, coronary arteries, and PVLs, are overlaid onto the fluoroscopy screen. The CT data remain merged to fluoroscopy with rotation of the C-arm, providing real-time 3D anatomic information during the procedure. CT-fluoroscopy fusion can facilitate access, wire crossing, and device deployment during PVL closure (**Figs. 4** and **5**). Currently, many catheterization laboratories may not be equipped

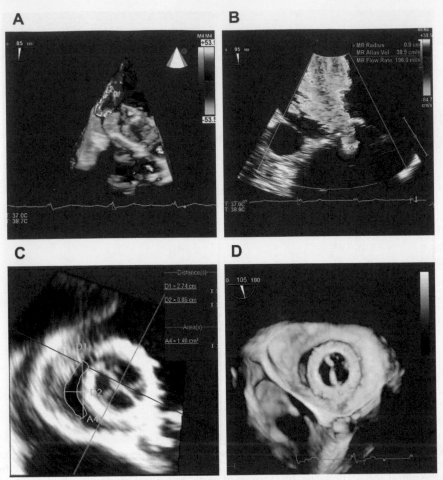

Fig. 2. Echocardiographic evaluation of a mitral PVL. (*A*) Three-dimensional color flow Doppler identifies para-valvular regurgitation and the annular location of the leak. (*B*) Two-dimensional color flow Doppler demon-strates flow through the PVL, and a proximal isovelocity surface area shell can be measured to estimate regurgitant volume. (*C, D*) Three-dimensional TEE evaluation of the PVL can further assess the size of the PVL, location around the prosthetic valve, and shape of the PVL to guide closure device selection.

with software for CT-fluoroscopy fusion, although commercially available software is available and may be used with increasing frequency in the future.

CLOSURE DEVICES

No devices for percutaneous PVL closure are approved by the US Food and Drug Administration. Currently, the most frequently used off-label devices for PVL closure in the United States are the Amplatzer family of devices (St. Jude Medical, St. Paul, MN, USA). These include the Amplatzer septal occluder (ASO), muscular VSD occluder (mVSD), ductal occluder (ADO), and vascular plugs II and IV (AVP-II and AVP-IV, respectively). These devices are constructed of nitinol and are circular in shape, with occlusive disks connected by a waist when 2 disks are present (ASO, mVSD, AVP-II), or a single disk attached to a cylindrical body in the case of the ADO. The AVP-IV consists of 2 conical-shaped pieces of nitinol mesh joined at the bases by a central articulation. Each device is available in multiple sizes. Outside the United States, the Amplatzer vascular plug III (AVP-III, CE marked in Europe) is an oblong-shaped device that may better conform to crescent- or oval-shaped PVLs. At the authors' institution, the AVP-II is currently the most frequently used device for PVL closure. Device selection is based on the size and shape of the leak and anatomic location, with the intent of oversizing the device to completely occlude the defect, without interference of mitral inflow, left ventricular outflow, or leaflet function. If using circular devices, larger leaks may be better occluded with

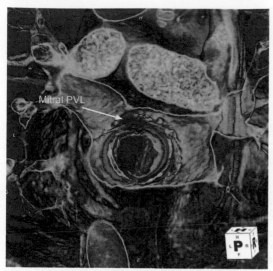

Fig. 3. Three-dimensional reconstructed CTA showing a mitral PVL. Cardiac CTA can provide reliable measurements of PVL size and location, and assessment of surrounding anatomy (mitral PVL, *white arrow*).

multiple smaller devices rather than a single larger device to achieve a closer approximation of a crescent- or irregularly shaped PVL, while avoiding valvular interference.[17] TEE or CTA imaging is used to identify the length and width of the PVL when choosing devices. The distance from the

PVL to the inner surface of the prosthetic frame or ring should be identified, and the devices should be selected accordingly to avoid extension beyond this point.[18] In the case of mechanical prosthetic valves, aggressive oversizing of a closure device may cause the device to extend beyond the inner edge of the prosthetic valve frame, resulting in obstruction of the prosthetic valve leaflet and significant valvular regurgitation or stenosis. Careful TEE examination should be performed before release to ensure adequate valvular function when closure devices are in place. TEE examination should be repeated after device release, because the position may shift slightly.

PATIENT PREPARATION

Percutaneous PVL closure in the cardiac catheterization laboratory is usually performed under general anesthesia for patient comfort and safety. The procedure may be lengthy, and prolonged TEE examination and possible management of complications are best handled while the patient is intubated. The authors recommend sterile surgical preparation and draping of the patient from neck to groin regardless of access route, with an antimicrobial incise drape applied to the chest if transapical access is performed. A well-functioning intravenous line or a venous sheath should be

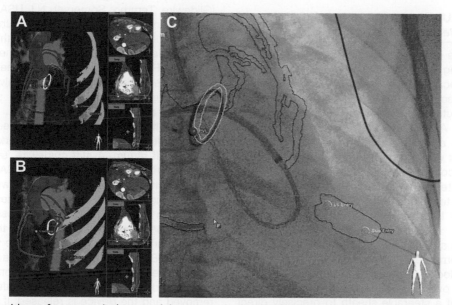

Fig. 4. CT guidance for transapical access. (*A*) CT data obtained before the procedure are reconstructed into 3D images. The intrathoracic structures are segmented (aorta and coronary arteries [*red*], ribs [*tan*], mitral prosthesis [*yellow*]). The mitral PVL (*red dot*) and planned skin and transapical puncture sites are marked (*green dots*). (*B*) A cylinder is constructed to connect the skin and transapical puncture sites (*purple*) in a line coaxial with the PVL. (*C*) The CT data are overlaid onto the live fluoroscopy screen and used to guide safe needle puncture of the left ventricular apex.

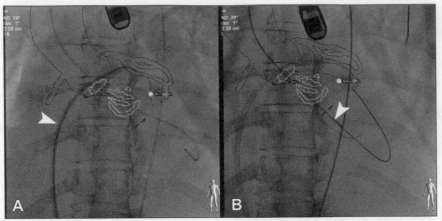

Fig. 5. Antegrade transseptal and retrograde aortic approaches for PVL closure in a patient with mitral and aortic PVLs, with CT-fluoroscopy fusion guidance. (*A*) A transseptal catheter is placed in the left atrium (*white arrowhead*). The PVL (*yellow dot*) has been crossed with a guidewire but cannot be advanced further because of tortuosity in the track. A second catheter is advanced across the aortic PVL (*red dot*) using a retrograde aortic approach and placed in the left ventricle. The outline of the aorta and coronary arteries in red are overlaid onto the fluoroscopy screen using CT-fluoroscopy fusion software (HeartNavigator, Phillips. Best, The Netherlands). (*B*) Through the catheter across the aortic PVL, the mitral PVL (*yellow dot*) is crossed retrograde with a guidewire (*white arrow head*). With the guidewire across both PVLs, a delivery sheath was advanced retrograde for sequential closure of the mitral and aortic PVLs.

placed at the start of the procedure, and an arterial line should be placed for monitoring. When available, procedures may be performed in a hybrid catheterization laboratory to facilitate surgical rescue in the event of a major complication.

TECHNIQUES FOR MITRAL PVL CLOSURE
Antegrade Transseptal Approach

Before the procedure, all echocardiographic and CT imaging studies should be reviewed to identify the leak location and review the surrounding anatomy. Based on the patient's specific anatomy and clinical factors, an initial access route should be planned. An antegrade transseptal approach combines a high degree of success in crossing the defect with the guidewire and a lower risk of bleeding complications than the retrograde transapical route. Transseptal access is obtained using standard techniques. For PVLs with a posterior or septal location (1–6 o'clock), a transseptal approach requires greater angulation of the guidewire after transseptal puncture to reach the defect compared with anterior and lateral PVLs (6–12 o'clock), and may be facilitated by a more posterior puncture of the interatrial septum and the use of a steerable sheath to precisely direct the guidewire toward the lesion, such as the Agilis sheath (St. Jude Medical, St. Paul, MN, USA) which may be flexed and rotated to probe the mitral annulus to locate the PVL. After obtaining transseptal access, heparin is administered to

achieve anticoagulation, with activated clotting times similar to those used for percutaneous coronary interventions. A 5 French catheter, such as a multipurpose, JR4, or Berenstein catheter (AngioDynamics, Latham, NY, USA), and a 0.035″ hydrophilic guidewire with an angled tip (Glidewire, Terumo, Somerset, NJ, USA) are telescoped through the transseptal sheath, and the mitral annulus is probed in the area of the PVL until the guidewire is advanced across the PVL (see **Fig. 5**A). TEE is then used to confirm the paravalvular course of the wire. When paravalvular location of the guidewire is confirmed, a delivery sheath is advanced across the PVL (**Fig. 6**A). One or multiple closure devices may be advanced into the left ventricle and the sheath is withdrawn into the left atrium. A stiff guidewire, such as an Inoue wire (Toray, New York, NY, USA), may be placed in the left ventricle as a safety wire (before withdrawing the sheath into the left atrium) in case the sheath must be readvanced across the PVL (see **Fig. 6**A). The closure devices are then pulled back toward the left atrium to occlude the defect (see **Fig. 6**B). TEE is used to assess the amount of residual regurgitation. If regurgitation is adequately reduced or eliminated, the safety wire is removed and the device is released. If the regurgitation is still significant, device position may be adjusted or the device may be removed and the process repeated with a different device or combination of devices until adequate reduction of regurgitation is achieved. After deploying the

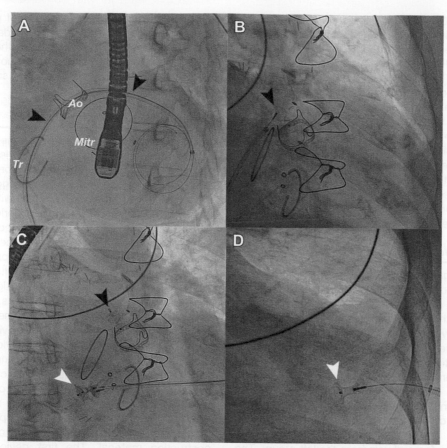

Fig. 6. Transseptal (*A, B*) and transapical (*C, D*) approaches to PVL closure in a patient with 2 mitral PVLs at 10 and 4 o'clock. (*A*) A transseptal catheter (*black arrowhead*) has been advanced across the 10 o'clock mitral PVL and placed in the left ventricle. The mitral prosthesis (Mitr), aortic prosthesis (Ao), and tricuspid annuloplasty ring (Tr) are visible on fluoroscopy. An AVP-II closure device and a stiff guidewire have been exteriorized into the left ventricle. (*B*) An AVP-II device is placed across the 10 o'clock mitral PVL (*black arrowhead*). (*C*) The 4 o'clock mitral PVL was crossed using a retrograde transapical approach, and 2 AVP-II devices are placed across the PVL (*white arrowhead*). The previously released AVP-II device across the 10 o'clock PVL is visible (*black arrowhead*). (*D*) An Amplatzer ductal occluder (ADO) is used to close the transapical puncture site after deployment of all PVL closure devices (*white arrowhead*).

closure device, TEE is used to confirm stability of device position and reassess valvular function. The sheath is then removed and a compressive mattress suture may be used for hemostasis of the femoral vein.

Retrograde Transapical Approach

The retrograde transapical approach for mitral PVLs provides the shortest and most direct route to approach the defect. This technique may be especially useful for posterior or septal PVLs, or cases in which closure of multiple PVLs at different locations around the prosthesis will be attempted. Preprocedural CTA is recommended for all transapical procedures, and is used to identify the puncture site at or near the left ventricular

apex such that it is coaxial to the defect and avoids puncture of the lung, right ventricle, papillary muscles, and coronary arteries during access.[19] The depth of the puncture site from the skin is identified, and longer needles may be used for transapical access in larger patients. The skin puncture site is approximated through palpation of the point of maximal intensity, and further identified on CTA in terms of distance from bony landmarks such as the ribs and sternum. Transapical access may be further facilitated by the use of CT-fluoroscopy fusion imaging, as described earlier (see **Fig. 4**). Once the operator has identified the skin puncture site, a 7-cm 21-gauge micropuncture needle is directed toward the left ventricle and intraventricular position is confirmed by contrast injection through the needle. A 0.018″ guidewire is advanced into the left ventricle and into the left atrium or aorta, and a 5 or 6 French radial sheath (Cook Medical, Bloomington, IL, USA) is advanced into the left ventricle. The sheath may be upsized as needed over a guidewire, and sheaths up to 12 French have been used with successful percutaneous closure of the entry site. Crossing of the defect, device deployment, and TEE assessment are performed using a similar technique as described earlier. After satisfactory device deployment (see **Fig. 6**C), the transapical access site is closed with the use of another Amplatzer device, usually an ADO or AVP-II device (see **Fig. 6**D). Larger sheath sizes may require a larger closure device.

Retrograde Aortic Approach

The retrograde aortic approach for mitral PVL closure is used infrequently because of the steep angulation required to direct the guidewire to the PVL from the left ventricle (see **Fig. 5**B). This technique may result in poor support for sheath advancement and device delivery. If the retrograde aortic approach is used, an arteriovenous rail is often created to facilitate device delivery. Formation of an arteriovenous rail is performed by obtaining transseptal access after the guidewire has crossed the PVL, and using a snare device to snare and exteriorize the guidewire through the femoral vein from the left atrium. The delivery sheath and device may then be delivered either retrograde or antegrade across the defect. During sheath advancement and device delivery, it is important to keep the guidewire looped in the left ventricle, because excessive tension on the wire may cause dysfunction and severe regurgitation of the mitral or aortic valve, which can be recognized by TEE.

Aortic PVLs

The fundamental technique for aortic PVL closure is similar to that for mitral PVLs, although specific factors for aortic leaks must be considered. At the authors' institution, the retrograde aortic approach is used most frequently (see **Fig. 4**B), followed by the antegrade transapical approach, and lastly the antegrade transseptal approach. When positioning closure devices across aortic PVLs, attention should be given to the prosthetic aortic valve leaflet function and the coronary arteries, because of the risk of interference with valve function or coronary flow by a closure device. Preprocedural CTA can identify the proximity of the PVL to the coronary arteries, and coronary angiography can be used during the procedure to assess coronary flow with the closure

devices in place. TEE assessment of prosthetic valve function during and after device deployment should be used to assess for prosthetic valve dysfunction. Creation of an arteriovenous rail, as described earlier, may provide extra support for device delivery.

Closure of Large PVLs

Smaller PVLs may be closed percutaneously with a single device in most cases. Larger leaks, however, may require 2 or more devices for adequate closure. If preprocedural imaging suggests that the leak may be inadequately closed with a single device, multiple devices can be exteriorized sequentially and pulled back simultaneously after the delivery sheath has been advanced through the defect. In some cases, the multiple devices may not adequately decrease regurgitation, and the devices may appear and feel tightly constrained within the PVL. In these cases, the presence of suture lines or tissue within the PVL may be preventing full expansion of the devices within the track of the defect. Individual device deployment on each side of the obstructing material may be required for adequate PVL closure. To facilitate this, a "hopscotch" technique can be performed. One device is first positioned across the PVL and, with the device not yet deployed, the PVL is crossed with a guidewire adjacent to the obstructing material. The first device is then released and the sheath is advanced across the PVL over the guidewire, adjacent to the first device. A second closure device is then positioned across the PVL and released. This process may be iterated until adequate closure is obtained.

Procedural Complications

Knowledge of potential complications and their management is essential when performing percutaneous PVL closure. The most frequent complications relate to device interference with the prosthetic valve, device embolization, and access-related bleeding complications.[5,6,18–22] Bileaflet and tilting-disk mechanical prosthetic valves present the highest risk of interference with closure devices. In some instances, the closure device may prohibit complete closure of a mechanical leaflet or disk, and lead to severe acute regurgitation. In other cases, a closure device may obstruct opening of the valve leaflet, which may lead to immediate hemodynamic instability. In either case, prompt recognition of leaflet dysfunction by TEE or fluoroscopy will allow device removal before deployment, and an alternative device may be used or the patient may require surgical PVL closure. Occasionally, the position of the closure device may shift immediately after deployment, and the device must be rapidly repositioned or removed. To remove a closure device, the authors use a Gooseneck snare (ev3 Endovascular, Plymouth, MN, USA) through a 6 French guide catheter to snare the pin of the closure device that was previously attached to the delivery cable.

Device embolization may occur if the closure device is undersized or deployed in an unstable position. In most cases, closure devices embolize to the iliac or femoral arteries, and can be located with fluoroscopy and retrieved using a Gooseneck snare or bioptome via femoral access. Device embolization is usually immediate, but can occur rarely up to several months after placement. The authors routinely perform CTA examination 6 months postprocedure to assess device stability.

If femoral access is used, bleeding complications from the arterial or venous access site may occur. If the transapical route is used, bleeding complications may include pericardial effusion, tamponade, or hemothorax.[23] Significant fluid accumulation may be seen on TEE in the pericardial or pleural space, and is treated with rapid placement of a pigtail drain in the pericardial or pleural space.

Less frequent procedural complications include coronary artery laceration or pneumothorax (with transapical access), coronary obstruction from closure devices, stroke, and air embolism. Worsening of hemolysis may occur postprocedure, and may decrease over time as the closure devices endothelialize. Reintervention or surgery may be necessary in some cases of severe hemolysis. Endocarditis of Amplatzer devices has also been reported after PVL closure.[20] Procedural death and the need for emergent cardiac surgery have each been reported to occur in up to 2% of cases.[5,6,19,20]

Outcomes with Percutaneous PVL Closure

Both technical success and clinical success with PVL closure have been reported. Technical success is typically defined as successful device deployment within the PVL, with improvement in regurgitation and lack of new prosthetic valve dysfunction. Clinical success is defined as improvement in congestive heart failure by at least 1 New York Heart Association grade and/or complete resolution of hemolysis. The largest reported series describe rates of technical success ranging from 77% to 86% and clinical success ranging from 67% to 77%.[5,6] The long-term outcomes in these series range from 86.5% survival at 18 months to an estimated survival of 64.3% at 3 years, with

lesser residual regurgitation associated with better long-term survival. Nonetheless, patients undergoing PVL closure are often of advanced age and have additional comorbidities, and noncardiac mortality is significant in these series.

SUMMARY

Percutaneous closure of PVLs in symptomatic patients offers a less-invasive option than surgical reoperation, with lower procedural morbidity. Newer imaging modalities, including 3D TEE and CTA with 3D/4D reconstruction, are important for preprocedural planning and intraprocedural guidance. Technical success is facilitated by operator experience, and may require the use of antegrade transseptal, retrograde aortic, or transapical access. Complication rates are low at experienced centers, but prompt recognition and management of potential complications is important when performing percutaneous PVL closure.

REFERENCES

1. Potter DD, Sundt TM 3rd, Zehr KJ, et al. Risk of repeat mitral valve replacement for failed mitral valve prostheses. Ann Thorac Surg 2004;78:67–72.
2. Bortolotti U, Milano A, Mossuto E, et al. The risk of reoperation in patients with bioprosthetic valves. J Card Surg 1991;6(Suppl 4):638–43.
3. Echevarria JR, Bernal JM, Rabasa JM, et al. Reoperation for bioprosthetic valve dysfunction. A decade of clinical experience. Eur J Cardiothorac Surg 1991;5:523–6.
4. Emery RW, Krogh CC, McAdams S, et al. Long-term follow up of patients undergoing reoperative surgery with aortic or mitral valve replacement using a St. Jude medical prosthesis. J Heart Valve Dis 2010; 19:473–84.
5. Ruiz CE, Jelnin V, Kronzon I, et al. Clinical outcomes in patients undergoing percutaneous closure of periprosthetic paravalvular leaks. J Am Coll Cardiol 2011;58:2210–7.
6. Sorajja P, Cabalka AK, Hagler DJ, et al. Long-term follow-up of percutaneous repair of paravalvular prosthetic regurgitation. J Am Coll Cardiol 2011; 58(21):2218–24.
7. De Cicco G, Russo C, Moreo A, et al. Mitral valve periprosthetic leakage: anatomical observations in 135 patients from a multicentre study. Eur J Cardiothorac Surg 2006;30(6):887–91.
8. Wasowicz M, Meineri M, Djaiani G, et al. Early complications and immediate postoperative outcomes of paravalvular leaks after valve replacement surgery. J Cardiothorac Vasc Anesth 2011;25:610–4.
9. Genoni M, Franzen D, Vogt P, et al. Paravalvular leak after mitral valve replacement: improved long-term

survival with aggressive surgery? Eur J Cardiothorac Surg 2000;17:14–9.

10. Skoularigis J, Essop MR, Skudicky D, et al. Frequency and severity of intravascular hemolysis after left-sided cardiac valve replacement with Medtronic hall and St. Jude medical prostheses, and influence of prosthetic type, position, size and number. Am J Cardiol 1993;71:587–91.

11. Qian Q, Nath KA, Wu Y, et al. Hemolysis and acute kidney failure. Am J Kidney Dis 2010;56(4):780–4.

12. Altarabsheh SE, Deo SV, Rihal CS, et al. Mitral paravalvular leak: caution in percutaneous occluder device deployment. Heart Surg Forum 2013;16(1):E21–3.

13. Shapira Y, Bairey O, Vatury M, et al. Erythropoietin can obviate the need for repeated heart valve replacement in high-risk patients with severe mechanical hemolytic anemia: case reports and literature review. J Heart Valve Dis 2001;10:431–5.

14. Zoghbi WA, Chambers JB, Dumesnil JG, et al. Recommendations for evaluation of prosthetic valves with echocardiography and Doppler ultrasound: a report from the American Society of Echocardiography's guidelines and standards committee and the task force on prosthetic valves. J Am Soc Echocardiogr 2009;22:975–1014.

15. Kronzon I, Sugeng L, Perk G, et al. Real-time 3-dimensional transesophageal echocardiography in the evaluation of post-operative mitral annuloplasty ring and prosthetic valve dehiscence. J Am Coll Cardiol 2009;53:1543–7.

16. Krishnaswamy A, Tuzcu EM, Kapadia SR. Three-dimensional computed tomography in the cardiac catheterization laboratory. Catheter Cardiovasc Interv 2011;77:860–5.

17. Rihal CS, Sorajja P, Booker JD, et al. Principles of percutaneous paravalvular leak closure. JACC Cardiovasc Interv 2012;5:121–30.

18. Kim MS, Casserly IP, Garcia JA, et al. Percutaneous transcatheter closure of prosthetic mitral paravalvular leaks: are we there yet? JACC Cardiovasc Interv 2009;2:81–90.

19. Pate GE, Al Zubaidi A, Chandavimol M, et al. Percutaneous closure of prosthetic paravalvular leaks: case series and review. Catheter Cardiovasc Interv 2006;68:528–33.

20. Hein R, Wunderlich N, Robertson G, et al. Catheter closure of paravalvular leak. EuroIntervention 2006;2:318–25.

21. Nietlispach F, Johnson M, Moss RR, et al. Transcatheter closure of paravalvular defects using a purpose-specific occluder. JACC Cardiovasc Interv 2010;3:759–65.

22. Shapira Y, Hirsch R, Kornowski R, et al. Percutaneous closure of perivalvular leaks with amplatzer occluders: feasibility, safety, and shortterm results. J Heart Valve Dis 2007;16:305–13.

23. Jelnin V, Dudiy Y, Einhorn BN, et al. Clinical experience with percutaneous left ventricular transapical access for interventions in structural heart defects a safe access and secure exit. JACC Cardiovasc Interv 2011;4:868–74.

A Practical Guide to the Use of Echocardiography in Assisting Structural Heart Disease Interventions

Ming-Sum Lee, MD, PhD[a],
Tasneem Z. Naqvi, MD, FRCP, MMM[b],*

KEYWORDS

- Echocardiography • Percutaneous intervention • Structural heart disease • TAVR • ASD

KEY POINTS

- Traditional imaging using fluoroscopy alone does not provide the necessary resolution to delineate intracardiac structures.
- Echocardiography allows detailed assessment of intracardiac pathology, aids in determining the suitability of that pathology for percutaneous intervention, guides the actual procedure through real-time imaging, and enables serial follow-up.
- Echocardiography has emerged as a fundamental imaging modality and is likely to remains in the forefront during percutaneous treatment of structural heart disease.

INTRODUCTION

Percutaneous intervention has emerged as an effective and less-invasive treatment option for patients with valvular heart disease who are poor surgical candidates. Echocardiography plays an integral role through all stages in the evaluation and treatment of patients undergoing percutaneous interventions.[1] Before the procedure, accurate assessment of cardiac anatomy using echocardiography is crucial in determining patient eligibility for the procedure. During catheterization, echocardiography is used in conjunction with fluoroscopy for procedural guidance. Unlike intracardiac catheters that are readily visualized with fluoroscopy, intracardiac structures require an imaging modality such as echocardiography for clear delineation. As an additional imaging modality beyond fluoroscopy, echocardiography helps improve the safety of the procedure. Because echocardiography uses ultrasound instead of radiation, the radiation exposure to the patient and operator is reduced, which is particularly important in patients who are young, who are pregnant, and in whom the use of radiographic contrast must be minimized. After the procedure, echocardiography is the most commonly used tool for patient follow-up, evaluating the percutaneously placed device or valve, and determining the effect of percutaneous intervention on cardiac remodeling over time.

This article focuses on the role of echocardiography in guiding the most commonly performed interventional procedures for structural heart disease, including percutaneous atrial septal defect (ASD) closure, transcatheter aortic valve replacement (TAVR), percutaneous repair of paravalvular leaks, percutaneous mitral valve edge-to-edge repair, and percutaneous placement of appendage occlusion devices.

[a] Division of Cardiology, Keck School of Medicine, University of Southern California, 1510 San Pablo Street, Los Angeles, CA 90033, USA; [b] Mayo Clinic, 13400 E. Shea Blvd, Scottsdale, AZ 85259, USA
* Corresponding author.
E-mail address: naqvi.tasneem@mayo.edu

Cardiol Clin 31 (2013) 441–454
http://dx.doi.org/10.1016/j.ccl.2013.04.004
0733-8651/13/$ – see front matter © 2013 Elsevier Inc. All rights reserved.

PERCUTANEOUS ASD CLOSURE

Closure of an ASD is recommended in all patients with evidence of right atrial and right ventricular enlargement, regardless of symptoms.[2] In patients with secundum ASD, percutaneous closure is currently the preferred treatment. Clinical trials comparing percutaneous versus surgical closure of ASD showed lower complication rates and shorter hospital stay with percutaneous closure, while achieving similar efficacy rates as surgical repair.[3,4] However, not all patients have the appropriate anatomy for percutaneous closure. Superior and inferior sinus venosus defects and septum primum defects are currently not amenable to percutaneous closure because of inadequate/deficient rims and the risk of encroachment by the device on adjacent cardiac structures. Transthoracic echocardiogram (TTE) provides evidence of shunting across the interatrial septum and is often able to diagnose a secundum ASD. Transesophageal echocardiogram (TEE) helps confirm ASD presence and location and defines patient eligibility through providing an accurate assessment of the size of ASD, identifying the margins of the ASD, and determining the relationship of the ASD with the adjacent cardiac structures.[5]

It is important to image the ASD and its rims in multiple different planes. The rims of the secundum ASD are named based on the adjacent structures: aortic, mitral, superior venacaval, inferior venacaval, and posterior. Having an adequate tissue rim of greater than 5 mm around the defect is ideal for percutaneous closure.[6] Having adequate inferior caval and superior caval rims is particularly important for successful closure, whereas deficiency of the aortic rim is well tolerated and usually does not preclude a percutaneous option. Complete assessment of all the rims is performed using different omniplane angles on TEE. The posterior and the mitral rims can be assessed with the TEE probe at 0° at the midesophageal level (**Fig. 1**A). The probe should be moved in and out to assess the rims at different levels. At 45° to 65°, the posterior and the aortic rims can be assessed (see **Fig. 1**B). This view also usually shows the maximum size of the defect. The TEE probe at an angle of 90° to 110° is usually best for imaging the superior venacaval and inferior venacaval rims (see **Fig. 1**C). Three-dimensional echocardiography should be used when available, because it enables imaging of the interatrial septum en face and provides a comprehensive view of the ASD in one image.

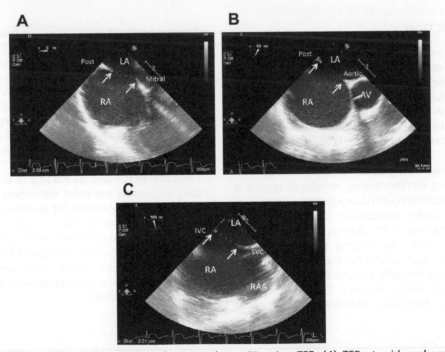

Fig. 1. Assessment of the different rims of a secundum ASD using TEE. (*A*) TEE at midesophageal level at 0° showing the margins of the ASD (*arrows*). The mitral rim (mitral) and the posterior rim (post) are clearly demonstrated. (*B*) At 50°, the aortic rim (aortic) and the posterior rim (post) are visualized (*arrows*). (*C*) TEE at 105° showing the typical bicaval view with the superior vena cava and inferior vena cava. The superior venacaval rim (SVC) and the inferior venacaval rim (IVC) can be assessed from this view (*arrows*). AV, aortic valve; IVC, inferior vena cava; RA, right atrium; RAA, right atrial appendage; RV, right ventricle; SVC, superior vena cava.

Anatomic findings that preclude a percutaneous option include large defects, insufficient septal rims, or insufficient left atrial size.[7] The most commonly used device is the Amplatzer Septal Occluder (St Jude Medical, St. Paul, MN). This is a self-expandable device made of nitinol wire mesh, with 2 flat discs and a connecting waist. The device is designed to straddle the atrial septal defect, with one disc on the left atrium and the other on the right. The waist diameter should match the diameter of the atrial defect diameter. Currently, Amplatzer devices with 4- to 38-mm waist diameters are available, excluding defects larger than 38 mm from closure with this device.

During the procedure, TEE visualizes the catheters and the guide across the defect. TEE allows visualization of the sizing balloon across the defect (**Fig. 2**A). Color flow Doppler can be used to size the defect and help select the correct-sized device through visualizing any residual flow across the defect around the balloon (see **Fig. 2**B). During device deployment, TEE confirms that the left atrial disc is in the left atrium adjacent to the defect. TEE helps evaluate whether any portion of the left atrial disk is pulled across the defect into the right atrium as the disk is pulled close to the defect, in which case the device is pulled back into the sheath and readvanced into the left atrium. Once the left atrial disc is appropriately positioned, the right atrial disc is released under TEE guidance. TEE confirms if the right atrial disc is located on the right side of the septum and has not been released into the left atrium or not moved across the defect into the left atrium after release. Presence of a thin rim of atrium septum in between the disk arms is confirmed by TEE before the device is released. Three-dimensional TEE imaging can be used to confirm correct position of the device (**Fig. 3**). The degree of residual ASD is also assessed. If a large residual leak is present, a larger sized ASD device is needed

to seal the defect. As long as the delivery cable has not be released, the Amplatzer device can be recaptured into the delivery sheath if the discs are not appropriately located or if a significant residual atrial septal defect is present. The device can then be repositioned or a larger device can be chosen. After deployment, 2-dimensional and color flow Doppler imaging of the interatrial septum is used to assess whether residual leaks are present and if a second device is needed. The immediate effects of device deployment on pulmonary artery pressure, tricuspid regurgitation, and right ventricular size and function can be assessed. During follow-up, TTE helps assess device stability. Any residual leak is assessed with color flow Doppler and saline contrast injection with and without the Valsalva maneuver. TTE helps evaluate the long-term effect of defect closure on cardiac remodeling, especially pulmonary pressure, and right ventricular size and function.

TRANSCATHETER AORTIC VALVE REPLACEMENT

TAVR is an effective therapy for patients deemed high risk for conventional surgery. The PARTNER trial showed that among high-risk patients with aortic stenosis, TAVR was associated with similar survival and symptom reduction as surgery for up to 2 years.[8] The 2 most commonly used valves are the SAPIEN valve (Edwards Lifesciences, Irvine, CA) and the CoreValve (Medtronic, Minneapolis, MN).[9] The SAPIEN valve is a bovine pericardial valve in a balloon-expandable cylindrical stainless steel frame. The valve is delivered through a transfemoral or transapical approach and placed inside the native valve through balloon expansion. The CoreValve is a porcine pericardial valve in a self-expanding Nitinol frame that can be delivered through the femoral artery or using

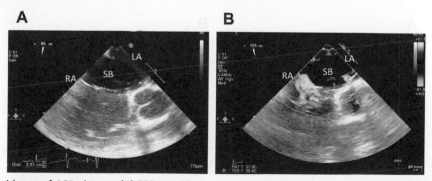

Fig. 2. TEE guidance of ASD closure. (*A*) TEE at midesophageal level at 80° showing an echolucent sizing balloon across the atrial septal defect. (*B*) An inflated sizing balloon is seen across the atrial septal defect. The neck of the fully inflated balloon is measured to size the ASD device. Interrogation of the interatrial septum using color flow Doppler shows no flow across the septum. LA, left atrium; RA, right atrium; SB, sizing balloon.

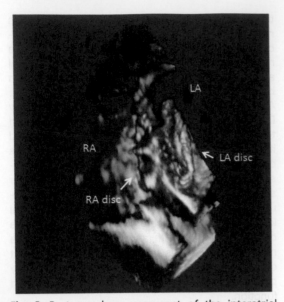

Fig. 3. Postprocedure assessment of the interatrial septum. Three-dimensional TEE imaging of the interatrial septum showing an Amplatzer septal occluder device straddling the atrial septal defect, with one disc on the left atrial side (LA disc) and the other disc on the right atrial side (RA disc). LA, left atrium; RA, right atrium.

a transaortic or subclavian approach. The Core-Valve has a larger profile compared with the SA-PIEN valve. Its frame is anchored within the aortic annulus, extends into the ascending aorta, and anchors in the ascending aorta above the coronary ostia.

Imaging with echocardiography is critical during preprocedure planning. TTE is the most well-established imaging modality for assessing the severity of aortic stenosis.[10] The echocardiographic criteria used in the PARTNER trial for SA-PIEN implantation are a peak transaortic velocity of 4 m/s or greater, a mean gradient of 40 mm Hg or greater, and a valve area of less than 0.8 cm^2.[11] In patients with low-gradient aortic stenosis with left ventricular dysfunction, dobutamine echocardiography using dobutamine doses of less than 20 µg/kg/min can be used to distinguish between true aortic stenosis and pseudo-severe aortic stenosis, which is defined as an increase in valve area by 0.2 cm^2 without an increase in aortic valve gradient.[12] The anatomy of the aortic valve should be examined. Transcatheter aortic valve replacement is usually not performed in patients with bicuspid aortic valve, because the irregularly shaped valvular orifice associated with bicuspid valve may predispose to incorrect deployment, and the fragile aortic wall predisposes to dissection during balloon expansion. A complete echocardiographic examination of the heart also helps identify other structural abnormalities, such as severe mitral regurgitation, severe tricuspid regurgitation, pulmonary hypertension, and left or right ventricular dysfunction, which are associated with higher procedural mortality and worse outcomes. A sigmoid-shape interventricular septum resulting from basal septal hypertrophy, or marked focal calcification of the left ventricular outflow tract or the basal anterior mitral leaflet may interfere with CoreValve deployment and cause valve displacement. The presence of thrombi in the left atrium or the left ventricle is a contraindication to the procedure. In patients with reduced left ventricular dysfunction, contrast-enhanced echocardiography should be performed to exclude left ventricular thrombus (**Fig. 4**A, B).

Accurate preprocedural aortic annular dimension measurements are important for the selection of appropriate valve prosthesis size. Erroneous measurements can lead to selection of inappropriate valve size, and in turn to serious complications such as valve embolization, perivalvular

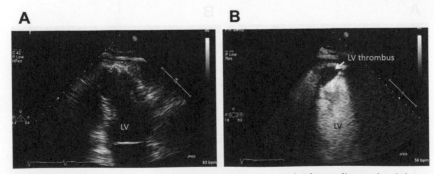

Fig. 4. Assessment of left ventricular thrombus using contrast-enhanced echocardiography. (*A*) An apical 2-chamber view on TTE showing aneurysmal dilatation of the left ventricular apex. The poor image quality precludes definitive exclusion of a left ventricular thrombus. (*B*) The same patient imaged using contrast-enhanced echocardiography. A thrombus is clearly seen at the left ventricular apex (*arrow*). LV, left ventricle.

leak, or rupture of the aortic annulus. With a SAPIEN device, a 23-mm prosthesis is generally used for aortic annular diameters of 18 to 21 mm, and a 26-mm prosthesis for annular diameters of 22 to 25 mm. The CoreValve comes in slightly larger sizes. The 26-mm CoreValve prosthesis is designed for patients with annular diameters of 20 to 23 mm, whereas the 29-mm prosthesis can be used in patients with annular diameters of 24 to 27 mm. The CoreValve has an upper segment that is anchored to the ascending aorta, and an ascending aortic diameter of greater than 43 mm precludes the use of this valve. Measurement of annular diameter with 2-dimensional TTE is performed in a parasternal long-axis view. The measurement is taken at the hinge points, which include the point of insertion of the right coronary cusp with the interventricular septum, and the

noncoronary cusp with the mitral annulus (from tissue–blood interface to blood–tissue interface) during systole (**Fig. 5**A). However, measurement using 2-dimensional TTE tends to underestimate the true aortic annular size compared with TEE,[13] which in turn tends to underestimate the annular size compared with computed tomography (CT). This finding is because the aortic annulus is elliptical, and the anteroposterior diameter measured with TTE is generally the shorter of the 2 diameters. Three-dimensional TTE may provide a more accurate assessment of aortic annular size (see **Fig. 5**C), but the low frame rate, lack of boundary resolution, and presence of blurred margins caused by calcification can make measurements difficult. When the measurements are near critical cutoff values, TEE should be performed to confirm annular size.

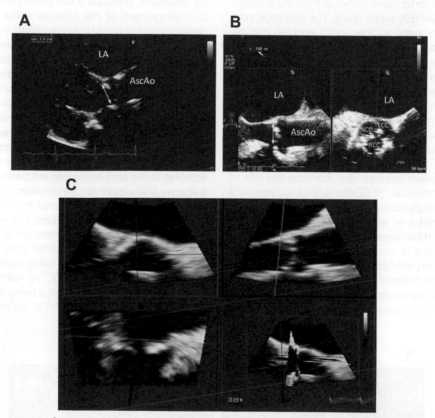

Fig. 5. Measurement of aortic annular diameter. (*A*) Measurement of aortic annular diameter with 2D TTE is performed in a parasternal long-axis view. The measurement is taken at the point of insertion of the aortic valve cusps during systole, from tissue–blood interface to blood–tissue interface (*white double arrow*). (*B*) Simultaneous biplane TEE imaging using orthogonal planes of the aortic valve at the midesophageal level. The aortic valve is in short axis on one plane. The second plane should bisect the commissure between the noncoronary cusp (NCC) and the left coronary cusp (LCC) on one side, and bisects the belly of the right coronary cusp (RCC) on the other side. The aortic annular diameter is taken from the long-axis view from tissue–blood interface to blood–tissue interface (*white double arrow*). (*C*) Three-dimensional TEE image of the aortic annulus. Using 3 multiplanar reconstruction planes, reconstructed orthogonal long and short axis views of the aortic annulus are obtained. AscAo, ascending aorta; LA, left atrium.

The preferred method to measure aortic annulus on TEE is using the biplane mode, with the aortic valve in short axis on one plane (usually obtained at 35°–55°). The second plane should bisect the commissure between the noncoronary cusp and the left coronary cusp on one side of the annulus, and bisect the belly of the right coronary cusp on the other side of the annulus (see **Fig. 5**B). This technique allows measurement of the annulus diameter at its greatest. The true annular plane should be nearly perpendicular to the long axis of the aorta. Bulky or irregular calcification of the aortic landing zone should be assessed and is associated with suboptimal valve deployment and perivalvular leaks. The distance of coronary ostia from the aortic annulus should be measured and the bulkiness of native valve leaflets should be noted, because low coronary ostia are susceptible to coronary occlusion either from the crushed bulky native aortic valve leaflet or from the superior rim of the SAPIEN valve stent. The distance from the coronary ostia to the aortic annulus can be measured at 110° to 130°. Three-dimensional TEE can be helpful, especially when measuring the distance from the left coronary ostium to the aortic annulus. Ideally, the distance should be greater than 10 mm for a 23-mm SAPIEN valve, and greater than 11 mm for a 26-mm valve. The risk of coronary occlusion should also be assessed through comparing the coronary ostia distance with the length of the coronary cusps. Heavily calcified sinuses also increase the risk of coronary occlusion. TEE also allows assessment of aortic calcification, because the presence of aortic atheroma is associated with a higher risk of stroke and peripheral embolization (**Fig. 6**A, B).

TEE imaging is useful for procedural guidance. During balloon valvuloplasty, TEE can guide positioning of the balloon and help determine if leaflet expansion is symmetric. The position of the aortic cusps and their relation with the coronary ostia can be monitored. During valve deployment, TEE is used to guide valve position (**Fig. 7**A, B). For SAPIEN valves, the valve should be roughly 50% to 60% above the annulus and 40% to 50% below. Valves that are too high may obstruct the coronary ostia, whereas valves that are too low are associated with leaflet overhang, abnormal flow convergence into the valve, and abnormal valve closure, which causes central regurgitation and risk of heart block, particularly with the CoreValve. For the CoreValve, the procedure can be performed in stages and the valve position can still be adjusted after initial release of the device from the sheath. The depth of a CoreValve in the left ventricular outflow tract is particularly important to assess, because the CoreValve has a large profile, and low deployment is associated with an increased risk of complete heart block.[14] The effect of the stent on the mitral valve complex anatomy should be assessed, because a low deployment can lead to impingement of the anterior mitral leaflet and development of mitral valve gradients (see **Fig. 7**C).

On complete deployment of the valve, the valve leaflets should be imaged to ensure all cusps are moving. Severe intravalvular regurgitation may occasionally occur with SAPIEN valves, because of inadequate expansion of one cusp. Assessing the presence, location, and severity of any perivalvular leaks is also important, because even a mild degree of leakage is associated with poor outcome (**Fig. 8**A, B).[8] For SAPIEN valves, paravalvular leaks should be judged below the stent, because leaks seen above the stent or in the middle of the stent may not translate into real leaks because of the skirt of the stent. The valve should be assessed in multiple planes, particularly using the short axis view of the aortic valve. Each leak must be imaged individually using specific angulation so that vena contracta, jet width, and the effective regurgitant orifice area using the proximal isovelocity surface area (PISA) method can be

A   **B**

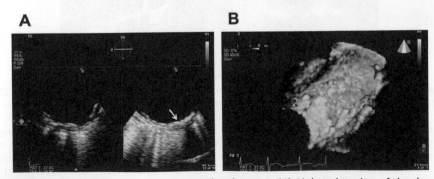

Fig. 6. Imaging of the descending aorta showing aortic atheroma. (*A*) Biplane imaging of the descending aorta showing multiple plaques in the descending aorta (*arrow*). (*B*) Three-dimensional imaging of the aorta showing multiple plaques.

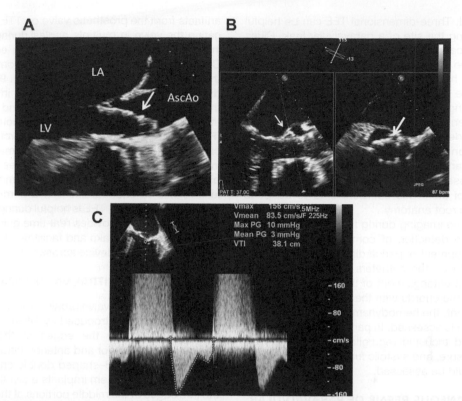

Fig. 7. Use of TEE to guide transcutaneous aortic valve replacement. (*A*) TEE image showing the position of a Cor-eValve (*arrow*) before release from the catheter. The relationship between the lower end of the valve with the basal septum and the anterior mitral leaflet is evaluated. The valve is positioned such that it does not impinge on the mitral valve apparatus. (*B*) Biplane image showing the CoreValve (*arrow*) after its release from the delivery catheter. The sinus of Valsalva can be seen posterior to the valve. (*C*) Assessment of the gradients across the mitral valve after transcutaneous aortic valve implantation by continuous wave Doppler. In this case, the peak transmi-tral gradient is 10 mm Hg and the mean transmitral gradient is 3 mm Hg. A low deployment of the aortic valve can lead to impingement of the anterior mitral leaflet and development of significant mitral valve gradients, and increases the risk of heart block with CoreValve. AscAo, ascending aorta; LA, left atrium; LV, left ventricle.

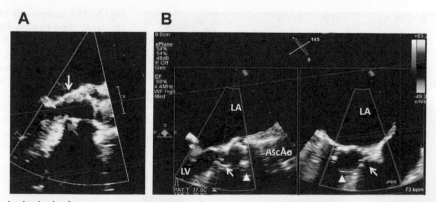

Fig. 8. Paravalvular leak after percutaneous aortic valve replacement. (*A*) TEE imaging showing 2 jets of paravalv-ular leak. A mild anterior leak (*blue arrow*) and a mild posterior leak (*white arrow*) are seen. (*B*) Biplane imaging showing trace perivalvular leak after placement of a CoreValve (*arrowhead*). Color flow Doppler is used to assess the exact location of the leak (*arrow*). AscAo, ascending aorta; LA, left atrium; LV, left ventricle.

measured. Three-dimensional TEE can be helpful in localizing the site of a paravalvular leak. Clues for significant paravalvular leaks are holodiastolic flow in the descending thoracic aorta, and rapid pressure half time. Echocardiographic findings should be combined with fluoroscopic assessment using aortic root angiography, and with assessment of left ventricular end diastolic pressure, to determine the hemodynamic effects of the leak on the left ventricle. For the CoreValve, it is important to allow approximately 10 minutes before assessment of a paravalvular leak so that the Nitinol stent has sufficient time to adapt to the aortic root anatomy.

Real-time imaging during the procedure allows immediate detection of complications, including the development of pericardial effusion, formation of thrombi on the catheters or periaortic hematoma, and entanglement of the mitral valve complex and the chords with the catheter. After valve deployment, the hemodynamic effect of valve implantation is assessed. In particular, the degree of mitral and tricuspid regurgitation, pulmonary artery pressure, and systolic function of both ventricles should be assessed.

PERCUTANEOUS REPAIR OF PARAVALVULAR LEAK

Paravalvular leaks are a complication after mechanical or bioprosthetic valve replacement in the mitral or aortic position. Hemodynamically significant paravalvular leaks or those resulting in hemolysis are usually treated with repeat surgery. Percutaneous closure of paravalvular leaks is a viable alternative in patients at high surgical operative risk who have appropriate anatomy. TEE is usually required for the assessment of paravalvular leaks because of reverberation and shadowing

artifacts from the prosthetic valve on TTE. Interrogating the valve in multiple angles during TEE is important, because the jets are often eccentric. Color flow Doppler can be used to confirm that the flow is outside the sewing ring (**Fig. 9**). Three-dimensional TEE is particularly helpful in defining the location and shape of the leaks and whether the leak is amenable to percutaneous repair (**Fig. 10**). Contraindications to percutaneous closure of perivalvular leaks include mechanical instability of the valve, such as those seen in large paravalvular tears; intracardiac thrombus; and leak related to endocarditis.[15] If a percutaneous approach is pursued, TEE is helpful during the procedure because it provides real-time guidance on the location of the leaks and facilitates the placement of the closure device across the defects.

PERCUTANEOUS MITRAL VALVE REPAIR

Percutaneous mitral valve repair mimics the edge-to-edge technique introduced by Alfieri,[16] wherein stitches appropriate the edges of the middle portion of the posterior and anterior mitral leaflets, creating a figure of 8–shaped double orifice. The Evalve MitraClip system implants a clip that holds the free edges of the middle portions of the 2 mitral leaflets together to reduce the degree of mitral regurgitation. The EVEREST II trial showed that percutaneous mitral valve repair is noninferior to surgical repair or replacement and is associated with lower procedural risk.[17] Percutaneous repair is less effective at reducing mitral regurgitation, although patients showed similar clinical improvement in symptoms and exercise capacity.

Patient selection is crucial in ensuring procedural success. The edge-to-edge repair technique is successful in reducing mitral regurgitation in 2 groups of patients: those with myxomatous

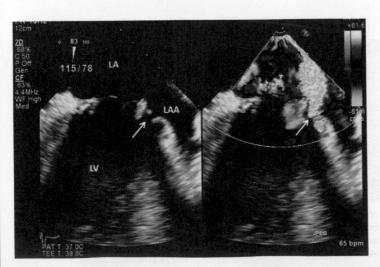

Fig. 9. TEE assessment of paravalvular leak. Side-by-side images of 2-dimensional and color flow Doppler showing a bioprosthetic valve in the mitral position. A gap is seen outside of the sewing ring on the 2-dimensional image (*arrow*). Color flow Doppler reveals significant paravalvular regurgitation through the gap (*arrow*). LA, left atrium; LAA, left atrial appendage; LV, left ventricle.

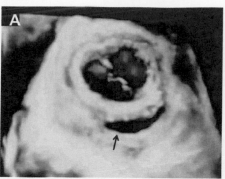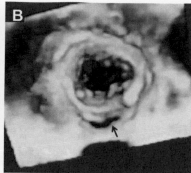

Fig. 10. Real-time 3-dimensional imaging with TEE showing a paravalvular defect. (*A*) Live 3-dimensional view from the left atrial perspective showing a bioprosthetic mitral valve and a large defect outside the sewing ring (*arrow*). (*B*) Three-dimensional view of the valve from the left ventricular perspective showing the same defect outside the sewing ring (*arrow*).

degeneration with prolapse or flail of the middle scallop of one of the mitral leaflets, and those with functional mitral regurgitation associated with left ventricular enlargement and systolic dysfunction. Percutaneous mitral repair is generally not effective in patients with rheumatic mitral regurgitation and restricted leaflet motion, those with prolapse that does not involve the middle scallops, or those in whom the middle scallops are heavily calcified.[18]

Preoperative echocardiography plays an important role in patient selection through determining the mechanism and quantifying the severity of mitral regurgitation. Using TEE, the mitral valve should be systematically mapped by imaging the valve in all 3 planes (upper esophageal, midesophageal, and lower esophageal) at 3 omniplane angles (0°, 60°, and 120°) to identify all scallops. The severity of mitral regurgitation should be quantified on a zoom midesophageal view of the regurgitant jet so that the diameter of the vena contracta and the aliasing radius to calculate regurgitant orifice area can be measured.[10] The PISA method may underestimate mitral regurgitation severity in the presence of multiple jets, in which case regurgitation severity may be assessed using the continuity equation.[10] Pulsed Doppler evaluation of the pulmonary vein flow pattern to identify systolic flow reversal and continuous-wave Doppler assessment of the density of the regurgitant jet provide useful adjunct data.

The origin of the mitral regurgitant jet must be assessed, because the clip is only effective when the regurgitant jet origin is associated with the A2 and P2 segments of the mitral valve. The clip has 2 arms that are roughly 8 mm long and 4 mm wide. Enough leaflet tissue must be present for the clip to grasp. Thus, a severe flail gap of more than 10 mm and marked restriction of leaflet motion with minimal leaflet surface contact in functional

MR are relative contraindications to the procedure. In the EVEREST trial, the echocardiographic inclusion criteria stipulate that for patients with a flail leaflet, the flail gap must be less than 10 mm and the flail width less than 15 mm (**Fig. 11**A, B).[19] For patients with function mitral regurgitation, the coaptation length must be 2 mm or greater and the coaptation depth less than 11 mm (see **Fig. 11**C).

TEE plays an important role during the procedure. During transseptal puncture, TEE allows visualization of the transseptal needle and guides the site at the interatrial septum where transseptal puncture is performed, which is aimed at the superior and posterior portion of the interatrial septum. This technique is important because catheter manipulation is difficult if the transseptal puncture site is too low and hence close to the mitral valve annulus, or too anterior and hence away from the plane of the mitral valve, which is a posterior cardiac structure. The bicaval view at 90° to 100° with simultaneous biplane imaging allows good visualization of the septum and all of the adjacent structures (**Fig. 12**). The midesophageal 0° four-chamber view is useful in assessing the distance of the transseptal puncture site to the valve plane.[18] A high puncture site is needed so that the device can approach the valve in the perpendicular manner.

TEE is also used to ensure that the bulky guide and device tip does not scrape the lateral wall of the left atrium or the pulmonary veins. After transseptal crossing, TEE imaging helps direct the delivery catheter so that it is aligned with the mitral regurgitant flow. The ideal position for deployment is where the clip splits the largest mitral regurgitant jet in two (**Fig. 13**C). The biplane view in a 3-dimensional imaging probe is particularly useful to guide placement of the clip above the MR jet. The clip arms must be

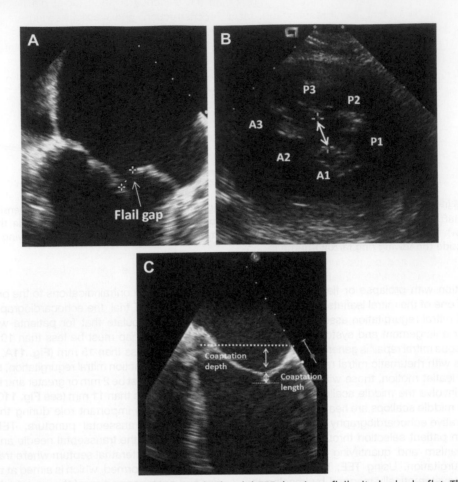

Fig. 11. Preprocedural TEE assessment of the mitral valve. (*A*) TEE showing a flail mitral valve leaflet. The flail gap (*arrow*) is measured as shown. For successful repair using the MitraClip, the flail gap should be less than 10 mm. (*B*) The flail width is most commonly measured on a transgastric short-axis view. The flail width is measured as shown (*double arrow*). The ideal flail width for successful percutaneous repair is less than 15 mm. The scallops of the anterior leaflet are labeled A1 to A3. Scallops of the posterior leaflets are labeled P1 to P3. (*C*) In functional mitral regurgitation, important anatomic features associated with procedural success are coaptation length of 2 mm or greater, and a coaptation depth of less than 11 mm. Measurements of coaptation depth and coaptation length are shown.

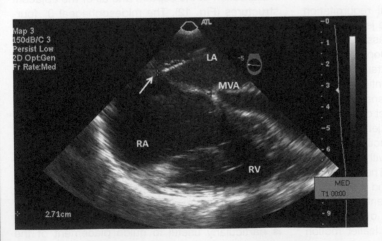

Fig. 12. TEE guidance of transeptal puncture. TEE allows visualization of the transseptal needle and guides the site at the interatrial septum where transseptal puncture is performed. The transseptal puncture site (*arrow*) should be far enough away from the mitral valve annulus (MVA) to provide enough room for manipulation of the catheter. The midesophageal 0° four-chamber view is useful for assessing the distance of the transseptal puncture site to the valve plane. In this case, the catheter is seen in the left atrium. The transseptal puncture site is measured to be 2.71 cm above the MVA. LA, left atrium; RA, right atrium; RV, right ventricle.

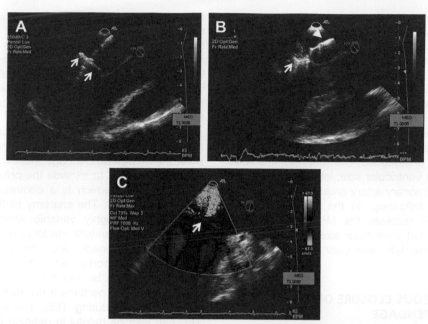

Fig. 13. Placement of the MitraClip under TEE guidance. (*A*) TEE allows visualization of the clip and the delivery apparatus. The 2 arms of the clip (*arrows*) can be clearly visualized above the mitral valve apparatus. (*B*) Real-time imaging during clip deployment showing that both the anterior and posterior mitral leaflets are grasped by the clip. The MitraClip (*arrow*) and the delivery catheter (*arrowhead*) can be seen. (*C*) Color flow Doppler showing the jet of mitral regurgitation. The ideal position for deployment is where the clip (*arrow*) splits the largest mitral regurgitant jet in two.

rotated to be perpendicular to the mitral coaptation line; this can be imaged using the transgastric short axis view of the mitral valve, or through using 3-dimensional echocardiography.[20] Real-time imaging during clip deployment helps ensure that the anterior and posterior mitral leaflets are grasped by the clip (see **Fig. 13**A, B). The immediate effect of clip closure on the degree of residual mitral regurgitation is reassessed (**Fig. 14**). The degree of mitral regurgitation should be quantified based on vena contracta width, PISA, regurgitant jet area on color flow Doppler, and pulmonary vein flow pattern. With the MitraClip (Abbott Laboratories, Abbott Park, IL) system, if the degree of mitral regurgitation remains severe, the clip can be everted and repositioned. If one clip is not sufficient, a second clip can be placed. Because placing more than one clip may result in mitral stenosis, the gradients across the valve should be assessed using continuous wave Doppler before releasing the clip, although mitral stenosis in general is not an issue in the presence of degenerative MR when leaflets are bulky.

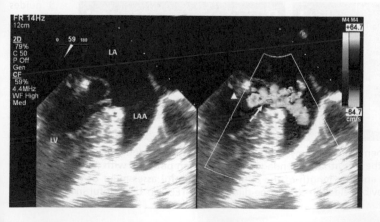

Fig. 14. Postassessment of the mitral valve by TEE showing residual mitral regurgitation. Side-by-side view with 2-dimensional and color flow Doppler showing significant residual mitral regurgitation (*arrow*) after placement of one MitraClip. The jet is eccentric and directed toward the left atrial appendage. The MitraClip is indicated by the arrowhead. In this particular case, a second clip was subsequently placed with good result. LA, left atrium; LAA, left atrial appendage; LV, left ventricle.

During the entire procedure, TEE monitoring helps with early identification of complications, such as thrombus formation on the catheters, development of pericardial effusion from left atrial puncture, injury to the mitral valve apparatus, or tangling of the mitral valve chords with the device.

Postprocedure follow-up includes a comprehensive TTE examination wherein the stability of the clip and the figure-of-8 appearance or double orifice of the mitral valve is confirmed and residual mitral regurgitation is assessed. The effect of mitral valve repair on left ventricular size, left ventricular function, and pulmonary artery pressure is also evaluated during follow-up. In the EVEREST II trial, patients who received the MitraClip showed a reduction in left ventricular size, which could be from favorable left ventricular remodeling after repair.[17]

PERCUTANEOUS CLOSURE OF THE LEFT ATRIAL APPENDAGE

Patients with atrial fibrillation who cannot tolerate anticoagulation have a significantly elevated risk of stroke. Because most thrombi in patients with nonvalvular atrial fibrillation are found in the left atrial appendage, obliteration of the left atrial appendage is performed with the goal of reducing stroke.[21] The Watchman (Atritech Inc, Plymouth, MN) left atrial appendage occlusion system is a self-expanding Nitinol device for percutaneous implantation to seal the communication between the left atrial appendage and the left atrium.[22] In the PROTECT-AF trial, patients with nonvalvular atrial fibrillation were randomized to the Watchman device or long-term warfarin. Patients who received the Watchman device had fewer hemorrhagic strokes, with a noninferior primary efficacy rate compared with warfarin.[23]

Placement of this device is performed under fluoroscopic and TEE guidance. Before the procedure, the left atrial appendage should be examined in multiple planes to exclude the presence of left atrial thrombus, which is a contraindication for device placement. The anatomy of the left atrial appendage is highly variable among patients (**Fig. 15**A–C). Therefore, measuring the width of the appendage neck and the length of the appendage is important so that an appropriately sized device can be selected. These measurements should be performed on multiple different imaging planes during TEE. Three-dimensional TEE can also be helpful in defining the anatomy (see **Fig. 15**D). During the procedure, TEE is helpful in guiding transseptal puncture. Real-time TEE imaging during device deployment helps ensure correct placement of the device at the appendage. After device release, TEE imaging is used to examine device stability. Color flow Doppler is performed to evaluate for leakage.

Like other procedures that require a transseptal puncture, the interatrial septum is examined to

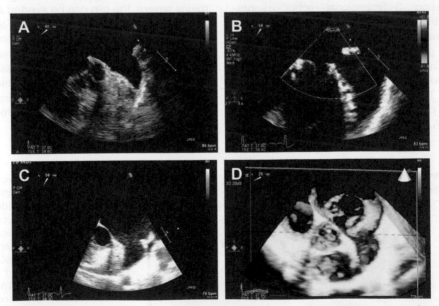

Fig. 15. Assessment of left atrial appendage anatomy by TEE. (*A–C*) Left atrial appendages from 3 different patients are shown. The anatomy of the left atrial appendage varies between patients, with marked difference in the width of the appendage neck and the length of the appendage. Careful assessment of the anatomy is important for appropriate closure device selection. (*D*) Three-dimensional TEE can be helpful in defining the anatomy of the left atrial appendage.

ensure the puncture did not result in a large atrial septal defect. A small residual defect is commonly seen, and often closes spontaneously over time.

SUMMARY

A percutaneous approach to the treatment of structural heart disease is expected to become increasingly common. Traditional imaging using fluoroscopy alone does not provide the necessary resolution to delineate intracardiac structures. Echocardiography allows the detailed assessment of intracardiac abnormalities, helps determine suitability for percutaneous intervention, guides the actual procedure through real-time imaging, and enables serial follow-up. It has emerged as a fundamental imaging modality and is likely to remain in the forefront during percutaneous treatment of structural heart disease.

REFERENCES

1. Zamorano JL, Badano LP, Bruce C, et al. EAE/ASE recommendations for the use of echocardiography in new transcatheter interventions for valvular heart disease. J Am Soc Echocardiogr 2011;24(9):937–65.
2. Warnes CA, Williams RG, Bashore TM, et al. ACC/AHA 2008 guidelines for the management of adults with congenital heart disease: a report of the American College of Cardiology/American heart Association Task Force on Practice guidelines (Writing Committee to Develop guidelines on the management of adults with congenital heart disease). Developed in Collaboration with the American Society of echocardiography, heart Rhythm Society, International Society for Adult congenital heart disease, Society for Cardiovascular angiography and interventions, and Society of thoracic Surgeons. J Am Coll Cardiol 2008;52(23):e143–263.
3. Du ZD, Hijazi ZM, Kleinman CS, et al. Comparison between transcatheter and surgical closure of secundum atrial septal defect in children and adults: results of a multicenter nonrandomized trial. J Am Coll Cardiol 2002;39(11):1836–44.
4. Jones TK, Latson LA, Zahn E, et al. Results of the U.S. multicenter pivotal study of the HELEX septal occluder for percutaneous closure of secundum atrial septal defects. J Am Coll Cardiol 2007; 49(22):2215–21.
5. Vaidyanathan R, Simpson JM, Kumar RK. Transesophageal echocardiography for device closure of atrial septal defects: case selection, planning, and procedural guidance. JACC Cardiovasc Imaging 2009;2(10):1238–42.
6. Cooke JC, Gelman JS, Harper RW. Echocardiologists' role in the deployment of the Amplatzer atrial

7. septal occluder device in adults. J Am Soc Echocardiogr 2001;14(6):588–94.
7. Tobis J, Shenoda M. Percutaneous treatment of patent foramen ovale and atrial septal defects. J Am Coll Cardiol 2012;60(18):1722–32.
8. Kodali SK, Williams MR, Smith CR, et al. Two-year outcomes after transcatheter or surgical aortic-valve replacement. N Engl J Med 2012;366(18):1686–95.
9. Webb JG, Wood DA. Current status of transcatheter aortic valve replacement. J Am Coll Cardiol 2012;60(6):483–92.
10. Bonow RO, Carabello BA, Chatterjee K, et al. 2008 focused update incorporated into the ACC/AHA 2006 guidelines for the management of patients with valvular heart disease: a report of the American College of Cardiology/American Heart Association Task Force on Practice Guidelines (Writing Committee to revise the 1998 guidelines for the management of patients with valvular heart disease). Endorsed by the Society of Cardiovascular Anesthesiologists, Society for Cardiovascular Angiography and Interventions, and Society of Thoracic Surgeons. J Am Coll Cardiol 2008;52(13):e1–142.
11. Smith CR, Leon MB, Mack MJ, et al. Transcatheter versus surgical aortic-valve replacement in high-risk patients. N Engl J Med 2011;364(23):2187–98.
12. Grayburn PA. Assessment of low-gradient aortic stenosis with dobutamine. Circulation 2006;113(5):604–6.
13. Messika-Zeitoun D, Serfaty JM, Brochet E, et al. Multimodal assessment of the aortic annulus diameter: implications for transcatheter aortic valve implantation. J Am Coll Cardiol 2010;55(3):186–94.
14. Bleiziffer S, Ruge H, Horer J, et al. Predictors for new-onset complete heart block after transcatheter aortic valve implantation. JACC Cardiovasc Interv 2010;3(5):524–30.
15. Bhindi R, Bull S, Schrale RG, et al. Surgery Insight: percutaneous treatment of prosthetic paravalvular leaks. Nat Clin Pract Cardiovasc Med 2008;5(3):140–7.
16. Maisano F, La Canna G, Colombo A, et al. The evolution from surgery to percutaneous mitral valve interventions: the role of the edge-to-edge technique. J Am Coll Cardiol 2011;58(21):2174–82.
17. Feldman T, Foster E, Glower DD, et al. Percutaneous repair or surgery for mitral regurgitation. N Engl J Med 2011;364(15):1395–406.
18. Silvestry FE, Rodriguez LL, Herrmann HC, et al. Echocardiographic guidance and assessment of percutaneous repair for mitral regurgitation with the Evalve MitraClip: lessons learned from EVEREST I. J Am Soc Echocardiogr 2007;20(10):1131–40.
19. Feldman T, Kar S, Rinaldi M, et al. Percutaneous mitral repair with the MitraClip system: safety and

midterm durability in the initial EVEREST (Endovascular Valve Edge-to-Edge REpair Study) cohort. J Am Coll Cardiol 2009;54(8):686–94.

20. Cavalcante JL, Rodriguez LL, Kapadia S, et al. Role of echocardiography in percutaneous mitral valve interventions. JACC Cardiovasc Imaging 2012;5(7): 733–46.

21. Blackshear JL, Odell JA. Appendage obliteration to reduce stroke in cardiac surgical patients with atrial fibrillation. Ann Thorac Surg 1996;61(2):755–9.

22. Sick PB, Schuler G, Hauptmann KE, et al. Initial worldwide experience with the WATCHMAN left atrial appendage system for stroke prevention in atrial fibrillation. J Am Coll Cardiol 2007;49(13): 1490–5.

23. Holmes DR, Reddy VY, Turi ZG, et al. Percutaneous closure of the left atrial appendage versus warfarin therapy for prevention of stroke in patients with atrial fibrillation: a randomised non-inferiority trial. Lancet 2009;374(9689):534–42.

Anesthesia for Structural Heart Interventions

Steven Haddy, MD, FACC

KEYWORDS

- Anesthesiology • Sedation • Complications • Monitoring • Practice standards
- Catheter-based techniques

KEY POINTS

- Complications arising from sedation in the CL/EPL are not uncommon.
- When they occur, these complications can be life-threatening.
- If more than "mild" sedation is planned, a qualified practitioner not involved in the procedure should be present to administer the sedation and monitor the patient.
- Anesthetic technique may impact the outcome of the procedure positively or negatively.

INTRODUCTION

Communication between the proceduralist and anesthesiologist is always important, but never more so than during procedures in the cardiac catheterization or electrophysiology laboratories (CL/EPL). A thorough understanding of the procedure is key to the safe conduct of any anesthetic; it is all the more important in the unfamiliar surroundings of the intervention suite. Unless a dedicated hybrid operating room is being used, the layout of the CL/EPL probably was not designed with the needs of the anesthesiologist in mind. The anesthesia machine and equipment may be well beyond arm's reach from the patient, there may not be ready access to the airway, and the anesthesiologist often must dodge the movements of the image intensifier. To make matters worse, unless the hospital's volume is high enough to justify dedicated cardiac anesthesia personnel, these cases may be assigned to junior members of the department under the incorrect but commonly held belief that if the patient requires only sedation, little can go wrong. Taking a moment or two to review the procedure's anticipated duration and potential complications with the anesthesiologist leads to a smoother and more pleasurable experience for all concerned. It is particularly helpful to notify the anesthesiologist when moments of especially painful stimulation will occur so that the patient's level of sedation and analgesia may be adjusted in advance.

STANDARDS OF CARE

The applicable standards of care regarding personnel and monitoring are determined by the depth of sedation, not by the location where the procedure will be done. The specific procedure being performed and the physical status of the patient also impact the sedation and monitoring requirements but to a lesser extent. Indeed, preventable complications are more common and more severe in remote locations than in the operating room.[1]

THE CONTINUUM OF SEDATION

Few topics in anesthesiology inspire as much controversy and are as misunderstood as the continuum from consciousness through sedation and ultimately to general anesthesia. The multiple terms used to describe sedation often overlap and cause confusion. These include local with sedation; monitored anesthesia care (this term

There are no conflicts of interest to disclose.

Department of Anesthesiology, Keck School of Medicine, University of Southern California, 1500 San Pablo Street, 4th Floor, Los Angeles, CA 90033, USA

E-mail address: haddy@med.usc.edu

Cardiol Clin 31 (2013) 455–465

http://dx.doi.org/10.1016/j.ccl.2013.04.005

sometimes is mistakenly believed to stand for minimal anesthesia care); local stand-by; light general anesthesia; twilight; and conscious sedation, moderate sedation, and heavy or deep sedation.

The American Society of Anesthesiologists (ASA)[2] sets out criteria defining the four stages of progression from sedation to general anesthesia as shown in **Table 1**. For practical purposes, the table can be divided in half. It is the progression from "moderate sedation/analgesia" to "deep sedation/analgesia" that is critical. This marks the transition from a patient who is able to maintain his or her own protective airway reflexes and respond appropriately to hypoxia and hypercarbia to one who cannot. Most sedation-related complications are caused by inadequate oxygenation or ventilation, and by aspiration lung injury.[1,3] Once the patient cannot reliably protect his or her own airway, clear away secretions, and maintain unassisted oxygenation and ventilation, monitoring must meet the same standards that apply to a patient under general anesthesia. This includes the presence of a qualified anesthesia practitioner skilled in airway management and anesthetic pharmacology who can recognize oversedation and make the appropriate physical or pharmacologic interventions. It is frighteningly easy to slip from moderate to deep sedation, even for the most experienced provider. The alarming speed at which this transition may occur, and the delays that may occur in detecting it, are among the major sources of anesthesia-related morbidity and mortality.

Practices Vary Widely

Practices vary widely among different institutions and even among different practitioners within an institution. Anesthesiologists, nurse anesthetists, nurses with special training in sedation, and proceduralists have all been used in various combinations to provide sedation and general anesthesia. The reasons most often cited for not using formal anesthesia services are cost and scheduling difficulties.[4] Although several large series[5,6] have been reported wherein nonanesthesia personnel were supervised by the proceduralist with minimal complications, it is worth noting that morphine, fentanyl, and midazolam were the agents most often used, and propofol was generally avoided.

COMPLICATIONS ARE NOT UNCOMMON

Since 1990, the ASA has maintained a closed claims database of anesthesia-related complications. The data come from the insurance industry and are carefully examined by a panel of anesthesiologists. These data have been extensively reviewed and commented on.[3,7] Among the consistent findings are the following:

1. Claims arising in remote locations (gastrointestinal laboratory, CL/EPL, or emergency room) are eight times more frequent than those arising in the operating room.
2. Thirty percent of complications were caused by an overdose of sedative or narcotic.
3. Fifty-four percent of the cases were judged to have been managed below the standard of care.
4. Thirty-two percent of the complications were judged to have been preventable with better monitoring.
5. The incidence of inadequate oxygenation or ventilation was sevenfold higher in remote locations compared with the operating room.
6. Complications resulting in death or severe disability were more likely to occur during cases performed outside the operating room.

Table 1
Continuum of the depth of sedation

	Minimal Sedation/ Anxiolysis	Moderate Sedation/ Analgesia	Deep Sedation/ Analgesia	General Anesthesia
Responsiveness	Normal response to verbal stimulation	Purposeful[a] response to verbal or tactile stimulation	Purposeful[a] response after repeated or painful stimulation	Unarouseable even with painful stimulus
Airway	Unaffected	No intervention required	Intervention may be required	Intervention usually required
Spontaneous ventilation	Unaffected	Adequate	May be inadequate	Frequently inadequate
Cardiovascular function	Unaffected	Usually maintained	Usually maintained	May be impaired

[a] Reflex withdrawal from painful stimulus is *not* considered a purposeful response.
Adapted from ASA Committee on Quality Management and Departmental Administration. Continuum of depth of sedation: definition of general anesthesia and levels of sedation/analgesia. Available at: http://www.asahq.org. Accessed May 20, 2013.

Cravero and coworkers[8,9] reviewed outcomes from two large series of pediatric sedations. Interventions (primarily airway interventions) were required in about 1 in 70 cases to prevent serious complications. In another large study in adults,[10] 40% of patients required some form of intervention to prevent or correct airway obstruction. The situation is further complicated in the CL/EPL because the image intensifier frequently limits access to the patient's head, making detection of hypoventilation and emergent interventions even more difficult.[4,11] Clearly, sedation for interventional procedures must be taken seriously.

THE FRIGHTENING EASE OF UNINTENDED PROGRESSION TO DEEP SEDATION

The unintended progression to deep sedation is especially quick and surreptitious when propofol is being used, whether alone or (worse) in combination with benzodiazepines and narcotics. Propofol is a potent respiratory depressant. The therapeutic dose can be quite close to a relative overdose that causes respiratory depression or hemodynamic compromise, and is closer still in debilitated patients and those with fragile cardiorespiratory status at baseline. This has led the ASA to issue the following recommendation, quoting from the Astra-Zeneca package insert for Dipravan (propofol):

"...propofol used for sedation or anesthesia 'should be administered only by persons trained in the administration of general anesthesia and not involved in the conduct of the surgical/diagnostic procedure.'"[12]

The level of stimulation during any procedure may vary greatly from minute to minute. Stimulation is the natural antagonist to the depressant effects of all sedatives and narcotics. An appropriate level of sedation/analgesia for electrical cardioversion one moment must be quite deep in the interest of patient comfort and amnesia, but often causes apnea, airway obstruction, and oxygen desaturation a moment later when there is virtually no stimulation. In such situations, the person providing the sedation must be immediately available, able to promptly recognize the problem, and intervene appropriately with physical or pharmacologic means.

PREOPERATIVE EVALUATION: DOES THE SITUATION REQUIRE AN ANESTHESIOLOGIST?

Although many procedures, such as diagnostic catheterizations, may be performed safely using minimal sedation under the direction of the proceduralist, some cannot. The decision to involve an anesthesiologist ideally should be made before the start of the procedure. Calling "stat" for someone to "make him hold still" or rescue a deteriorating patient is a recipe for disaster. Some points to consider are

1. Many of the patients are ASA class 3 or 4 (**Box 1** for definitions) by virtue of their heart disease alone. Virtually all have additional significant comorbidities; diabetes, hypertension, chronic obstructive lung disease, peripheral vascular disease, and obesity are the most commonly encountered. Significant comorbidities complicate the situation and increase the risks of sedation. Patients with significant debilitation may be oversedated by the "usual" doses of any agent.

2. Paradoxic agitation in response to sedatives is more common in the elderly. In addition, delayed metabolism and elimination in this population is commonly associated with perioperative delirium, which prolongs hospitalization and increases morbidity.

3. Inability to lie flat for a prolonged period because of dyspnea or the discomfort of the hard angiography table is not uncommon.

4. Patients at increased risk for airway obstruction or difficult mask ventilation (eg, edentulous or heavily bearded patients) benefit from a proactive approach to airway management. Similarly, the epidemic of obesity and its associated obstructive sleep apnea predispose to airway obstruction, desaturation, hypercarbia, and pulmonary hypertension.

5. Intubation should not be feared. Even with the most severe lung disease, few patients truly become chronically ventilator dependent from intubation alone. More commonly, it is the

---

Box 1
ASA physical status classification system

ASA Physical Status 1: A normal healthy patient

ASA Physical Status 2: A patient with mild systemic disease

ASA Physical Status 3: A patient with severe systemic disease

ASA Physical Status 4: A patient with severe systemic disease that is a constant threat to life

ASA Physical Status 5: A moribund patient who is not expected to survive without the operation

ASA Physical Status 6: A declared brain-dead patient whose organs are being removed for donor purposes

events occurring while they are intubated (surgery, deterioration of their medical condition, and so forth) that prevent subsequent weaning from mechanical ventilation. The more hemodynamically unstable the patient, the less they tolerate even brief episodes of hypoxia or hypercarbia. When the hemodynamics are deteriorating, having a controlled airway and not having to worry about oxygenation and ventilation simplifies much of the management.

6. Patients with dementia, developmental delay, or severe anxiety frequently require more sedation than average to tolerate even relatively painless procedures.

7. During emergent or technically difficult procedures on unstable patients, the presence of an anesthesiologist allows the cardiologist to concentrate on the procedure.

PREOPERATIVE FASTING

The current ASA guidelines for preoperative fasting[13] are outlined in **Table 2**. It should be remembered that these apply to otherwise normal patients. Patients with diabetic stasis or gastroesophageal reflux, pregnant patients, and any patient who has received narcotics do not have normal gastric emptying and should either fast longer or have airway protection by intubation if more than the mildest sedation is planned. Antacids, proton-pump inhibitors, and drugs to promote gastric emptying should not be relied on to protect against aspiration, nor does their use allow the recommended fasting periods to be shortened.

Table 2 Preoperative fasting guidelines	
Clear liquids	2 h
Light meal[a]	6 h
Full meal[b]	8 h

Preoperative antacids, gastrointestinal stimulants, and pharmacologic blockade of gastric acid secretion cannot be relied on to shorten the above times and are not recommended routinely for patients not at increased risk of gastric aspiration.

[a] eg, toast and clear liquid (tea/coffee without milk or cream).

[b] eg, meal containing fatty food, milk, cream, etc.

Data from Apfelbaum J. Practice guidelines for preoperative fasting and the use of pharmacologic agents to reduce the risk of pulmonary aspiration: application to healthy patients undergoing elective procedures an updated report by the American Society of Anesthesiologists Committee on Standards and Practice Parameters. Anesthesiology 2011;114(3):495.

GENERAL CONCERNS

CL/EPLs typically were not designed with the requirements of general anesthesia in mind. Hybrid operating rooms (although clearly not perfect) are preferred for all but the most superficial procedures. General physical requirements are outlined in **Box 2**.

OUTPATIENT PROCEDURES

Although requirements vary by institution and practice location, in addition to the usual concerns, for patients having outpatient procedures the issues outlined in **Box 3** must be addressed. Patients with comorbidities, such as obesity hypoventilation syndrome, diabetes, and seizure disorders, are at increased risk for complications after discharge either from residual sedation or interruption of their medication regimen. They require special instructions and closer follow-up.

RADIATION SAFETY

Too few anesthesiologists are knowledgeable about radiation safety, which is unfortunate. One study[14] showed that the average yearly radiation dose to the anesthesiologists at a hospital doubled after an EPL was opened, although all doses remained well below the allowable limits. Indeed, because of the way many procedure suites are arranged, the dose to the anesthesiologist may well be greater than that to the cardiologist.

Anesthesiologists cannot impact the amount of radiation used, but can significantly decrease their own exposure through the appropriate use of shielding and distance. They should be encouraged to use appropriate personal and fixed shields, including protective eyewear. In addition, the radiation dose delivered to anesthesiologists has been shown to be directly related to the number of drug interventions made, probably because they came out from behind shields and got closer to the patients at these times.[15] Extension tubing and some forethought can significantly limit this exposure. Anesthesia personnel who visit the CL/EPL infrequently often do not have radiation safety badges, nor do they know where the badges should be worn. Both of these situations are easy to correct and are an integral part of an institution's overall radiation safety program.

GENERAL PRINCIPLES OF SEDATION
Respiratory Depression

All narcotics, benzodiazepines, and hypnotics (propofol, thiopental, methohexital) are respiratory depressants, and when combined their effects are

---

Box 2
Physical requirements for safely delivering sedation and general anesthesia

1. Oxygen: There must be a sufficient number of conveniently located oxygen outlets, remembering that the anesthesiologist and perfusionist (should cardiopulmonary bypass be required) cannot share them. While anesthesia can be administered using the tanks on the anesthesia machine, this is not ideal and requires increased vigilance to prevent loss of oxygen pressure - especially if general anesthesia is being administered since most anesthesia ventilators are powered by oxygen pressure.

2. Suction: The anesthesiologist needs suction that can access the patient's head. This must be separate from those for the cardiologist/surgeon, and perfusionist, each of whom need their own.

3. Access to a difficult-airway cart and malignant hyperthermia cart must be readily available.

4. Monitors: Monitors must be visible to the anesthesiologist and the cardiologist.

5. Electricity: Sufficient electrical outlets connected to the hospital's emergency generator system for the anesthesia monitors, anesthesia machine, cardiopulmonary bypass machine, cardiopulmonary bypass heater/cooler, and cell saver must be available.

6. Waste gas disposal: If inhalational anesthesia is to be used, a mechanism for waste gas removal from the procedure suite must be available.

7. Blood administration: Warmers, tubing, and so forth must be available. If the likelihood of blood administration is high, a mechanism for promptly getting the blood to the procedure room or a "cooler" system to keep blood in the interventional suite is needed.

8. Communications: A reliable method to promptly summon help or unanticipated equipment from other areas of the hospital close enough to the anesthesiologist so that he or she does not have to lose contact with the patient is essential.

9. Drugs: Both the usual anesthetic agents and drugs for resuscitation must be immediately available.

10. Airway and other devices: Access to the airway management devices usually found in the anesthesiologist's cart must be immediately available.

11. Recovery: A location to recover the patient, appropriately staffed, until they are able to be discharged to their usual nursing unit, or go home.

Box 3
Additional requirements for outpatient procedures

1. Transportation: Patients who have received sedation should not drive for 24 hours

2. Adult supervision: Many practitioners require the presence of an adult to accompany the patient at the time of discharge

3. Must be able to ambulate without dizziness, significant pain, or nausea

4. Stable hemodynamics: No bleeding or significant hematoma formation at vascular access sites or elsewhere

5. Specific written instructions must be given to the patient

6. Contact information in case of emergency

7. Necessary prescriptions for pain, nausea, and coexisting medical conditions should be given before discharge

---

at least additive, if not synergistic.[10] Those drugs that are thought not to depress respiratory drive (dexmedetomidine, ketamine, etomidate) can still lead to respiratory complications because of airway obstruction, aspiration, or laryngospasm. Etomidate combines minimal respiratory depression with markedly stable hemodynamics. It's action to depress adrenal corticoid production makes it unsuitable for infusion. However, there are few data to support a significant negative impact on outcome from a single induction dose, making etomidate quite useful for induction of general anesthesia. It also finds use in cardioversion, and in the management of many hemodynamically unstable patients. Hypercarbia is also depressant to the central nervous system, additive to other sedatives, and when high enough can cause unconsciousness on its own. The time to onset and peak effects varies among patients and among drugs, sometimes significantly. It is important to allow enough time to pass to see the full respiratory depressant effects before a second dose of any sedative is given. Patients with low cardiac output may have significantly prolonged circulation times. This is particularly important because the level of stimulus (which protects against the depressant effects of these drugs) is quite variable in some types of cases. Intense stimulation (eg, defibrillation or alcohol injection) might punctuate a long period of minimal stimulation.

Supplemental Oxygen and the Need for Capnography

Virtually all patients receive supplemental oxygen during their procedures. Supplemental oxygen helps prevent arterial desaturation as measured by pulse oximetry and is generally thought to increase the margin of safety during sedation. However, increasing the Pao$_2$ allows a longer period of apnea to ensue before arterial desaturation falls low enough to prompt intervention.[17,18] Apneic episodes that are missed by anesthesia providers and proceduralists are reliably detected by capnography,[17–19] which has been shown to improve outcomes during endoscopy.[20] Remembering that 40% of CL/EPL patients required some form of airway intervention[10] it is not surprising that capnography has been recommended as a standard of care during cases involving moderate and deep sedation and general anesthesia since 2011.[2] Qualitative capnography does not require intubation. Special nasal cannulae and masks are available for use with capnographs, although they are not essential. Considering that it is easy, noninvasive, and a proved method to detect airway obstruction and hypoventilation, it is difficult to justify not using capnography in all but the most minimal of sedations. The need for airway intervention by definition means the patient has reached at least the level of deep sedation.

Carbon Dioxide Retention

Virtually all sedatives displace the carbon dioxide response curve to the right, even in the absence of airway obstruction. Increased carbon dioxide is well known to increase pulmonary artery pressures, especially in patients with preexisting pulmonary hypertension of whatever cause. Many of these patients are in a tenuous hemodynamic state going into the procedure and are easily thrown into frank right heart failure.

Fire and Chemical Burns

Accumulation of alcohol-based preparation solutions can potentially lead to combustion whenever cautery or laser energy is used. Increased oxygen concentration around the head (from the patient's oxygen mask) further increases the risk. Solutions must not be allowed to pool either on the patient or on the drapes.

Hypothermia

Core temperature decrease during procedures is largely caused by redistribution of heat to the peripheral thermal compartment during the first 4 hours of a procedure. Hypothermia impairs wound healing; increases oxygen consumption (especially if shivering occurs); induces coagulopathy; and changes the kinetics of enzymatic reactions. Measures shown to be effective in preventing unintended hypothermia include warming intravenous fluids, forced-air warming blankets, a heater-humidifier for the anesthesia circuit if the patient is intubated, and a prewarming routine. Prewarming decreases the gradient from core to peripheral thermal compartment.[21] This can be particularly valuable because often forced-air warming blankets cannot be used during the procedure because of the large surface area that needs to be kept sterile. One hour of prewarming largely prevents the heat loss caused by redistribution occurring during the first 4 hours of a procedure.

Pressure Injury

Radiologic procedure tables are hard and have minimal padding. Elderly debilitated patients often have minimal subcutaneous tissue. Some diagnostic and therapeutic procedures may take 6 to 8 hours to complete. All of these conditions predispose patients to pressure injuries, including skin damage and nerve compression syndromes. When possible, padding should be used, especially over areas known to be at risk, and occasional changes in the position of pressure points, such as the patient's heels, should be considered.

SPECIFIC PROCEDURES
Coronary Interventions

In all but the sickest patients, coronary interventions are usually performed with minimal or mild sedation under the direction of the cardiologist. Patients in shock or requiring mechanical support definitely benefit from the presence of an anesthesiologist, allowing the cardiologist to focus on the technical aspects of the procedure. Here again, intubation should not be considered only when sedation "fails" but rather as a prophylactic measure against further hemodynamic deterioration, which may result from hypoxia or hypercarbia.

Ventricular-assist Device Insertion

Nonpulsatile ventricular-assist devices may render noninvasive blood pressure and pulse oximetry inaccurate or completely unusable. Invasive blood pressure monitoring is usually required. If transesophageal echocardiography (TEE) is required (eg, to aid septostomy), the patient likely requires intubation. During percutaneous ventricular-assist device placement, TEE is often helpful to look at cannula position and helps prevent recirculation during venovenous extracorporeal membrane oxygenation.

Shunt Closure

Either TEE or intracardiac echocardiography can be used to assist placement of atrial or ventricular septal defect closure devices. Sedation is acceptable if intracardiac echocardiography is used, but it must be deep enough to ensure that the patient does not move at a critical moment. This level of sedation may not be tolerated by patients with preexisting pulmonary hypertension, who may progress to right ventricular failure if they develop hypercarbia and respiratory acidosis. Whenever a shunt is suspected, the anesthesiologist should be informed so that extra attention can be given to removing any air from the intravenous tubing. Left-to-right shunts frequently reverse on induction of anesthesia (or even moderate sedation) because of the decreased systemic vascular resistance that results from many anesthetic medications, such as propofol. Air-trapping filters are available and should be considered.

Transvascular Aortic Valve Implantation

Currently, transvascular aortic valve implantation (TAVI) is restricted to patients whose physical status renders them ineligible or at very high risk for conventional aortic valve replacement. However, their comorbidities should not be considered a contraindication to general anesthesia. The author has been impressed with the stability of most patients undergoing TAVI under general anesthesia. However, TAVI performed under sedation is more common in Europe. In a recent review[22] half of the institutions in Europe reported using sedation as their primary technique compared with about 5% of US institutions. Reported advantages include better hemodynamic stability, faster procedure times, and the ability to assess the patient's neurologic status.[23] Most institutions using sedation use transthoracic echocardiography rather than TEE. The reported rate of conversion to general anesthesia is 7% to 20% in various studies.[22] Again, the level of sedation required

may lead to hypoventilation, hypoxia, and hypercarbia. TAVI is best performed in a "hybrid" operating room because the potential for requiring the sudden institution of cardiopulmonary bypass is always present. A dedicated echocardiographer should be present to allow the anesthesiologist to concentrate on the hemodynamics of the patient.

An arterial catheter is placed before induction for continuous blood pressure measurement. Central venous access is very useful for drug administration and pacing, but in any event good venous access is imperative because major complications related to arterial access are possible. Leakage around and through arterial sheaths can be significant and is largely hidden because it frequently drips down between the patient's legs. The anesthesiologist should be informed if unusual bleeding occurs. A pulmonary artery catheter is rarely necessary because there is usually minimal blood loss; cardiac filling and function can be assessed with echocardiography.

Intentional rapid pacing to decrease cardiac output and forward flow during deployment of the valve often leads to ischemia, especially in hypertrophied ventricles. Having a vasopressor (norepinephrine is usually favored) immediately available is critical. A small bolus of vasoconstrictor just before pacing helps promptly restore perfusion pressure when pacing is discontinued. These insults to ventricular function are cumulative, and more ventricular depression and the need for more support should be anticipated as the number or duration of pacing bursts increases. Occasionally, more aggressive pharmacologic support is required.

Although most TAVIs are placed using the femoral artery, other access sites are also used in cases of severe atherosclerosis or small femoral arteries. If a transapical approach is used, general anesthesia is required because a subxyphoid incision is necessary. In addition, one-lung ventilation with deflation of the left lung may be necessary to allow the surgeon access to a quiet operative field. When required, this is accomplished using either an endobronchial tube or a bronchial blocker. Either technique requires fiberoptic confirmation of tube position. Some institutions find one-lung ventilation unnecessary and use a single lumen tube for all cases. One-lung ventilation causes increases in pulmonary artery pressure and can lead to arterial desaturation, both of which increase the chance of right ventricular failure. Direct puncture of the ascending aorta through a small right thoracotomy incision is another surgical approach to TAVI that also requires one-lung ventilation. Blood loss may be massive, should the surgeon lose control of the aortotomy or the insertion sheath be displaced.

Although this patient population is often elderly and frail, most patients are extubated in the operating room and spend only 24 hours in the intensive care unit. The use of agents with short durations of action and rapid elimination helps minimize postoperative delirium, which can cause major morbidity in the elderly.

Mitral Valve Repair

Because mitral valve repairs are performed using venous rather than arterial access, the potential for bleeding at the access sites is reduced. However, cardiac tamponade resulting from attempted septal puncture and the necessity for cardiopulmonary bypass remain. Because TEE is used to guide the procedure, intubation usually is necessary.

Electrophysiology Procedures

Patients presenting for electrophysiology procedures frequently have depressed ejection fraction and multiple comorbidities. Procedures may vary widely in terms of duration and complexity.

Atrial Fibrillation Ablation

Atrial fibrillation (AF) ablations can be lengthy and require deep sedation for patient comfort. Airway obstruction must be avoided because the cardiac and chest wall movement that accompanies heavy snoring can make mapping difficult. Even the regular chest wall motion associated with mechanical ventilation can prove to be a hindrance. Smaller tidal volumes provide some relief, but some physicians have resorted to high-frequency jet ventilation (HFJV) to further decrease respiratory movement.[24] HFJV[24] may decrease catheter movement by decreasing respiratory motion and decreasing fluctuations in left atrial volume. Studies have demonstrated decreased procedural time[24,25] and improved outcomes.[26] Because inhalational agents cannot reliably be delivered with HFJV, a total intravenous anesthetic technique (usually remifentanil and propofol) is used. If there is concern about phrenic nerve stimulation or injury the anesthesiologist should be asked to avoid or minimize nondepolarizing muscle relaxants to verify the preservation of diaphragmatic function.

Some facilities use magnetic resonance imaging to assist with mapping, which adds an additional level of complexity to the anesthetic management. The magnetic resonance imaging suite requires specialized equipment for anesthetic administration that is compatible with the strong magnetic field used.[27]

Pacing-induced arrhythmias may cause hemodynamic deterioration. Catecholamines, such as isoproterenol, which are often used to induce tachyarrhythmias, have the additional potential to cause an increase in anesthetic requirements and may cause the patient to become too lightly sedated at an inappropriate time.[28–30] Monitoring electromechanical association to ensure adequate perfusion during arrhythmias is necessary either by arterial line or pulse oximetry.

Ablation around the pulmonary veins can lead to esophageal thermal injury, and esophageal temperature monitoring is recommended for patients under general anesthesia. Ablation systems that use saline irrigation to cool the catheter can result in significant volume administration during these lengthy procedures, and the anesthesiologist should be kept informed of the amount of irrigation used. If an oral contrast agent is used to decrease the risk of esophageal injury, either the airway must be protected with an endotracheal tube or the patient must be awake enough to protect himself or herself from aspiration. The risk of esophageal injury is thought to be higher in patients under general anesthesia.[31,32] If the right pulmonary veins are to be treated, the potential for phrenic injury is increased and it may be helpful to minimize neuromuscular blockade to allow continuous monitoring of diaphragmatic function.

Patients in chronic AF may be anticoagulated and frequently undergo TEE before cardioversion to detect intracardiac thrombus. Manipulation of the airway and other invasive procedures are more prone to bleeding complications in the anticoagulated patient.

Unfortunately, our understanding of the effects of anesthetic medications, inhaled and intravenous, on cardiac conduction is far from complete. Sedation of any kind decreases endogenous catecholamine release, potentially reducing the likelihood that arrhythmias may be induced for the purposes of diagnosis or ablation. Isoflurane (an halogenated ether) and propofol are equally acceptable for radiofrequency ablation of supraventricular tachycardia, but isoflurane can increase the refractoriness of accessory pathways and possibly interfere with the evaluation and ablation of accessory bypass tracts.[28] Sevoflurane, a newer halogenated ether, does not affect sinus node, AV node, or accessory pathway function.[28] Desflurane, another newer halogenated ether, causes increased heart rate but does not impact the ability to induce or map arrhythmias.[33] Propofol has little effect on conduction or SA/AV node function, but prolonged infusions during AF ablation cases have been associated with a constellation of symptoms including rhabdomyolysis, acute metabolic acidosis, renal failure, and cardiac failure, which have become known as propofol infusion syndrome.[34]

Most anesthetics (with the exception of propofol) have the potential to prolong the QT interval.[35] However, virtually all have been used in patients with congenital QT syndrome for electrophysiologic (EP) studies and other types of surgery. Opioids have no effect on the QT interval.

Opioids may increase parasympathetic tone and thereby decrease heart rate. Remifentanil in particular can cause bradycardia or nodal rhythms. Dexmedetomidine may interfere with EP studies because of central sympatholysis and its effects on cardiac alpha-2A receptors. The sedative effect of dexmedetomidine is not associated with respiratory depression unless it is combined with opioids or sedatives, which it potentiates. It has been shown to decrease the incidence of AF after cardiac surgery and to terminate tachyarrhythmias after congenital heart surgery.[36,37]

Ketamine is an N-methyl-D-aspartate antagonist with sedative and analgesic properties. Although a direct myocardial depressant, it is associated with increased heart rate and blood pressure by increasing central sympathetic outflow. These effects are dose dependent and not usually a problem at the doses required to sedate or supplement narcotics and local infiltration. Similarly, the often-cited visual or auditory hallucinations are infrequent at low doses and when ketamine is combined with midazolam.

MUSCLE RELAXANTS

Succinylcholine prolongs the QT interval through autonomic effects and potassium release, and is best avoided unless rapid control of the airway is critical. Vecuronium and cisatracurium do not prolong the QT interval.[35] Reversal of neuromuscular blockade, when necessary, is accomplished with atropine or glycopyrrolate combined with neostigmine or edrophonium. All of these drug combinations have been shown to prolong the QT interval in healthy subjects but rarely to induce arrhythmias. They should be used with caution in patients at risk for QT-related arrhythmias.

ANTIEMETICS

Droperidol and ondansetron have been implicated in prolonged QT syndromes and arrhythmias.[38,39] Unfortunately, few equally effective alternative antiemetics exist.

CARDIOVERSION

This procedure is typically preceded by TEE to rule out atrial thrombus. The depth of sedation required to afford patient comfort during the electrical stimulus clearly renders the patient unable to maintain his or her own airway and is equivalent to a general anesthetic. All of the standards applicable to deep sedation or general anesthesia should apply.

PACEMAKER/IMPLANTABLE CARDIOVERTER-DEFIBRILLATOR INSERTION

Although usually accomplished under mild sedation with local infiltration, deeper levels (equivalent to general anesthesia) are required if the defibrillation thresholds are to be tested. The literature indicates that multiple defibrillation threshold tests are well tolerated[40] but hemodynamic deterioration may ensue. Complications including perforation, vascular injury, and arrhythmias may be encountered. If resynchronization therapy is to be instituted, TEE may be used to optimize function and intubation may be required.

LASER LEAD EXTRACTION

The removal of pacemaker leads old enough to undergo fibrosis and become adherent to the endocardium has the potential to cause massive bleeding, tamponade, acute tricuspid regurgitation, and vascular injury. Although significant complications occur in less than 1% of cases, many institutions prefer to perform these in the operating room or hybrid room. Good venous access is critical and invasive pressure monitoring is useful to promptly detect hemodynamic changes. Because TEE is often used to follow the course of the procedure and detect complications, intubation is often required.

ALCOHOL SEPTAL ABLATION

Alcohol septal ablation essentially produces an iatrogenic myocardial infarction as a minimally invasive modality for treatment of hypertrophic obstructive cardiomyopathy. The injection of alcohol into the septal perforator induces controlled infarction of the hypertrophied septum, and abolishes the outflow tract obstruction. The cardiac catheterization can be performed under local infiltration and minimal sedation. However, the alcohol injection into the septum is painful and anxiety provoking, frequently requiring deep sedation.

SUMMARY

Virtually all surgical procedures are becoming less invasive necessitating the development of new, unfamiliar, and continually evolving techniques and approaches. Although the advantages to the patient are well documented, these minimally invasive procedures often must be performed in the setting of unfamiliar and even potentially hostile environments. The need for close interdepartmental cooperation and collaboration between anesthesiology and cardiology are obvious, and will only increase over time.

REFERENCES

1. Bhananker SM, Posner KL, Cheney FW, et al. Injury and liability associated with monitored anesthesia care: a closed claims analysis. Anesthesiology 2006;104(2):228–34.

2. Committee of Origin. Standards and Practice Parameters. Standards for basic anesthesia monitoring. ASA Website 2011. Available at: http://www. asahq.org/For-Members/Standards-Guidelines-and-Statements.aspx. Accessed April 20, 2013.

3. Metzner J, Posner KL, Lam MS, et al. Closed claims' analysis. Best Pract Res Clin Anaesthesiol 2011; 25(2):263–76.

4. Gaitan BD, Trentman TL, Fassett SL, et al. Sedation and analgesia in the cardiac electrophysiology laboratory: a national survey of electrophysiologists investigating the who, how, and why? J Cardiothorac Vasc Anesth 2011;25(4):647–59.

5. Geiger MJ, Wase A, Kearney MM, et al. Evaluation of the safety and efficacy of deep sedation for electrophysiology procedures administered in the absence of an anesthetist. Pacing Clin Electrophysiol 1997; 20(7):1808–14.

6. Kezerashvili A, Fisher JD, DeLaney J, et al. Intravenous sedation for cardiac procedures can be administered safely and cost-effectively by non-anesthesia personnel. J Interv Card Electrophysiol 2008;21(1):43–51.

7. Metzner J, Posner KL, Domino KB. The risk and safety of anesthesia at remote locations: the US closed claims analysis. Curr Opin Anaesthesiol 2009;22(4):502–8.

8. Cravero JP, Blike GT, Beach M, et al. Incidence and nature of adverse events during pediatric sedation/anesthesia for procedures outside the operating room: report from the Pediatric Sedation Research Consortium. Pediatrics 2006;118(3): 1087–96.

9. Cravero JP, Beach ML, Blike GT, et al. The incidence and nature of adverse events during pediatric sedation/anesthesia with propofol for procedures outside the operating room: a report from the Pediatric Sedation Research Consortium. Anesth Analg 2009;108(3):795–804.

10. Trentman TL, Fassett SL, Mueller JT, et al. Airway interventions in the cardiac electrophysiology laboratory: a retrospective review. J Cardiothorac Vasc Anesth 2009;23(6):841–5.

11. Shook DC, Savage RM. Anesthesia in the cardiac catheterization laboratory and electrophysiology laboratory. Anesthesiol Clin 2009;27(1):47–56.

12. ASA Committee on Ambulatory Surgical Care. Statement on safe use of propofol committee of origin: ambulatory surgical care (Approved by the ASA House of Delegates on October 27, 2004, and amended on October 21, 2009). American Society of Anesthesiologists (ASAHQ ORG);2013(1/22):1.

13. Apfelbaum J. Practice guidelines for preoperative fasting and the use of pharmacologic agents to reduce the risk of pulmonary aspiration: application to healthy patients undergoing elective procedures an updated report by the American Society of Anesthesiologists committee on standards and practice parameters. Anesthesiology 2011;114(3):495.

14. Katz J. Radiation exposure to anesthesia personnel: the impact of an electrophysiology laboratory. Anesth Analg 2005;101(6):1725.

15. Anastasian ZH, Strozyk D, Meyers PM, et al. Radiation exposure of the anesthesiologist in the neurointerventional suite. Anesthesiology 2011;114(3):512–20.

16. Hug CC. MAC should stand for Maximum anesthesia caution, not minimal anesthesiology care. Anesthesiology 2006;104(2):221–3.

17. Fu ES, Downs JB, Schweiger JW, et al. Supplemental oxygen impairs detection of hypoventilation by pulse oximetry. Chest 2004;126(5):1552–8.

18. Gerstenberger PD. Capnography and patient safety for endoscopy. Clin Gastroenterol Hepatol 2010; 8(5):423–5.

19. Soto RG, Fu ES, Vila HJ, et al. Capnography accurately detects apnea during monitored anesthesia care. Anesth Analg 2004;99(2):379–82.

20. Qadeer MA, Vargo JJ, Dumot JA, et al. Capnographic monitoring of respiratory activity improves safety of sedation for endoscopic cholangiopancreatography and ultrasonography. Gastroenterology 2009;136(5):1568, 76; [quiz: 1819–20].

21. Leslie K, Sessler DI. Perioperative hypothermia in the high-risk surgical patient. Best Pract Res Clin Anaesthesiol 2003;17(4):485–98.

22. Bufton KA, Augoustides JG, Cobey FC. Anesthesia for transfemoral aortic valve replacement in North America and Europe. J Cardiothorac Vasc Anesth 2013;27(1):46–9.

23. Behan M, Haworth P, Hutchenson N, et al. Percutaneous aortic valve implants under sedation: our initial experience. Catheter Cardiovasc Interv 2008; 72(7):1012–5.

24. Raiten J, Elkassabany N, Mandel JE. The use of high-frequency jet ventilation for out of operating room anesthesia. Curr Opin Anaesthesiol 2012; 25(4):482–5.

25. Goode JS Jr, Taylor RL, Buffington CW, et al. High-frequency jet ventilation: utility in posterior left atrial catheter ablation. Heart Rhythm 2006;3(1):13–9.

26. Di Biase L, Conti S, Mohanty P, et al. General anesthesia reduces the prevalence of pulmonary vein reconnection during repeat ablation when compared

with conscious sedation: results from a randomized study. Heart Rhythm 2011;8(3):368–72.

27. Karlik SJ, Heatherley T, Pavan F, et al. Patient anesthesia and monitoring at a 1.5-T MRI installation. Magn Reson Med 1988;7(2):210–21.

28. Sharpe MD, Cuillerier DJ, Lee JK, et al. Sevoflurane has no effect on sinoatrial node function or on normal atrioventricular and accessory pathway conduction in Wolff-Parkinson-White syndrome during alfentanil/midazolam anesthesia. Anesthesiology 1999;90(1):60–5.

29. Smith MM, Andrzejowski JC. Decrease in bispectral index preceding signs of impending brain death in traumatic brain injury. J Neurosurg Anesthesiol 2010;22(3):268–9.

30. Andrzejowski J, Sleigh JW, Johnson IA, et al. The effect of intravenous epinephrine on the bispectral index and sedation. Anaesthesia 2000;55(8): 761–3.

31. Di Biase L, Saenz LC, Burkhardt DJ, et al. Esophageal capsule endoscopy after radiofrequency catheter ablation for atrial fibrillation: documented higher risk of luminal esophageal damage with general anesthesia as compared with conscious sedation. Circ Arrhythm Electrophysiol 2009;2(2): 108–12.

32. Calkins H, Kuck K, Cappato R. 2012 HRS/EHRA/ECAS expert consensus statement on catheter and surgical ablation of atrial fibrillation: recommendations for patient selection, procedural techniques, patient management, and follow-up, definitions, endpoints, and research trial design. J Interv Card Electrophysiol 2012;33:171.

33. Schaeffer M, Snuyder A, Morrision J. An assessment of desflurane for use during cardiac electrophysilogical study and radiofrequency ablation of supraventricular dysrhythmias in children. Paediatr Anaesth 2000;10:155.

34. Cravens GT, Packer DL, Johnson ME. Incidence of propofol infusion syndrome during noninvasive radiofrequency ablation for atrial flutter or fibrillation. Anesthesiology 2007;106(6):1134–8.

35. Kies SJ, Pabelick CM, Hurley HA, et al. Anesthesia for patients with congenital long QT syndrome. Anesthesiology 2005;102(1):204–10.

36. Chrysostomou C, Beerman L, Shiderly D, et al. Dexmedetomidine: a novel drug for the treatment of atrial and junctional tachyarrhythmias during the perioperative period for congenital cardiac surgery: a preliminary study. Anesth Analg 2008;107(5): 1514–22.

37. Chrysostomou C, Morell VO, Wearden P, et al. Dexmedetomidine: therapeutic use for the termination of reentrant supraventricular tachycardia. Congenit Heart Dis 2013;8(1):48–56.

38. Shafer S. Safety of patients reason for FDA black box warning on droperidol. Anesth Analg 2004; 98(2):551.

39. Charbit B, Albaladejo P, Funck-Brentano C, et al. Prolongation of QTc interval after postoperative nausea and vomiting treatment by droperidol or ondansetron. Anesthesiology 2005;102(6):1094.

40. Gilbert T, Gold M, Shorofsky S. Cardiovascular responses to repetitive defibrillation during implantable dardioverter-defibrillator testing. J Cardiothorac Vasc Anesth 2002;22:180.

Role of Cross-Sectional Imaging for Structural Heart Disease Interventions

João L. Cavalcante, MD[a],*, Paul Schoenhagen, MD[b]

KEYWORDS

- Structural heart disease interventions • Transcatheter therapies • Cross-sectional imaging
- Cardiac computed tomography • Cardiac magnetic resonance

KEY POINTS

- Transcatheter therapies in structural heart disease represent the new alternative therapeutic approach for patients with significant comorbidities.
- Direct visualization of the surgical field is traded for careful advanced preprocedural planning and intraprocedural decision making, which relies on image guidance.
- This article describes the role of cross-sectional imaging, with particular focus on multidetector computed tomography and cardiac magnetic resonance, for detailed assessment and preprocedural planning of aortic, mitral, and pulmonic valve interventions.

 Video of three-dimensional multi-planar reconstruction/reformatting of the aortic valve with cine loop assessing leaflet motion and aortic valve opening; and a video of dynamic intraprocedural CT angiography with fluoroscopy fusion/overlay allowing best angle assessment for prosthesis deployment accompany this article at http://www.cardiology.theclinics.com/

INTRODUCTION

Transcatheter interventions represent a new paradigm for treating patients with structural heart disease. For valvular disease, transcatheter aortic valve replacement (TAVR) has emerged as the new standard of care for symptomatic patients with severe aortic stenosis who are deemed inoperable or of high surgical risk.[1] Direct visualization of the surgical field is traded for careful advanced preprocedural planning and intraprocedural decision making, which relies on image guidance. Cross-sectional imaging, particularly using multidetector computed tomography (MDCT) angiography, has played a central role in evaluating patients for TAVR at 3 distinct stages: patient/device selection, intraprocedural guidance, and in the follow-up of selective cases.

This article describes the role of cross-sectional imaging, with particular focus on MDCT and cardiac magnetic resonance (CMR), for the detailed assessment and preprocedural planning of aortic, mitral, and pulmonic valve interventions. Recent insights obtained from advanced cardiovascular imaging, which have improved its safety and efficacy, are also highlighted.

IMAGING ACQUISITION, RECONSTRUCTION, AND ANALYSIS WITH MDCT

The use of MDCT for 3-dimensional cardiovascular imaging has become possible because of fast gantry rotation time and a large number of detector rows arranged with narrow collimated widths. A 360° rotation of the x-ray tube requires between 270 and 350 ms with state-of-the-art scanners, and

---

Disclosures: None of the authors have any relevant disclosures related to the content of this article.
[a] Advanced Cardiovascular Imaging, Heart & Vascular Institute, University of Pittsburgh Medical Center, University of Pittsburgh, Scaife Hall, S-571, 200 Lothrop Street, Pittsburgh, PA 15213, USA; [b] Cleveland Clinic, Imaging Institute and Heart & Vascular Institute, Desk J1-4, 9500 Euclid Avenue, Cleveland, OH 44195, USA
* Corresponding author.
E-mail address: cavalcantejl@upmc.edu

Cardiol Clin 31 (2013) 467–478
http://dx.doi.org/10.1016/j.ccl.2013.04.006
0733-8651/13/$ – see front matter © 2013 Elsevier Inc. All rights reserved.

determines the temporal resolution. The best temporal resolution (75 ms) can be achieved using dual-tube technology. Data covering the entire heart, synchronized to the heartbeat, are acquired within a single breath hold. Because of the extensive and rapid motion of valvular structures during the cardiac cycle, use of state-of-the-art scanners (at a minimum 64-slice technology) is critical for imaging in the context of valvular interventions. Retrospective echocardiogram gating allows reconstruction at multiple points throughout the cardiac cycle and subsequent dynamic 4-dimensional display of cardiac and valvular motion. However, retrospective gating is associated with higher radiation exposure, whereas in prospective echocardiogram-triggered acquisitions, data are acquired only during a prespecified cardiac phase. Because the x-ray tube is turned on only in this limited window, significantly reduced radiation dose is achieved. A comprehensive review of the specifics of scanner technology, image acquisition parameters, and settings can be found elsewhere.[2–4]

After a 3-dimensional imaging dataset is acquired, images can be reconstructed, with slice thickness ranging from 0.5 to 3 mm depending on the specific cardiac application. For the purpose of TAVR planning, several other postprocessing algorithms can be used for image reconstruction, such as multiplanar reconstruction/reformatting (MPR), maximum intensity projection, volume-rendered imaging, and cine/4-dimensional imaging (**Fig. 1**, Video 1). Ideally the imaging data should be stored and available for review as an integral part of the patient's electronic medical record.[5]

CROSS-SECTIONAL IMAGING IN PATIENT SELECTION FOR TAVR

In the United States, 2 bioprosthesis are currently available for TAVR implants, which are very distinct in their profile design and delivery characteristics (**Fig. 2**). Although the Edwards Sapien THV or XT models (Edwards Lifesciences, Irvine, CA, USA) are balloon-inflatable bioprostheses requiring rapid pacing for deployment, the CoreValve (Medtronic, Minneapolis, MN, USA) is a self-expandable bioprosthesis that extends up to the sinotubular

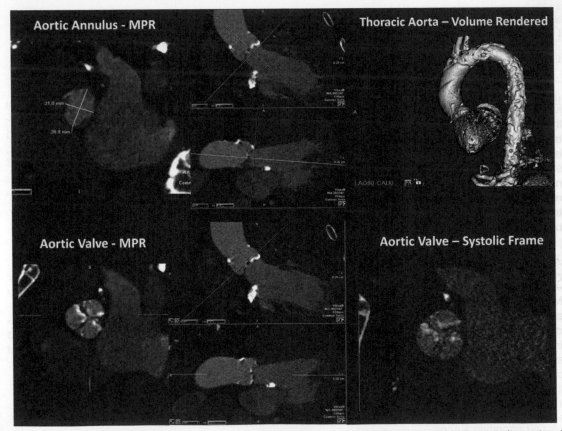

Fig. 1. Three-dimensional dataset reconstruction of the aortic annulus and aortic valve using a 3-dimensional dataset from MDCT with MPR. Volume rendering projection of the thoracic aorta shows significant calcification involving the aortic arch and descending segments.

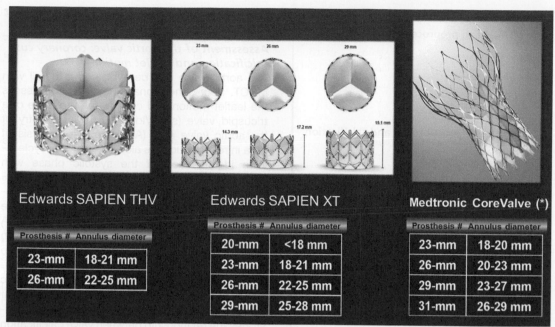

Edwards SAPIEN THV

Prosthesis #	Annulus diameter
23-mm	18-21 mm
26-mm	22-25 mm

Edwards SAPIEN XT

Prosthesis #	Annulus diameter
20-mm	<18 mm
23-mm	18-21 mm
26-mm	22-25 mm
29-mm	25-28 mm

Medtronic CoreValve (*)

Prosthesis #	Annulus diameter
23-mm	18-20 mm
26-mm	20-23 mm
29-mm	23-27 mm
31-mm	26-29 mm

Fig. 2. Bioprosthesis currently available in the United States for transcatheter aortic valve implantation. (*) Height and Width of the sinuses and the Asc Aorta diameter should carefully measured. If Asc Aorta >45 mm and/or aortic annular diameter <20 or >27 mm, this device should not be implanted. (Corevalve image *Courtesy of* Medtronic, Inc., Minneapolis, MN. The CoreValve® System is not commercially available in all countries and is an investigational device in other countries such as the US. CoreValve is a registered trademark of Medtronic CV Luxembourg S.a.r.l. Edwards SAPIEN Transcatheter Heart Valve and Edwards SAPIEN XT Transcatheter Heart Valve images *courtesy of* Edwards Lifesciences LLC, Irvine, CA. Edwards SAPIEN, and SAPIEN XT are trademarks of Edwards Lifesciences Corporation.)

junction and typically does not require rapid pacing for its delivery. Because of its profile, the Medtronic CoreValve requires measurements of the height and width of the aortic sinus and dimensions of the aorta at the sinotubular junction. A minimum trans-sinus dimension of 27 mm is required, and the ascending aorta must be less than 43 mm in diameter. The CoreValve has not been tested or approved for transapical implant.

Assessment of Aortic Annulus Size, Calcification, and Morphologic Characteristics

MDCT has multiple roles in the preprocedural assessment for TAVR (**Box 1**). One of the most important is aortic annulus sizing.[6] Traditionally this measurement has been obtained by 2-dimensional echocardiography and extrapolated to be a circle for calculation of the aortic valve area using the continuity equation. However, cross-sectional imaging has shown the annulus more frequently assumes an ellipsoid/oval shape with 2 diameters (major and minor).[7] Therefore, underestimation of the annular size can commonly occur with standard 2-dimensional unidimensional planar

measurement in either transthoracic or transesophageal imaging. Advances in transesophageal imaging with full-volume 3-dimensional datasets have allowed, similar to MDCT, MPR, which has improved correlation with MDCT[8] (**Fig. 3**) with better prediction of annular coverage and lower incidence of paravalvular aortic regurgitation (PVAR). Jilaihawi and colleagues[9] suggest that using 3-dimensional datasets as the gold standard for annular measurements might reduce the incidence of serious PVAR by approximately 15%.

Therefore, MDCT measurements of the aortic annulus should be performed using MPR with double-oblique transverse images and measuring the 2 distinct diameters of the annulus (see **Fig. 1**).[6] Other groups have proposed using the aortic annulus perimeter measurement and dividing it by π (3.14) for the "averaged" annular dimension, which seems to be less susceptible to the dynamic changes of the cardiac cycle.[10]

Growing evidence shows that prosthesis undersizing is an independent predictor of PVAR.[1,9,11] However, even with routine oversizing of the implanted valve by 1 to 2 mm, moderate-to-severe PVAR is still observed in 10% to 15% of patients

Box 1
Role of MDCT in preprocedural assessment

Aorta

- Annulus size
- Aortic root
  - ○ Calcification
  - ○ Sinotubular junction size and calcification
- Coronary ostia
  - ○ Location
  - ○ Distance from leaflets
- Aortic tortuosity and dimensions
- Aortic atheroma

Procedural access

- Iliac arteries
  - ○ Caliber
  - ○ Atherosclerosis
  - ○ Calcification
  - ○ Tortuosity
- Transapical
  - ○ Entry into the left ventricle

Intraprocedural guidance

- Correct angiographic planes

postprocedure and associated with adverse outcomes.[11,12] This finding suggests that other variables could be also important in the genesis of PVAR and should be further evaluated.

Additional Information Obtained by MDCT at the Preprocedural Stage

Assessment of the aortic valve: coronary cusp calcification and leaflet motion

The aortic valve can be evaluated in detail with MDCT. Four-dimensional cine loops can assess the leaflet motion and confirm the presence of a tricuspid valve (see Video 1). For planimetry of the aortic valve area (AVA), detailed analysis of data in reconstructions along the cardiac cycle allows identification of the systolic phase with maximum valve opening (typically a 20%–30% R wave to R wave [R-R] interval). In this reconstruction, a plane perpendicular to the valve plane is placed at the leaflet tips to measure the AVA using planimetry.[13] Direct planimetry of AVA with MDCT has been shown to provide reproducible results compared with transthoracic and transesophageal echocardiography and magnetic resonance imaging.[14,15] Functional valvular assessment with MDCT is possible and demonstrates the relationship between valve calcification and leaflet motion. The extent and severity of aortic valve calcification play an important role in TAVR deployment requiring repeat maneuvers during implantation, and have been associated with increased degrees of PVAR.[16,17]

Coronary artery location and height of coronary ostia

Knowledge about the relationship between aortic valve leaflet height and distance between the insertion of the left/right coronary cusp and the coronary ostia is important to avoid coronary complications. The risk of coronary occlusion is low but

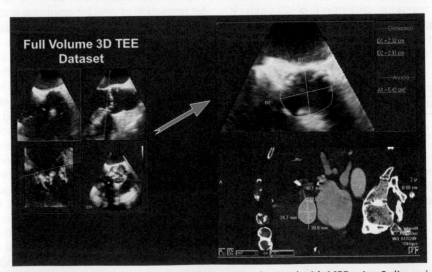

Full Volume 3D TEE Dataset

Fig. 3. Good accuracy when comparing annular measurements obtained with MPR using 3-dimensional transesophageal dataset versus MDCT data. TEE, transesophageal echocardiogram.

difficult to assess because it depends on the bulk-iness of the native leaflets, height of the coronary ostia, and dimensions of the sinus of Valsalva. At this point, no definite criteria exist to exclude patients based on the risk of coronary obstruction; however, a distance less than 10 mm between the aortic annulus and coronary ostia may identify patients with increased risk.[18] In these patients, perideployment placement of a guidewire in the left main should be considered to ensure access in the case of complications.

Definition of aortic plane for TAVR deployment

Optimal positioning of the prosthetic valve during TAVR with precise coaxial alignment of the stent valve along the centerline of the aortic valve plane is crucial to avoid procedural complications, such as prosthetic embolization, coronary ostial obstruction, PVAR, and conduction disturbance.[19] Aortic root orientation is typically assessed using multiple repeat catheter aortograms in 1 or 2 orthogonal planes before starting the procedure or during the preprocedural diagnostic angiogram. Kurra and colleagues[20] described the role of MDCT in predicting 2-dimensional angiographic projections orthogonal to the aortic valve plane, simplifying the subsequent implantation of the percutaneous valve. Double-oblique transverse multiplanar reconstructions are performed at the level of the root and then rotated through a series of any angles (**Fig. 4**).[21]

Recently Samim and colleagues[22] demonstrated that automated prediction of annulus plane angulation using MDCT allowed safe deployment of balloon-expandable prostheses with a low rate of valve malpositioning and regurgitation. This approach was performed without an aortogram in most patients, therefore shortening both procedure time and contrast use.

Aortic dimensions and extent of calcification of the ascending aorta and arch

The presence of significant aneurysmal dilation is considered a contraindication for TAVR. The extent of atherosclerotic plaque is likely associated with complications, including stroke post-surgical aortic valve replacement.[23] Aortic arch calcification also seems to be associated with increased embolic risk, especially in those undergoing TAVR via a transfemoral approach.[24] In addition, MDCT can also identify patients with porcelain aorta, defined as an extensive, circumferential calcification of the entire ascending aorta extending into the proximal aortic arch.[25] These patients represent a higher-risk cohort in whom surgical aortic cross-clamping is not feasible. They should be considered for alternative TAVR approaches, such as via the subclavian artery or a transapical and even transaortic route, as shown recently by Bapat and colleagues.[26]

Assessment of Ileofemoral Access and Deciding Suitability of Transfemoral Route

Given the advanced age and comorbidities, peripheral vascular disease is common in older patients being evaluated for TAVR procedures. Because of the large diameter of the delivery sheaths (≥18 French), appropriate vascular access is critical. Small luminal diameter, dense and circumferential and/or horseshoe calcification, and severe tortuosity are common in this

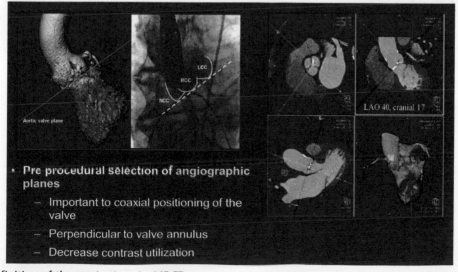

Fig. 4. Definition of the aortic plane by MDCT.

patient population and increase the risk of access site complications and central embolization. Therefore, MDCT plays an important role in assessing the safety and feasibility of performing TAVR via the transfemoral access route (**Fig. 5**).

Kurra and colleagues[27] reported that at least one-third of patients with critical aortic stenosis had unfavorable iliofemoral arteries, with most having minimal luminal diameters of 8 mm. In these patients, alternative access approaches may include via a surgical side graft on the iliac arteries, or subclavian or transapical access.

INTRAPROCEDURAL MONITORING: THE ROLE OF FUSIONAL IMAGING

Growing interest has been shown in the use of intraprocedural dynamic computed tomography (CT) to improve imaging guidance during TAVR implantations. The raw dataset is acquired through rotational angiography under rapid ventricular pacing using the C-arm of the fluoroscopy system. Angiography requires 15 mL of contrast agent, which is comparable to the amount used during one root angiography. Afterward, 3-dimensional reconstruction can be performed using the Siemens Syngo Aortic ValveGuide (Siemens AG, Forchheim, Germany) software prototype. Images are overlaid on the fluoroscopy to guide TAVR implantation using the precise angulation and depth into the aortic annulus (**Fig. 6**, Video 2).[28]

ROLE OF MDCT IN POST-TAVR FOLLOW-UP

A potential important role of MDCT in the follow-up of patients who underwent TAVR is assessing prosthesis deployment and conformation in relationship to the landing zone and native aortic annulus. Delgado and colleagues[13] verified that post-TAVR with balloon-expandable prosthesis (Sapien), circular deployment was achieved in most patients (86%) in such a way that the prosthesis remodeled the annulus. A more noncircular deployment was associated with higher degrees of calcification and paravalvular regurgitation. Schultz and colleagues[29] noted that in self-expandable TAVR prostheses (CoreValve), some degree of incomplete apposition occurred in up to 61% patients, with only 50% having circular conformation, suggesting that the annulus remodeled the prosthesis. Hence, although the role of MDCT post-TAVR remains investigational, it would be reasonable to consider in the follow-up of selected patients, in particular those with significant PVAR.

POTENTIAL ROLE OF CMR IMAGING IN PATIENTS BEING EVALUATED FOR TAVR

The role of CMR imaging in the context of TAVR procedures has recently been described. CMR is a noninvasive, radiation-free imaging modality that allows detailed visualization of cardiac structures and functional assessment, including wall

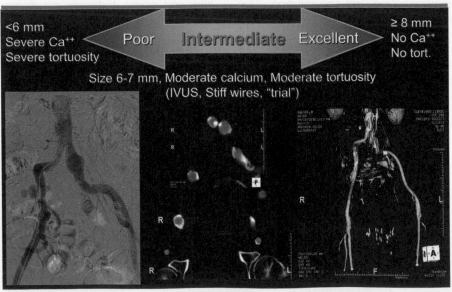

Fig. 5. MDCT evaluation of feasibility for transfemoral access in TAVR. Ca++, calcification; IVUS, intravenous ultrasound; tort, tortuosity.

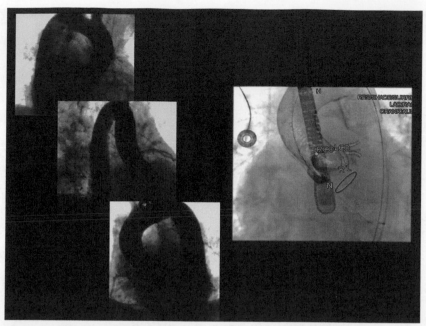

Fig. 6. Intraprocedural rotational CT angiography dataset is obtained and later coregistered in the fluoroscopy, aiding proper selection of aortic plane and TAVR bioprosthesis position coaxial to the native aorta. L, left coronary cusp; LCO, left coronary ostium; N, non-coronary cusp; R, right coronary cusp; RCO, right coronary ostium.

motion analysis, quantification of cardiac function, and myocardial tissue characterization. Similar to MDCT, CMR also provides imaging with exquisite spatial resolution and ability for 3-dimensional MPR (**Fig. 7**). Another advantage of CMR imaging over MDCT is that no iodinated contrast is needed for adequate visualization of the cardiovascular structures. This advantage can become particularly important in elderly patients with decreased renal function in which the risk of contrast-induced nephropathy in increased. In these patients, magnetic resonance imaging sequences without contrast administration can be pursued (Gadolinium contrast would be contraindicated in these patient because of the potential risk of nephrogenic systemic fibrosis).

Direct comparison of CMR imaging and MDCT measurements of the aortic root and aortic annulus has shown close agreement.[30,31] The severity of PVAR was associated with increasing annulus diameter on both CMR imaging and MDCT.[30] In addition, magnetic resonance angiography with gadolinium and true fast imaging using steady-state free-precession sequences enables characterization of the vessel wall and accurate assessment of the severity of iliac artery stenosis.[32] In the postprocedural period, assessment of CMR imaging may provide incremental value.[33]

In patients with renal insufficiency, 3-dimensional echocardiogram-gated nonenhanced magnetic resonance angiography seems to be an alternative to MDCT to characterize the proximal aorta, allowing accurate measurements, but also to evaluate the aortoiliofemoral system. A comprehensive review of these techniques is beyond the scope of this article, but can be found elsewhere.[34]

However, CMR has 2 potential shortcomings in patients undergoing TAVR: (1) calcifications of cardiac structures are not well seen by this technique, and (2) CMR is contraindicated and not approved for use in patients with cardiac devices such as permanent pacemakers and defibrillators.

ROLE OF CROSS-SECTIONAL IMAGING IN TRANSCATHETER MITRAL VALVE AND PULMONIC VALVE PROCEDURES

In the context of transcatheter valve procedures, 3-dimensional imaging generally allows a detailed understanding of the mitral valve apparatus, including the mitral annulus, valve leaflets, and chordae tendineae/papillary muscles (**Fig. 8**).[35] Real-time 3-dimensional, full-volume acquisition with transesophageal echocardiography allows imaging of the entire annular volume, including

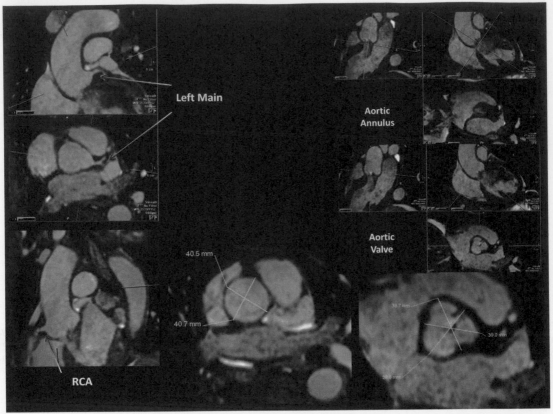

Fig. 7. Three-dimensional dataset reconstruction of the aortic annulus and aortic valve using 3-dimensional dataset from CMR with MPR. This dataset was obtained without gadolinium and with the free-breathing (non-enhanced echocardiogram-gated 3-dimensional steady-state free-precession magnetic resonance angiography). RCA, right coronary artery.

the valve over full cardiac cycles.[36] The complex anatomic structure of the mitral annulus determines valve function, but the interactions are incompletely understood. Most emerging MDCT data, therefore, describe mitral annular anatomy (**Fig. 9**).

Accurate definition of mitral annular geometry is critical for preoperative planning in the context of recently introduced transcatheter approaches for ring annuloplasty.[37] The goal of these devices, which are placed in the coronary sinus (CS), is to change the anterior-posterior dimension by displacing the posterior mitral valve leaflet forward, improving leaflet coaptation and therefore reducing mitral regurgitation severity. Schofer and colleagues[38] showed the feasibility of percutaneous reduction of functional mitral regurgitation using a novel CS-based mitral annuloplasty device in patients with heart failure, which translated into improved quality of life and exercise tolerance.

Several MDCT studies have described the relationship among the CS, mitral annulus, and

coronary arteries. In most patients, the CS courses superiorly to the mitral annulus, whereas the circumflex artery courses between the CS and the mitral annulus in 68% to 97% of the patients, depending on coronary dominance.[37,39] Similar findings were also seen with CMR imaging.[40] These data raise concern for potential coronary ischemia induced by a CS-based device. Hence, MDCT may provide useful information in selecting potential candidates for percutaneous mitral annuloplasty via a coronary sinus approach.

Transcatheter pulmonic valve replacement with a Melody valve bioprosthesis (Medtronic, Minneapolis, MN, USA) was recently approved in the United States for placement in dysfunctional right ventricular outflow tract conduits and moderately severe pulmonary regurgitation. Given the young age of this cohort (median, 19 years), all patients underwent CMR imaging before transcatheter pulmonic valve replacement, and most also 6 months after. Core laboratory measurements demonstrated significant reduction of pulmonic regurgitation (regurgitation

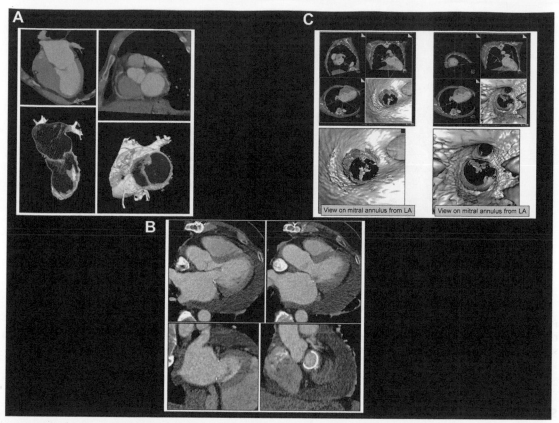

Fig. 8. Visualization of the mitral annulus. (*A*) MPR and volume-rendered (VR) images of the mitral annulus. Because of the complex saddle-shaped configuration of the mitral annulus, representation in a single MPR can be challenging. (*B*) Position of a surgically placed C-shaped mitral annular ring. (*C*) VR images (endoscopic views) of the mitral annulus, as seen from the left atrium (*left panels*) and left ventricle (*right panel*).

Fig. 9. MDCT shows significant mitral annular calcification involving both annuli and medial commissure. Desc Ao, Descending Aorta.

fraction decreased from 26.7% to 1.8%), with significant decrease in right ventricular end-diastolic volumes, albeit with unchanged right ventricular systolic function.[41]

ROLE OF MDCT IN PERCUTANEOUS CLOSURE OF PATENT FORAMEN OVALE AND ATRIAL SEPTAL DEFECTS

Advances in real-time 3-dimensional transesophageal echocardiography have enabled excellent preoperative imaging evaluation and intraprocedural guidance in percutaneous interventions related to patent foramen ovale and atrial septal defects.[42] Need for intravenous contrast, radiation exposure, and streak artifacts created after device implantation have decreased the up-front use of MDCT for these specific purposes.[43] MDCT, however, can still be considered to have an adjunctive role for selected patients in evaluating pulmonary venous drainage and/or those presenting with residual left-to-right shunting (**Fig. 10**).

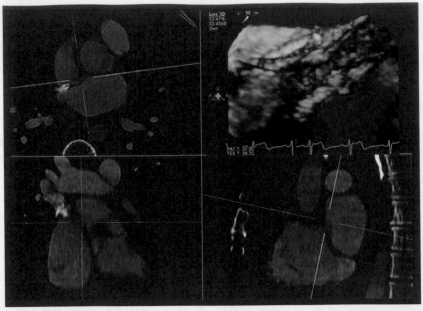

Fig. 10. MDCT of patient after surgical repair of sinus venosus atrial septal defect presenting with residual left-to-right shunting and right-sided chamber enlargement. No anomalous pulmonary vein drainage is noted, but a sizable patent foramen ovale is observed, for which percutaneous closure was performed (*top right*).

SUMMARY

Precise preoperative and intraoperative imaging is critical for valvular interventional procedures. Complementing standard echocardiography and catheterization, novel 3-dimensional imaging modalities, including CMR, MDCT, and 3-dimensional transesophageal echocardiography, acquire volumetric datasets, allowing subsequent 3-dimensional reformatting, display, and visualization in unlimited planes. In the context of MDCT imaging and radiation exposure, alternative imaging modalities are important to consider given the differences in the patient populations undergoing aortic versus mitral/pulmonic procedures.

The data suggest an emerging role for 3-dimensional imaging for novel surgical and transcatheter approaches. Evidence-based data showing a favorable risk/benefit impact of these imaging techniques are quickly increasing, but more prospective data are needed, particularly comparing the utility of different imaging modalities and showing clinical impact of image guidance in the context of these procedures.

SUPPLEMENTARY DATA

Supplementary data related to this article can be found online at http://dx.doi.org/10.1016/j.ccl.2013.04.006.

REFERENCES

1. Webb JG, Wood DA. Current status of transcatheter aortic valve replacement. J Am Coll Cardiol 2012;60: 483–92.
2. Halliburton SS. Recent technologic advances in multi-detector row cardiac CT. Cardiol Clin 2009; 27:655–64.
3. Leipsic J, Gurvitch R, Labounty TM, et al. Multidetector computed tomography in transcatheter aortic valve implantation. JACC Cardiovasc Imaging 2011; 4:416–29.
4. Achenbach S, Delgado V, Hausleiter J, et al. SCCT expert consensus document on computed tomography imaging before transcatheter aortic valve implantation (TAVI)/transcatheter aortic valve replacement (TAVR). J Cardiovasc Comput Tomogr 2012;6:366–80.
5. Schoenhagen P, Falkner J, Piraino D. Transcatheter aortic valve repair, imaging, and electronic imaging health record. Curr Cardiol Rep 2013;15:319.
6. Kasel AM, Cassese S, Bleiziffer S, et al. Standardized imaging for aortic annular sizing: implications for transcatheter valve selection. JACC Cardiovasc Imaging 2013;6:249–62.
7. Schoenhagen P, Kapadia SR, Halliburton SS, et al. Computed tomography evaluation for transcatheter aortic valve implantation (TAVI): imaging of the aortic root and iliac arteries. J Cardiovasc Comput Tomogr 2011;5:293–300.

8. Ng AC, Delgado V, van der Kley F, et al. Comparison of aortic root dimensions and geometries before and after transcatheter aortic valve implantation by 2- and 3-dimensional transesophageal echocardiography and multislice computed tomography. Circ Cardiovasc Imaging 2010;3:94–102.

9. Jilaihawi H, Kashif M, Fontana G, et al. Cross-sectional computed tomographic assessment improves accuracy of aortic annular sizing for transcatheter aortic valve replacement and reduces the incidence of paravalvular aortic regurgitation. J Am Coll Cardiol 2012;59:1275–86.

10. Hamdan A, Guetta V, Konen E, et al. Deformation dynamics and mechanical properties of the aortic annulus by 4-dimensional computed tomography: insights into the functional anatomy of the aortic valve complex and implications for transcatheter aortic valve therapy. J Am Coll Cardiol 2012;59:119–27.

11. Genereux P, Head SJ, Hahn R, et al. Paravalvular leak after transcatheter aortic valve replacement: the new Achilles' heel? A comprehensive review of the literature. J Am Coll Cardiol 2013;61:1125–36.

12. Kodali SK, Williams MR, Smith CR, et al. Two-year outcomes after transcatheter or surgical aortic-valve replacement. N Engl J Med 2012;366:1686–95.

13. Delgado V, Ng AC, van de Veire NR, et al. Transcatheter aortic valve implantation: role of multi-detector row computed tomography to evaluate prosthesis positioning and deployment in relation to valve function. Eur Heart J 2010;31:1114–23.

14. Pouleur AC, le Polain de Waroux JB, Pasquet A, et al. Aortic valve area assessment: multidetector CT compared with cine MR imaging and transthoracic and transesophageal echocardiography. Radiology 2007;244:745–54.

15. Feuchtner GM, Dichtl W, Friedrich GJ, et al. Multislice computed tomography for detection of patients with aortic valve stenosis and quantification of severity. J Am Coll Cardiol 2006;47:1410–7.

16. Haensig M, Lehmkuhl L, Rastan AJ, et al. Aortic valve calcium scoring is a predictor of significant paravalvular aortic insufficiency in transapical-aortic valve implantation. Eur J Cardiothorac Surg 2012;41:1234–40.

17. Ewe SH, Ng AC, Schuijf JD, et al. Location and severity of aortic valve calcium and implications for aortic regurgitation after transcatheter aortic valve implantation. Am J Cardiol 2011;108:1470–7.

18. Masson JB, Kovac J, Schuler G, et al. Transcatheter aortic valve implantation: review of the nature, management, and avoidance of procedural complications. JACC Cardiovasc Interv 2009;2:811–20.

19. Tuzcu EM. Transcatheter aortic valve replacement malposition and embolization: innovation brings solutions also new challenges. Catheter Cardiovasc Interv 2008;72:579–80.

20. Kurra V, Kapadia SR, Tuzcu EM, et al. Pre-procedural imaging of aortic root orientation and dimensions: comparison between X-ray angiographic planar imaging and 3-dimensional multidetector row computed tomography. JACC Cardiovasc Interv 2010;3:105–13.

21. Gurvitch R, Wood DA, Leipsic J, et al. Multislice computed tomography for prediction of optimal angiographic deployment projections during transcatheter aortic valve implantation. JACC Cardiovasc Interv 2010;3:1157–65.

22. Samim M, Stella PR, Agostoni P, et al. Automated 3D analysis of pre-procedural MDCT to predict annulus plane angulation and C-arm positioning: benefit on procedural outcome in patients referred for TAVR. JACC Cardiovasc Imaging 2013;6:238–48.

23. Kurra V, Lieber ML, Sola S, et al. Extent of thoracic aortic atheroma burden and long-term mortality after cardiothoracic surgery: a computed tomography study. JACC Cardiovasc Imaging 2010;3:1020–9.

24. Szeto WY, Augoustides JG, Desai ND, et al. Cerebral embolic exposure during transfemoral and transapical transcatheter aortic valve replacement. J Card Surg 2011;26:348–54.

25. Kappetein AP, Head SJ, Genereux P, et al. Updated standardized endpoint definitions for transcatheter aortic valve implantation: the Valve Academic Research Consortium-2 consensus document. J Am Coll Cardiol 2012;60:1438–54.

26. Bapat VN, Attia RQ, Thomas M. Distribution of calcium in the ascending aorta in patients undergoing transcatheter aortic valve implantation and its relevance to the transaortic approach. JACC Cardiovasc Interv 2012;5:470–6.

27. Kurra V, Schoenhagen P, Roselli EE, et al. Prevalence of significant peripheral artery disease in patients evaluated for percutaneous aortic valve insertion: preprocedural assessment with multidetector computed tomography. J Thorac Cardiovasc Surg 2009;137:1258–64.

28. Kempfert J, Noettling A, John M, et al. Automatically segmented DynaCT: enhanced imaging during transcatheter aortic valve implantation. J Am Coll Cardiol 2011;58:e211.

29. Schultz CJ, Weustink A, Piazza N, et al. Geometry and degree of apposition of the CoreValve ReValving system with multislice computed tomography after implantation in patients with aortic stenosis. J Am Coll Cardiol 2009;54:911–8.

30. Jabbour A, Ismail TF, Moat N, et al. Multimodality imaging in transcatheter aortic valve implantation and post-procedural aortic regurgitation: comparison among cardiovascular magnetic resonance, cardiac computed tomography, and echocardiography. J Am Coll Cardiol 2011;58:2165–73.

31. Koos R, Altiok E, Mahnken AH, et al. Evaluation of aortic root for definition of prosthesis size by

magnetic resonance imaging and cardiac computed tomography: implications for transcatheter aortic valve implantation. Int J Cardiol 2012; 158:353–8.

32. Iozzelli A, D'Orta G, Aliprandi A, et al. The value of true-FISP sequence added to conventional gadolinium-enhanced MRA of abdominal aorta and its major branches. Eur J Radiol 2009;72:489–93.

33. Stahli BE, Bunzli R, Grunenfelder J, et al. Transcatheter aortic valve implantation (TAVI) outcome according to standardized endpoint definitions by the Valve Academic Research Consortium (VARC). J Invasive Cardiol 2011;23:307–12.

34. Miyazaki M, Lee VS. Nonenhanced MR angiography. Radiology 2008;248:20–43.

35. Shanks M, Delgado V, Ng AC, et al. Mitral valve morphology assessment: three-dimensional transesophageal echocardiography versus computed tomography. Ann Thorac Surg 2010;90:1922–9.

36. Cavalcante JL, Rodriguez LL, Kapadia S, et al. Role of echocardiography in percutaneous mitral valve interventions. JACC Cardiovasc Imaging 2012;5: 733–46.

37. Tops LF, Van de Veire NR, Schuijf JD, et al. Noninvasive evaluation of coronary sinus anatomy and its relation to the mitral valve annulus: implications for percutaneous mitral annuloplasty. Circulation 2007; 115:1426–32.

38. Schofer J, Siminiak T, Haude M, et al. Percutaneous mitral annuloplasty for functional mitral regurgitation: results of the CARILLON Mitral Annuloplasty Device European Union Study. Circulation 2009; 120:326–33.

39. Choure AJ, Garcia MJ, Hesse B, et al. In vivo analysis of the anatomical relationship of coronary sinus to mitral annulus and left circumflex coronary artery using cardiac multidetector computed tomography: implications for percutaneous coronary sinus mitral annuloplasty. J Am Coll Cardiol 2006;48:1938–45.

40. Chiribiri A, Kelle S, Kohler U, et al. Magnetic resonance cardiac vein imaging: relation to mitral valve annulus and left circumflex coronary artery. JACC Cardiovasc Imaging 2008;1:729–38.

41. McElhinney DB, Hellenbrand WE, Zahn EM, et al. Short- and medium-term outcomes after transcatheter pulmonary valve placement in the expanded multicenter US melody valve trial. Circulation 2010; 122:507–16.

42. Bartel T, Muller S. Contemporary echocardiographic guiding tools for device closure of interatrial communications. Cardiovasc Diagn Ther 2013;3:38–46.

43. Ko SF, Liang CD, Yip HK, et al. Amplatzer septal occluder closure of atrial septal defect: evaluation of transthoracic echocardiography, cardiac CT, and transesophageal echocardiography. AJR Am J Roentgenol 2009;193:1522–9.

Index

A

ACP. *See* Amplatzer Cardiac Plug (ACP)

AF. *See* Atrial fibrillation (AF)

Alcohol septal ablation
  as structural heart intervention, 463

Amplatzer Cardiac Plug (ACP)
  in LAA occlusion, 374–375
    postprocedure care, 380
    preprocedural considerations, 379
    procedure, 379

Amplatzer family of septal occluder devices
  for PVO closure, 406

Anesthesia/anesthetics
  for structural heart interventions, **455–465**
    AF ablation, 462–463
    alcohol septal ablation, 463
    antiemetics, 463
    cardioversion, 463
    complications related to, 456–457
    continuum of sedation in, 455–456
    coronary interventions, 460
    electrophysiology procedures, 462
    general concerns, 458
    general principles of sedation, 458–460
      capnography, 460
      carbon dioxide retention, 460
      fire and chemical burns, 460
      hypothermia, 460
      pressure injury, 460
      respiratory depression, 458–460
      supplemental oxygen, 460
    introduction, 455
    laser lead extraction, 463
    mitral valve repair, 462
    muscle relaxants, 463
    outpatient procedures, 458
    pacemaker/implantable cardioverter-
      defibrillator insertion, 463
    preoperative evaluation, 457–458
    preoperative fasting, 458
    radiation safety, 458
    shunt closure, 461
    standards of care, 455
    TAVI, 461–462
    unintended progression to deep sedation, 457
    ventricular-assist device insertion, 461

Antegrade transseptal approach

  in percutaneous PVL closure, 436–437

Antiemetics
  for structural heart interventions, 463

Aortic stenosis (AS), **327–336**
  calcification in, 329
  chronic inflammation in, 329
  introduction, 327
  lipid deposition in, 328–329
  pathologic considerations in, 327–328
  treatment of, 329–333
    BAV in, 329–333. *See also* Balloon aortic
      valvuloplasty (BAV), in AS

AS. *See* Aortic stenosis (AS)

ASDs. *See* Atrial septal defects (ASDs)

Atrial fibrillation (AF)
  mortality data, 363
  prevalence of, 363
  stroke due to, 363

Atrial fibrillation (AF) ablation
  anesthesia for, 462–463

Atrial septal defects (ASDs), 393
  anatomy related to, 387, 401–403
  closure of, **385–400**
    catheterization laboratory setup for, 389
    complications of, 394–397
    for defects with deficient rims, 393
    devices for, 387–389
    future directions in, 398
    indications for, 385–387
    for large defects, 392
    MDCT in, 476
    for multifenestrated defects, 394
    for multiple defects, 394
    patient follow-up, 397–398
    patient preparation for, 389
    patient selection for, 385–387
    percutaneous, 389–392. *See also*
      Percutaneous ASD closure
    postprocedure care, 397
    rates of, 385
    troubleshooting Chiari network and redundant
      eustachian valves, 394

Atrial septum
  anatomy of, 387, 401–403
  embryology of, 401–403

Atrioventricular block
  TAVR using Edwards SAPIEN transcatheter heart
    valves and, 347

Cardiol Clin 31 (2013) 479–483
http://dx.doi.org/10.1016/S0733-8651(13)00060-X
0733-8651/13/$ – see front matter © 2013 Elsevier Inc. All rights reserved.

Printed and bound by CPI Group (UK) Ltd, Croydon, CR0 4YY

03/10/2024

01040378-0015